Caregiving
Research • Practice • Policy

Ronda C. Talley, Series Editor

An official publication of
The Rosalynn Carter Institute for Caregiving

For further volumes:
http://www.springer.com/series/8274

Editorial Board

Ronda C. Talley • Ruth McCorkle
Walter F. Baile
Editors

Cancer Caregiving in the United States

Research, Practice, Policy

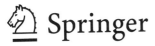 Springer

Editors
Dr. Ronda C. Talley
Western Kentucky University
Bowling Green, KY, USA

Ruth McCorkle
School of Nursing
Yale University
New Haven, CT, USA

Walter F. Baile
Department of Behavioral Science
M.D. Anderson Cancer Center
University of Texas
Houston, TX, USA

ISSN 2192-340X   ISSN 2192-3418 (electronic)
ISBN 978-1-4614-3153-4   ISBN 978-1-4614-3154-1 (eBook)
DOI 10.1007/978-1-4614-3154-1
Springer New York Dordrecht Heidelberg London

Library of Congress Control Number: 2012934957

Printed on acid-free paper

Springer is part of Springer Science+Business Media (www.springer.com)

To my grandfather, Jim, F. McCoy; my father, Jack Howard Talley; and my Kiwi, Francis Michael Fearon; and to the women who cared for them when they battled cancer. My grandfather survived and lived to 100 years of age. My Father and Kiwi did not, and we lost them far too young to this devastating disease. We, the caregivers, still mourn.

Ronda C. Talley

To the caregivers of the past, present, and future—and to my greatest caregiver, my mother, Virginia McCorkle.

Ruth McCorkle

To Beth, who is always there through thick and thin.

Walter F. Baile

Foreword

From its inception in 1987, the Rosalynn Carter Institute for Caregiving (RCI) has sought to bring attention to the extraordinary contributions made by caregivers to their loved ones. I grew up in a home that was regularly transformed into a caregiving household when members of my family became seriously ill, disabled or frail with age, so my interest in the issue is personal. In my hometown of Plains, Georgia, as in most communities across our country, it was expected that family members and neighbors would take on the responsibility of providing care whenever illness struck close to home. Delivering such care with the love, respect, and attention it deserves is both labor-intensive and personally-demanding. Those who do so represent one of this nation's most significant yet underappreciated assets in our health delivery system.

When the RCI began, "caregiving" was found nowhere in the nation's health lexicon. Its existence was not a secret but rather simply accepted as a fact of life. In deciding on the direction and priorities of the new institute, we convened groups of family and professional caregivers from around the region to tell their personal stories. As I listened to neighbors describe caring for aged and/or chronically ill or disabled family members, I recognized that their experiences reflected mine. They testified that, while caregiving for them was full of personal meaning and significance and could be extremely rewarding, it could also be fraught with anxiety, stress, and feelings of isolation. Many felt unprepared and most were overwhelmed at times. A critical issue in the "field" of caregiving, I realized, was the need to better understand the kinds of policies and programs necessary to support those who quietly and consistently care for loved ones.

With the aging of America's Baby Boomers expecting to double the elderly population in the next 20 years, deinstitutionalization of individuals with chronic mental illnesses and developmental disabilities, a rising percentage of women in the workforce, smaller and more dispersed families, changes in the role of hospitals, and a range of other factors, caregiving has become one of the most significant issues of our time. Caregiving as an area of research, as a focus and concern of policy-making, and as an area of professional training and practice has reached a new and unparalleled level of importance in our society and indeed globally.

As we survey the field of caregiving today, we now recognize that it is an essential component of long-term care in the community, yet also a potential health risk for those who provide care. The basic features of a public health approach have emerged: a focus on populations of caregivers and recipients, tracking and surveillance of health risks, understanding the factors associated with risk status, and the development and testing of the effectiveness of various interventions to maximize benefits for both the recipients of care and their providers.

The accumulated wisdom from this work is represented in the volumes that make up the Springer Caregiving Series. This series presents a broad portrait of the nature of caregiving in the United States in the twenty-first century. Most Americans have been, are now, or will be caregivers. With our society's increasing demands for care, we cannot expect a high quality of life for our seniors and others living with limitations due to illness or disability unless we understand and support the work of caregivers. Without thoughtful planning, intelligent policies, and sensitive interventions, there is the risk that the work of family, paraprofessional, and professional caregivers will become intolerably difficult and burdensome. We cannot let this happen.

This volume focuses on the caregiving demands for family and loved ones of someone diagnosed with cancer. At each stage of the disease's progression from diagnosis to treatment to struggles with rehabilitation, recuperation, remission, and potentially recurrence, both the person with the diagnosis and the family encounter specific challenges. Among these, obviously are the emotional distress experienced by all involved following the diagnosis and progressing across all that follows in fighting against the disease, maintnaing hope, and preparing for both the best and worst outcomes. Part of that distress is the sense that above all one must spare the person with cancer any sense of the diagnosis' impact on loved ones. Beyond its emotional demands, cancer also presents caregivers with a broad array of comprehensive caregiving. The chapters within this volume will inform readers of the complexity of caregiving for this far too prevalent and highly feared diagnosis.

Readers of this series will find hope and evidence that improved support for family and professional caregivers lies within our reach. The field of caregiving has matured and, as evidenced in these volumes, has generated rigorous and practical research findings to guide effective and enlightened policy and program options. My hope is that these volumes will play an important role in documenting the research base, guiding practice, and moving our nation toward effective polices to support all of America's caregivers.

Rosalynn Carter

Contents

About the Editors

Ronda C. Talley, PhD, MPH is Professor of Psychology at Western Kentucky University. Her prior work experience includes providing leadership on caregiving issues and organizational development as Executive Director of the Rosalynn Carter Institute for Caregiving; working with national government groups to promote caregiving issues as Associate Director of Legislation, Policy, and Planning/Health Scientist for the Centers for Disease Control and Prevention, U.S. Department of Health and Human Services; and promoting the science and practice of psychology in the schools as Associate Executive Director of Education and Director of School Policy and Practice at the American Psychological Association. Dr. Talley, as Adjunct Associate Professor, taught ethics and legal issues in school psychology at the University of Maryland, College Park. Dr. Talley received the Outstanding Alumni Award from Indiana University and the Jack Bardon Distinguished Service Award from the Division of School Psychology of the American Psychological Association. She serves on the national board of the American Association of Caregiving Youth. Dr. Talley may be reached at 1906 College Heights Boulevard, GRH 3023, Bowling Green, KY 42101; by telephone at (270) 745-2780; or via e-mail at Ronda.Talley@wku.edu.

Ruth McCorkle, PhD, FAAN is the Yale University Florence S. Wald Professor of Nursing and Professor of Epidemiology and former Director of the Center for Excellence in Chronic Illness Care. In addition, Dr. McCorkle is currently the Director of the Psycho-oncology program at the Smilow Cancer Hospital at Yale New Haven Hospital. She has won numerous awards recognizing her outstanding contributions to nursing science, cancer leadership, and psycho-oncology. Dr. McCorkle was elected both to the American Academy of Nursing and the Institute of Medicine. She has received the Nurse Scientist of the Year Award by the American Nurses Association, the Distinguished Research Award from the Oncology Nursing Society, and the Bernard Fox Memorial Award from the International Psycho-Oncology Society. In 2011, she received the Holland Distinguished Leadership Award from the American Psychosocial Oncology Society (APOS), the highest award given in the field of psycho-oncology. Dr. McCorkle was the first non-medical training grant award recipient from the National Cancer Institute (NCI) and is thus credited with opening the door for other non-medical researchers to secure funding for training from the NCI. Dr. McCorkle may be reached at the Yale University School of Nursing, 100 Church Street South, P.O. Box 9740, New Haven, CT 06536-0740; by phone at (203) 737-5501; or via e-mail at Ruth.McCorkle@yale.edu.

Walter F. Baile, MD is Professor of Behavioral Science and Director of the Program in Interpersonal Communication and Relationship Enhancement (I*CARE) in the Department of Faculty Development at The University of Texas M. D. Anderson Cancer Center. Dr. Baile has brought his talents in teaching communication skills to many parts of the world and has led workshops and other teaching programs in Japan, Italy, Germany, and other sites around the world. Currently, he participates in a National Cancer Institute sponsored program to train oncologists to teach communication skills. Dr. Baile produced "On Being an Oncologist," a video for cancer clinicians starring the actors William Hurt and Megan Cole and is author of over 150 scientific papers, book chapters, and abstracts on clinician-patient communication. Dr. Baile's latest project is development of the MD Anderson Library of Communication Skills in Oncology, a repository of video and contemporary educational tools to drive home the important messages of how to communicate with cancer patients. He can be reached at The University of Texas M. D. Anderson Cancer Center, 1515 Holcombe Blvd., Box 135, Houston, Texas 77030-4009; by phone at (713) 745-4116; or via e-mail at wbaile@mail.mdanderson.org.

Contributors

Joann Aaron, MA is a Scientific Editor/Medical Writer, Department of Community Oncology, The University of Texas M.D. Anderson Cancer Center. With more than 20 years of experience, Ms. Aaron has written and edited book chapters, articles, reviews, abstracts, grants and protocols. Joann had in-depth experience compiling detailed scientific and medical information in the areas of general oncology, neuro-oncology, phase I clinical trials, community oncology control and prevention trials, clinical and research focused manuscripts, posters, slide presentations, letters of intent, and other scientific materials. She may be reached at The University of Texas M.D. Anderson Cancer Center, 1515 Holcombe Blvd., Houston, TX 77030; or by phone at (877) MDA-6789.

Lodovico Balducci, MD is board-certified in medical oncology/hematology. He serves as Professor of Oncology and Medicine, University of South Florida College of Medicine, and Program Leader, Senior Adult Oncology Program, Department of Interdisciplinary Oncology, University of South Florida College of Medicine, and medical director of Affiliates and Referring Physician Relations at the H. Lee Moffitt Cancer Center. Dr. Balducci is nationally and internationally recognized for his contributions to geriatric oncology. Recent awards and recognition include the 17th annual Claude Jacquillat Award for Achievement in Clinical Oncology (Paris); the 2009 Nimmo Visiting Professorship in Adelaide, Australia; the 2009 Mehdi Tavassoli Memorial Lecture in Jackson, Miss.; the first American Society of Clinical Oncology B.J. Kennedy Award in 2007; the American Community Cancer Center recognition for outstanding clinical research in 2006; and the first Paul Calabresi Memorial Lecture for the International Society of Geriatric Oncology in 2005 (Rome, Italy). Dr. Balducci may be reached at the H. Lee Moffitt Cancer Center, 12902 Magnolia Drive, Tampa, FL 33612; by telephone at (813) 979–3822; or via e-mail at Balducci@moffitt.usf.edu.

Dee M. Baldwin, PhD, RN, FAAN is Director, School of Nursing, at the University of North Carolina at Charlotte. An expert in health promotion and women's well-ness, her scientific work addresses the promotion of breast health in older African American women and issues related to early detection and screening and health lit-eracy. Dr. Baldwin is the principal investigator for several studies on the promotion of breast health for older African American women, and has developed a model for encouraging low-income African American women to participate in breast and cervical cancer early detection and screening. She may be reached at the University of North Carolina at Charlotte, 9201 University City Blvd., CHHS 449B, Charlotte, NC 28223-0001; by phone at (704) 687–7953; or via e-mail at dbaldwi5@uncc.edu.

Robert Bergamini, MD is President of Unity Physician Hospital Organization and a physician who is board-certified in both pediatrics and pediatric hematology/oncology. His research interests focus on immune suppressor regulation. Dr. Bergamini may be reached at 607 S. New Ballas Road, Suite 2415, St. Louis, MO 63141; by phone at (314) 251–6986; or via e-mail at drbobstl@yahoo.com.

Kenneth R. Burns, PhD, RN is Professor and Chair of the Division of Nursing at Martin Methodist College. He may be reached at 433 West Madison Street, Pulaski, Tennessee 38478; by telephone at (931) 424–7395; or via e-mail at kburns@martinmethodist.edu.

Marilyn Frank-Stromborg, CNP, EdD, JD, FAAN is Special Court Administrator, Drug Court Coordinator for the DeKalb County Courthouse. She may be reached at 133 West State Street, Sycamore, Illinois 60178; by phone at (815) 895–7224; or via e-mail at mstromborg@dekalbcounty.org.

Barbara Given, PhD, RN, FAAN is the Associate Dean for Research and University Distinguished Professor, College of Nursing, Michigan State University. Her research and contributions to the nursing profession have won her various awards, including the Life Time Achievement Award, College of Nursing Alumni Association, as well as the Elizabeth McWilliams-Miller Award for Excellence in Research. She may be reached at Michigan State University, School of Nursing, B515-C West Fee Hall, East Lansing, MI 48824-1315; by phone at (517) 432–9159; or via e-mail at Barb.Given@hc.msu.edu.

Myra Glajchen, DSW is the Director of the Institute for Education and Research in Pain and Palliative Care, Department of Pain Medicine and Palliative Care, Beth Israel Medical Center. Dr. Glajchen created Beth Israel's Family Caregiver Program and as its Principal Investigator, has guided the development and dissemination of the program's deliverables and research studies. Among her accomplishments are development of the Brief Assessment Scale for Caregivers (BASC), creation of an award-winning website for caregivers, and publication of the widely acclaimed Caregiver Resource Directory. Dr. Glajchen is currently Principal Investigator for two studies, one on medication adherence for cancer and chronic pain patients and their caregivers; the other, a project to increase recognition of palliative care needs among patients and their caregivers in the Emergency Department through assessment, referral, clinical intervention and professional education. She may be reached at the Center at First Avenue at 16th Street, Baird Hall, Room 12BH23, New York, NY 10003; by phone at (212) 844.1472; or via e-mail at mglajchen@chpnet.org.

Carol D. Goodheart, EdD is a scholar–practitioner in independent practice in Princeton, New Jersey. Her career integrates practice, research, and service to psychology. Dr. Goodheart works at the intersection of physical and mental health, practice and science, humanism and scholarship. Dr. Goodheart was the 2010 President of the American Psychological Association and currently serves on its Board of Directors. As APA President, she founded the APA Presidential Task Force on Caregivers, which developed a "Family Caregiver Briefcase for Psychologists" to assist psychologists in recognizing, assessing, and addressing the needs of a broad group of family caregivers across the life span. Dr Goodheart earned awards as a Fellow of the American Psychological Association, a Distinguished Practitioner in the National Academy of Psychology, a Registrant in the National Register of Health Service Providers in Psychology, and the recipient of national and state Psychologist of the Year Awards from Psychologists in Independent Practice and from the New Jersey Psychological Association, as well as the recipient of the Distinguished Psychologist Award for lifetime contributions to psychotherapy from the Division of Psychotherapy of the American Psychological Association. Dr. Goodheart may be contacted at 114 Commons Way, Princeton, NJ 08540; by telephone/fax at (609) 987–8844; or via e-mail at carol@drcarolgoodheart.com. Additional information may be found on her website at www.DrCarolGoodheart.com.

Karrie Cummings Hendrickson, PhD, RN is a Clinical Coordinator for Finance and Decision Support at Yale-New Haven Health System and an Associate Research Scientist at Yale School of Nursing. Dr. Hendrickson may be reached at Decision Support, Yale-New Haven Health System, 20 York St., New Haven, CT 06510; by phone at 203-688-5214; or via e-mail at karrie.hendrickson@yale.edu.

Barry J. Jacobs, PsyD is the Director of Behavioral Sciences for the Crozer-Keystone Family Medicine Residency Program of Springfield, PA, and an adjunct faculty member of the Temple University School of Medicine, the University of Pennsylvania School of Nursing, and the Institute for Graduate Clinical Psychology of Widener University. A clinical psychologist and family therapist, Dr. Jacobs is the author of *The Emotional Survival Guide for Caregivers—Looking After Yourself and Your Family While Helping an Aging Parent*, which focuses on the story of two sisters in their fifties struggling to take care of their cancer-stricken, 80-year-old mother. He is also the editor of the "In Sickness and Health" column for the journal *Families, Systems and Health* and writes an advice column for "Take Care!", the newsletter of the National Family Caregivers Association. Dr. Jacobs may be reached at 1260 E. Woodland Avenue, Springfield, PA 19094; by phone at (610) 690-4490; or via e-mail at barry.jacobs@crozer.org.

Dale L. Kaufman, MPH, MA is a speechwriter at the Centers for Medicare and Medicaid Services in the U.S. Department of Health and Human Services. A career government employee, Ms. Kaufman formerly served as Senior Public Health Writer at U.S. Department of Veterans Affairs and Senior Speechwriter at the Office of Justice Programs, U.S. Department of Justice. Ms. Kaufman may be reach at the Centers for Medicare and Medicaid Services, 200 Independence Avenue S.W., 309D-02, Washington, DC, 20201; by telephone at (202) 260–1420; or via e-mail at Dale.Kaufman@cms.hhs.gov.

Sheryl LaCoursiere, PhD, FNP-BC, APRN is a Clinical Assistant Professor at the University of Massachusetts Boston and Lecturer at Yale School of Medicine, Center for Medical Informatics. She was previously a Department of Defense Postdoctoral Fellow in Breast Cancer at Yale School of Nursing. Dr. LaCoursiere's research interests include informatics and technology, and the use of the Internet for health communication and intervention, particularly for chronic illnesses across the life-span. Other research interests include complementary and alternative medicine, as well as family care and geriatrics. Dr. LaCoursiere developed a Theory of Online Social Support, which is being used internationally, as well as the Attitudes Toward Online Healthcare (ATOHC) scale, which has been studied with various chronic conditions. She may be reached at the University of Massachusetts Boston, 42 Middleway East, Waterbury, CT 06708; by phone at (203) 910-0052; or via e-mail at sheryl.lacoursiere@gmail.com.

Ann O'Mara, PhD, RN, MPH is Program Director, Community Oncology and Prevention Trials Research Program, Division of Cancer Prevention, National Cancer Institute, 6130 Executive Blvd., EPN 2010, Bethesda, MD 20892-7340. Dr. O'Mara previously served as a Cancer Prevention Fellow with the National Institute of Health. She may be reached at DHHS/NIH/NCI/DCP, MS-7340, Rockville MD 20892; by phone at (301) 402–5336; or via e-mail at omaraa@mail.nih.gov.

Mary Elizabeth Paulk, MD is Professor at the University of Texas Southwestern Medical Center. Dr. Paulk received the 2000 Soros Foundation Project on Death in America Faculty Scholar Award to support research in end-of-life care and the 2005 Champion of End-of-Life Care Award honoring Texans making an outstanding contribution to improving the quality of end-of-life care. She may be reached at the Division of General Internal Medicine, 5323 Hines Boulevard, Dallas, TX 75390-8889; by phone at (214) 648–0288; or via e-mail at Elizabeth.paulk@UTSouthwestern.edu.

Christina M. Puchalski, MD, MS, FACP is Christina Puchalski, MD, MS is the Founder and Executive Director of the George Washington Institute for Spirituality and Health (GWish) and a Professor of Medicine and Health Sciences at The George Washington University School of Medicine, where she has pioneered novel and effective educational and clinical strategies to address the spiritual concerns common in patients facing illness. Dr. Pulaski has received numerous awards including the Healthcare Foundation of New Jersey's Faculty Humanism in Medicine Award and the 2009 George Washington University Distinguished Alumni Award. She is a Fellow of the American College of Physicians and a member of the Alpha Omega Alpha (AΩA) medical honor society. Dr. Pulaski may be reached at The George Washington University, School of Medicine and Health Sciences, 2131 K St, NW, 5th floor, Washington, DC 20037; by phone at(202) 994–6220: or via e-mail at hcscmp@gwumc.edu.

Victoria H. Raveis, MA, MPhil, PhD is a Research Professor and Director of the Cardiology and Comprehensive Care Center in the College of Dentistry at New York University and Director of the university's Psychosocial Research Unit on

Health, Aging and the Community. She may be reached at 380 Second Avenue, Suite 301, New York, NY 10010; by phone at (212) 998–9805; or via e-mail at victoria.raveis@nyu.edu.

Christine M. Schrauf, PhD, RN, MBA has many years of experience as a medical nurse, with clinical, education, and administrative roles in the specialty of hemodialysis care. She has held nursing faculty positions during her early career and recent doctoral education. Her areas of knowledge and interest also include health policy and ethical dimensions of end-of-life care, topics of focus in recent presentations and publications. Her research addresses state support systems for informal family caregivers caring for loved ones at home. Professional memberships include Sigma Theta Tau, the American Nephrology Nurses Association, and the American Nurses Associations. She may be reached at Elms College Division of Nursing, 291 Springfield St. BH 431, Chicopee, MA 01030; by phone at (413) 265–2417; and via e-mail at schraufc@elms.edu.

Martin L. Smith, STD is Director of Clinical Ethics in the Department of Bioethics at the Cleveland Clinic. Previously, he served as Chief of Clinical Ethics and as an Associate Professor in the Department of Critical Care at The University of Texas M.D. Anderson Cancer Center. Dr. Smith's areas of research include ethics consultation, end-of-life issues, institutional ethics committees, medical mistakes, and informed consent. He may be reached at the Cleveland Clinic, Center for Ethics, Humanities and Spiritual Care, Mail Code JJ60, 9500 Euclid Avenue, Cleveland, OH 44195 or by phone at (216) 445–2769.

Phyddy Tacchi, RN, CNS, LMFT, LPC is a Clinical Nurse Specialist in the Department of Psychiatry, The University of Texas M.D. Anderson Cancer Center. As a psychiatric advanced practice nurse who specializes in the emotional difficulties patients and caregivers encounter in adjusting to living a life with cancer, Ms. Tacchi's interests include a focus on the emotional strengths and challenges of the family caregiver; working with couples struggling with the impact the cancer experience has placed upon their relationship; and training staff to enhance their communication skills during difficult conversations with patients and families using innovative role training techniques. She may be reached at the The University of Texas, M.D. Anderson Cancer Center, 1515 Holcombe Blvd, Houston, TX 77030; or by phone at (713) 792–6600.

Diana J. Wilkie, PhD, RN, FAAN is Professor and Harriet H. Werley Endowed Chair for Nursing Research in the Department of Biobehavioral Health Science College of Nursing, University of Illinois at Chicago. Dr. Wilkie is an internationally-known pain specialist with a special emphasis on palliative and end-of-life care in cancer and other life-threatening illnesses. She has many publications about pain, and her research program on pain has been continuously funded since 1986. Currently, she is conducting two randomized clinical trials testing the effects of massage and effects of computerized pain tools on clinical outcomes and several pilot studies. Dr. Wilkie may be reached at 845 South Damen Avenue (MC802), Chicago, IL 60612-7350; via phone at(312) 413–5469; or by e-mail at diwilkie@uic.edu.

Chapter 1
Caring for a Loved One with Cancer: Professional and Family Issues

Ruth McCorkle, Ronda C. Talley and Walter Baile

Caring for a Loved One with Cancer: Professional and Family Issues

The evolution of the healthcare system over the past few decades has resulted in shorter hospital stays and greater numbers of invasive, out-patient procedures for most patients. This change in healthcare delivery has resulted in more family members being thrust into the role of caregiver (Cawley and Gerdts 1988; Conkling 1989; Yost et al. 1993).

Historically and transculturally, there have always been a role for family caregivers although the role went largely unrecognized by health practitioners, researchers, and advocates. Although some caregiving research was conducted in the 1970s, it focused largely on the caregivers for individuals with dementia. Caregiving as a national issue came to the forefront in the early 1990s and found a champion in former First Lady Rosalynn Carter, who has a long-term interest in caring for the mentally ill. Over the years, the literature has evolved to address caregiver needs and concerns in many areas, including informational needs; psychological, physical, and spiritual health outcomes; race and gender disparities; and evidence-based support

---

The findings and conclusions in this chapter are those of the authors and do not necessarily represent the views of the Centers for Disease Control and Prevention.

R. McCorkle (✉)
School of Nursing, Yale University, 100 Church Street South, New Haven,
CT 06536-0740, USA
e-mail: Ruth.McCorkle@yale.edu

R. C. Talley
Centers for Disease Control and Prevention, Western Kentucky University,
1906 College Heights Boulevard, Bowling Green, KY 42101, USA
e-mail: Ronda.Talley@wku.edu

W. Baile
M. D. Anderson Cancer Center, University of Texas, Houston, TX 77230-1402, USA
e-mail: wbaile@mdanderson.org

R. C. Talley et al. (eds.), *Cancer Caregiving in the United States,*
Caregiving: Research, Practice, Policy,
DOI 10.1007/978-1-4614-3154-1_1, © Springer Science+Business Media, LLC 2012

and education strategies. Now a wide range of professional and family caregivers as well as professional advocacy organizations collaborate on caregiving-related health delivery, research, education, and policy concerns.

This increased attention to the needs of caregivers is timely. The level of technical, psychological, and physical support now demanded of family caregivers is unprecedented (Ganz 1990). The responsibility for complex patient care may reside with the family member without regard for adequacy of resources or sufficiency of preparation. Subsequently, family caregivers can suffer a myriad of physical, mental, social, and spiritual consequences which may, in turn, adversely affect the ill family member.

Definitions of Caregiving, Family Caregiver, and Professional Caregiver

To define *caregiving*, we turned to several well-known caregiving researchers and advocacy groups. The National Family Caregivers Association (NFCA n.d.) defines caregiving as the necessary physical and mental health support to care for a family member. One description of informal or family caregiving that has been widely accepted over time was offered in 1985 by Horowitz (1985), who indicated that informal care involves four dimensions: *direct care* (helping to dress, managing medications); *emotional care* (providing social support and encouragement); *mediation care* (negotiating with others on behalf of the care receiver); and *financial care* (through managing fiscal resources, including gifts or service purchases). The challenges of actually providing informal or family caregiving have been attributed to the level of intensity and physical intimacy required to provide care; the amount of burden, distress, and role strain that care engenders for the caregiver, and the skill required to master care tasks.

Relatedly, the Administration on Aging (n.d.) defines a *caregiver* as "anyone who provides assistance to another in need." The National Alliance for Caregiving and the American Association of Retired Persons (NAC/AARP 2009) define caregiving as caring for an adult family member or friend. However, most definitions of caregiving adopt a life span perspective that includes children and youth as both caregivers and care recipients.

More specifically, *family caregiver* is defined by the Health Plan of New York and NAC (n.d.) as a person who cares for relatives and loved ones. MetLife and NAC (2006) expanded on this definition by specifying additional qualifiers, stating that a family caregiver is "a person who cares for relatives and loved ones who are frail, elderly, or who have a physical or mental disability." Similarly, the NFCA (n.d.) added that family caregivers provide a vast array of emotional, financial, nursing, social, homemaking, and other services on a daily or intermittent basis. The NFCA advocates for the term *family caregiver* to be defined broadly and to include friends and neighbors who assist with care by providing respite, running errands, or doing a range of other tasks that support the caregiver and care recipient. In this book, we will use the terms *informal caregiver* and *family caregiver* interchangeably and employ the comprehensive NFCA definition of *family caregiver* to refer to caring relatives, friends, and neighbors of all ages across the life span (see *Intergenerational Caregiving*, this series).

Caregiving can have different meanings to individuals, depending on their relationship to the patient, the roles they take on as caregiver, the point in the disease trajectory, the predicted outcome for the patient, the support they receive from other family members and friends, and their cultural and religious background. Thus, definitions have to be individualized to each situation.

Caregiving is a process that occurs across the life span. It begins with infant care, changes to meet the development needs of children and adolescents, and continues as we enter adulthood and mid-life. This process concludes with end-of-life care, including bereavement care. When we look at caregiving across the continuum of life, it becomes easy to see why it is an issue that involves all people, regardless of race, gender, socioeconomic status, disability condition, or age. As noted in *The Multiple Dimensions of Caregiving and Disability*, the second book in the Rosalynn Carter Institute for Caregiving book series, "Caregiving is an activity in which we will all engage at some time(s) in our lives" (Crews and Talley 2011).

Throughout the book, we use the term *professional caregivers* to refer to paid care providers such as physicians, nurses, social workers, psychologists, case managers, hospice workers, home health aides, and many others. The designation as professional caregiver excludes family caregivers who may receive funds to provide care from new and emerging sources, such as the Medicaid Cash and Counseling Demonstration Program.

Our Nation's Caregivers

One of the most recent comprehensive reports that examined caregivers was done by the NAC and the AARP (NAC/AARP 2009). In the report, *Caregiving in the United States*, it is estimated there are 43.5 million caregivers in the nation, 3.5 million of whom care for individuals with cancer. The family caregiver population is heterogeneous: approximately 67% are female, 59% married, 55% employed, and 34% have a high school education or less.

Caregivers of a Loved One with Cancer

According to a recent report by the American Cancer Society (Cancer Statistics 2012), 577,000 deaths from cancer are projected to occur in the United States in 2012. An estimated 76% (or over 400,000) of these deceased patients had been cared for by a family member in the prior year(s). With the growing trend toward more cancer treatments provided on an ambulatory basis, much of the responsibility of care has shifted from healthcare professionals to patients and their families. In light of the large number of family caregivers for patients with cancer who confront circumstances that may pose a considerable risk to both their physical and mental health, we have undertaken this book to address the broad range of issues that we understand about caregiving, including what we know and what we do not know.

Caregiver Psychological Cost

The diagnosis of cancer has been well recognized as a major stressor that imposes disruption and disorganization for not only the person with cancer, but also for the caregiver (Montazeri et al. 1996). During the diagnostic phase, the person with cancer and the family caregiver face existential concerns that force an evaluation of their futures and life goals (Weisman and Worden 1976). The task of caring for the patient involves incorporation of a variety of complex skills which frequently fall on the spouse and other family members who may not be prepared, willing, or able to take on these tasks. Caregivers often find themselves physically, emotionally, and financially drained (Stetz 1987), which can make the care burdensome. Several studies have described the burden of family, however, these studies have primarily been limited to Caucasian populations and women (Northouse et al. 2006).

Caregiving Fiscal Cost

The cost associated with family caregiving to individuals with cancer was conservatively estimated at US$ 1 billion annually in 2001 (Hayman et al. 2001). Based on a sample of 7,443 individuals who participated in the Asset and Health Dynamic Study (AHEAD) survey, this accounts solely for direct patient care hours valued at US$ 8.17/hour. The cost of family caregiving far exceeds US$ 1 billion when one considers the health and social consequences incurred by the caregiver. The most frequently cited sources of caregiver compromise are: psychological impairment (Grunfeld et al. 2004; Kurtz et al. 2004); mood disturbance (Soothill et al. 2001); sleep disturbance (Carter 2003; Carter and Chang 2000); fatigue (Jensen and Given 1993); impaired immune function (Kiecolt-Glaser et al. 1991); decline in personal health status (Lee et al. 2003; Vitaliano et al. 1993); social isolation (Cameron et al. 2002); feelings of helplessness and lack of control (Goldstein et al. 2004); and insufficient skill to manage the ill family member's symptoms (Nijboer et al. 1999).

In a qualitative study of 15 family caregivers, Strang and Koop (2003) found that several factors facilitated or interfered with caregiver coping. One factor that interfered with caregiver coping is the competence, or the ability to provide care, of the professional caregiver. When professional caregivers were less than competent, they added to rather than reduced the caregiving burden. The economic cost of providing family care in the home also places a significant burden on caregivers. With the shift toward community-based care, a number of costs have shifted to the patient and caregiver. Out-of-pocket financial expenditures include medications, transportation, home medical equipment, supplies, and respite services. These costs are nonreimbursable and often invisible, however, are very real to families who are trying to provide care on a fixed income.

Caregiver Health Costs

Several studies attribute caregiving to a decline in personal health. The Caregiver Health Effects Study (Schulz and Beach 1999), a prospective population-based study, examined the relationship between spousal caregiving demands and all-cause mortality at four years. Using a study population of 392 spouse caregivers and 427 matched noncaregivers, and controlling for demographic and physical health status predictors, results at a four year follow-up revealed a 63% higher mortality risk among family caregivers experiencing strain (56.5% of caregivers) versus noncaregivers. Family caregiver s who did not experience strain (43.5% of caregivers) had mortality rates similar to noncaregivers. The authors concluded that the experience of mental or emotional strain among family caregivers is an independent risk factor for mortality. Additional studies unanimously conclude that chronic stress of caregiving contributes to cardiovascular disease (Lee et al. 2003; Vitaliano et al. 1977); neuroendocrine dysfunction (Irwin et al. 1997); and impaired immune function (Kiecolt-Glaser et al. 1991).

The psychological toll of caring for a family member with cancer has been well documented over the years (Grov et al. 2005; Grunfeld et al. 2004; Kurtz et al. 2004; Laizner et al. 1993). Anxiety and depression are the most often cited cancer family caregiver impairments, with prevalence estimates for depression ranging from 12 (Grunfeld et al. 2004) to 30% (Blanchard et al. 1997) and estimates for anxiety at 35% (Grunfeld et al. 2004). In several studies, the cancer family caregiver's mental health burden exceeded that of the cancer patient (Harding and Higginson 2003; Higginson and Wasde 1990; Soothill et al. 2001; Wingate and Lackey 1989). Anxiety, depression, stress, and tension have all been shown to increase as the patient's functional status declines and as the patient approaches death (Given et al. 2004; Grov et al. 2005; Grunfeld et al. 2004; Kurtz et al. 1994, 2004; Harding and Higginson 2003). A metaanalysis of the relationship between psychological distress of cancer patients and their caregivers (Hodges et al. 2005) indicates a mutuality of distress response in the dyad.

As the caregiver literature has matured, predictor variables for mental health issues among cancer family caregivers have been identified. Caregiver depression appears to be especially sensitive to: (a) sleep deprivation (Carter and Chang 2000); (b) perceived burden of caregiving (Schulz and Beach 1999; Lee et al. 2003); (c) caregiver shift in role; (d) responsibility level; (e) leisure activity (Williamson et al. 1998); (f) lifestyle interference; and (g) social isolation (Cameron et al. 2002; Goldstein et al. 2004); all of which are modifiable risk factors. Sleep disturbance and fatigue among family caregivers have been minimally investigated, possibly because they are an obvious and assumed dysfunction implied in the role of caregiver (Carter 2003; Carter and Chang 2000). In one study, the investigators discovered that although family caregivers were prescribed sleep medication they were reticent to take it for the fear that it would prevent them from carrying out their caregiver responsibilities. Predictably, strongly significant positive correlations were found between caregiver sleep problems and caregiver level of depression.

For many cancer family caregivers, physical and psychological outcomes appear to be mediated by perceptions of caregiving burden weighed against the positive aspects of the role (Glajchen 2004; Goldstein et al. 2004; Hudson 2004; Kurtz et al. 2004; Nijboer et al. 1999). Notably, perceived burden and the associated strain are not associated with the number of hours one devotes to caregiving, or the severity of the patient's symptoms (Kurtz et al. 2004). Instead, perception of burden seems to be most influenced by lifestyle interference (Cameron et al. 2002), social isolation and restriction in activity due to caregiver responsibilities (Williamson et al. 1998), and low self-efficacy or feelings of inadequacy when performing caregiving tasks (Nijboer et al. 1999).

Although much of the literature addresses the negative consequences of being a family caregiver, recently attention has been given to the rewards and satisfaction available to family caregivers (Hudson 2004). These include the protective effects of perceiving value and meaning in the caregiving role (Haley et al. 2003), a sense of accomplishment, and a better relationship with the care recipient, as well as personal growth and family cohesion (Cawley and Gerdts 1988; MacVicar and Archbold 1976; Wellisch et al. 1978). However, caregiving remains associated with negative consequences, particularly when care provision is perceived as an encumbrance to the caregiver. During the caregiving phase, when positive perceptions predominate over negative ones, it is possible that the benefits to the caregiver may extend to the bereavement experience (Koop and Strang 2003). The general health status of cancer caregivers tends to mirror that of adults with disabilities. Both groups display more risky health behaviors, such as alcohol and tobacco use, are less likely to make and keep routine medical visits, and have poorer perceptions of their health status (King et al. 1994). Burton et al. (1997) found that caregivers with a high level of involvement with the care recipient (defined as caring for an individual with at least one impairment in activities of daily living [ADLs]) reported not having enough time to exercise or recuperate from illness, and forgetting to take prescribed medications. All of these may have negative health consequences. For instance, caregiving has been overall linked to decreased physical health for the caregiver (Schulz and Beach 1999; Vitaliano and Katon 2006) and an increase in caregiver mortality rates (Irwin et al. 1997).

Clinicians should be mindful of how their personal views and concerns about cancer affect communication with cancer patients and family caregivers, especially at key decision-making and transition points along the continuum of care. It is essential for healthcare professionals to establish structured dialogue among patients, family members, and other professional caregivers regarding treatment goals and expectations. Within patient- and caregiver-centered care paradigms, it is necessary to separate and clarify the values, thoughts, and emotional reactions of care providers, patients, and families.

Social support has been consistently found to influence a person's psychosocial adjustment to cancer. The ability and availability of significant others to deal with diagnosis and treatment can significantly affect the patient's self-perception. Regardless of the type of cancer, individuals who receive a cancer diagnosis experience a heightened need for interpersonal support. Those who are able to maintain close connections with family and friends during the course of illness are more likely to cope effectively with the disease than those who are not able to maintain such relationships (Burton et al. 1997; Glajchen 2004).

Living with a chronic illness, such as cancer, often requires continuing care and management by a team of specialists. Care is usually provided through follow-up visits to ambulatory or out-patient clinics and consulting rooms rather than through hospitalization. The burden that caregiving places on the family highlights the family's needs and the importance of offering support and information that can help reduce caregiver burden. Helping to arrange respite care for the patient also aids in relieving caregiver burden.

During times of transition between the stages of disease and treatment, family members often have increasing responsibilities, assuming duties previously performed by the care recipient, and coordinating and potentially delivering care in the home. Family members' level of distress and methods of dealing with that distress, in fact, may vary throughout the illness trajectory from initial diagnosis through subsequent therapy to the point when viable treatment options have been exhausted. The increasing responsibilities of the family caregiver in the face of limited external support and the consequences of caregiving for the patient and family raise important challenges for professional caregivers.

Family members must cope with their emotional responses to the cancer diagnosis and cope with the physical, social, and financial dimensions of providing care. With a cancer diagnosis, family caregivers are now expected to play a major role in assisting with the management of the disease, treatment, and treatment-related side effects. Cancer and its treatment may alter family identity, roles, communication patterns, and daily functioning. These changes can occur over an extended period of time as family caregivers deal with unfamiliar situations and demands as cancer treatment continues, as the disease progresses, or as the patient recovers and survives.

When changes in patients' conditions are due to remissions and exacerbations, this necessitates changes in the family caregivers' care responsibilities and role demands. Change adds stress, and constant adaptations require more work, negotiation, and adjustment of family members. In addition, at some points in the care trajectory, the caregiver role may require observation and supervision only, while at other points (e.g., end-of-life) total physical care may be needed. Further, the caregiving role may be assumed by some caregivers for only a few weeks, while others may serve in this role for many months or years. In addition, there may be greatly varying demands in intensity across diverse caregiving situations as the patient's disease and treatment status changes.

The literature includes a number of studies describing strategies to help caregivers cope with living with cancer and its consequences (Pasacreta and McCorkle 2000). The interventions include a range of educational, psychoeducational, support, and skill-building strategies targeted at the patient and family caregiver as a dyad and at family caregivers alone. The value of providing information to cancer caregivers has been reported consistently in the research literature. Reported with equally consistent frequency, however, is the difficulty that caregivers have in obtaining information from healthcare professionals, particularly physicians and nurses. Despite the fact that it is often difficult to obtain, caregivers report that information is a critical element in helping them to cope with the patient's illness. Times when caregivers appear to be in the greatest need of information are: (a) at the time of diagnosis; (b) during hospitalizations, especially at the time of surgery; (c) at the start of new treatments; (d) at the time of recurrence; and (e) during the dying phase.

In addition to learning about the physical aspects of the illness, caregivers need to be informed about the emotional aspects of the illness and recovery. Caregivers want to know what to expect regarding the emotional aspects of the illness both for themselves and the patient. In this manner, caregivers can be reassured proactively that their own and the patient's psychological distress is to be expected and is not a sign of poor coping.

Sources of support for family caregivers have lagged far behind than those provided for patients. In particular, caregiving spouses report little support from health professionals, often due to limited contact with physicians and nurses in hospital and out-patient settings. However, within the last 5 years, support interventions have been developed to provide direct psychological services to family caregivers, often by different disciplines (e.g., social workers, psychologists, chaplains, nurses).

Longitudinal studies of caregiver adaptation to the cancer caregiving role are needed to explore the complex interactions of caregiver physical and mental health, including how usual self-care and health-promotion practices are altered given the continuous and ever-evolving role of caregiving. Interventions and clinical trials that assist the caregiver to engage in activities that promote health and build physiological resilience must be explored, including exercise programs, good nutrition guidance, social activation, regular sleep, and self-monitoring their physical and emotional health.

Professionals need to be taught how to assess caregivers' capacity to provide care in light of the patients' actual and anticipated needs. Professional caregivers need to have the knowledge and skills to facilitate family caregiver's role acquisition and to determine when emotional distress extends beyond expected levels and warrants treatment. Family caregivers need to be included in the patient's plan of care and kept informed about what to expect. Once professionals grasp that family caregivers can play a critical role in enhancing patient clinical outcomes, they may be more willing to assess the caregiver's health and emotional capacity to provide care as a partner in the process. When professional caregivers form partnerships with family caregivers, together they can achieve the clinical outcomes they desire for the patient with cancer and the caregivers themselves.

Genesis of the Rosalynn Carter Institute Caregiving Book Series

The development of this book was sponsored by Johnson & Johnson (J&J), an international healthcare business leader. With J&J funding, the Rosalynn Carter Institute convened a series of 10 expert panels to address a wide variety of caregiving issues. These included disability; Alzheimer's disease; cancer; mental health; life span caregiving; rural caregiving; intergenerational caregiving; education, training, and support programs for caregivers; interdisciplinary caregiving; and building community caregiving capacity. The result of the collaboration with expert panelists has culminated in the Rosalynn Carter Institute for Caregiving Book Series with Dr. Ronda Talley serving as the series editor. We launched the book series in 2008 with the release of *The Multiple Dimensions of Caregiving and Disability*. The second release in the series was *Education, Training, and Support Programs for Caregivers*. The third release in the series was *Rural Caregiving*. This volume, *Caring for a Loved One with Cancer: Professional and Family Issues*, is the fourth volume to be released in the series.

Contents and Organization of *Caring for a Loved One with Cancer: Professional and Family Issues*

Caring for a Loved One with Cancer: Professional and Family Issues is divided into three main sections that address different areas of caregiver impact. These include: (1) issues affecting the care triad, i.e., patient, family, and healthcare professional; (2) issues in providing quality care, including education, support, end-of-life issues, and (3) cross-cutting issues impacting caregivers and caregiving, including issues of faith, economics, legal concerns, ethics, and cancer care policy and advocacy. Each chapter provides an overview of the current status of the topic across four areas: practice, research, education/training, and policy/advocacy, then offers recommendations for future action in these areas. The closing chapter summarizes issues raised across the chapters and offers a call for action in each area.

Issues Affecting the Care Triad

This section addresses specific care-related issues that have an impact on the patient, the family, and the healthcare team.

Wilkie In her chapter, Wilkie discusses the needs of the patient with cancer, their caregivers, and the family unit by addressing the issues relevant during the diagnostic period. She suggests implementing a model of simultaneous care during this period, a system that addresses development of a plan for both the treatment phase and palliative care. Within this approach to the diagnostic period, the author further describes the various roles that the professional caregiver might assume in response to the dynamics of the patient and family. These include the role of consultant, collaborator, or guide. Adoption of any one of these roles should reflect the patient and their family's desired level of autonomy or support during the various phases of illness. These roles are explored in terms of the cancer care team, which might take on these various responsibilities, and the types of training that are available for assuming multiple aspects of care.

The emphasis of this chapter is specifically on providing family-centered care, particularly assessment of the family's values and priorities, as well as their ability to manage the patient's illness and treatment. Issues regarding training in family assessment are explored.

McCorkle and Given This chapter provides a summary of the growing body of literature addressing the impact of cancer on family caregivers. Family caregivers experience both physical and emotional distress, as well as a lack of knowledge and support to provide care to their loved ones. The authors explore the emotional distress of family caregivers and the various factors that influence it, such as severity and duration of illness, physical status of the patient, and the amount of care devoted to cancer care. A variety of interventions aimed at helping caregivers are described, and their limitations noted.

Goodheart Goodheart discusses the impact of economic and ethnic disparities in the United States and the significant impact of these factors on healthcare and health status among different socioeconomic and ethnic groups in this country. In turn, these disparities have an impact on caregiving situations among individuals and families. As examples, she describes instances of disparity in the rates of cancer for African American s and Whites, and high rates of uninsured Latinos. The author also cautions against creating stereotypes that mask individual differences within cultural or ethnic groups.

Although literature addressing disparities related to cancer care and caregiving is limited, there is a large amount of information available that can be applied to cancer, and Good heart summarizes this. Research on health disparities and caregivers outlines a large number of significant outcomes for minority caregivers. These include decreased work hours; compromised health status; variability in resilience and knowledge; and increased reliance on religion for support, resourcefulness, and hospice use when compared to the general population. In each of these areas, there may be a positive or negative association, such as increased resilience and resourcefulness, however, poorer health status among African American caregivers. Another area of disparity is the unequal cancer treatment given to African American or Hispanic/Latino individuals. Gender disparities are also present, with women typically receiving less caregiving than men. In addition to these factors, individuals from minority groups also experience barriers to care. These include inadequate access to services due to poverty, language and cultural barriers, and health professionals' knowledge and attitudes.

Baile, Kettler, and Aaron Baile et al. discuss the importance of promoting collaboration between the patient, family, and healthcare treatment team to optimize care for both the cancer patient and their caregivers. They introduce the notion of creating a

have similar needs to caregivers of adult cancer patients; however, the overriding concerns of parents are different, focusing on providing emotional support to the child and having accurate information. One unique aspect of this group is the strain that caring for a child with cancer places on the marital relationship. Another group that is discussed is young caregivers of individuals with cancer.

Jacobs A significant number of cancer patients become long-term survivors and may present caregivers with additional burdens beyond those discussed in the previous chapters. Much progress has been made in the areas of clinical care, research, and advocacy for cancer patients in terms of short-term survival. Once they have survived their cancer, however, these individuals may experience chronic illness-related burdens, such as uncertainty of recurrence, physical impairments related to treatment, and potential loss of identify and self-esteem.

In addition, there has been little research and few interventions designed for caregivers to assist family members who are long-term cancer survivors. A number of factors related to long-term cancer survivors have an impact on the caregiver. For example, the greater the severity and course of disease, the more distress felt by the family, especially the primary caregiver. This is particularly true for childhood cancer survivors and their caregivers. The authors discuss obstacles that can impair family support systems, including shifts in family roles, breakdown of communication among family members, preexisting negative relationships among family members and friends, and willingness of caregivers to accept support.

Balducci and LaCoursiere End-of-life caregiving issues are addressed by Balducci and LaCoursiere. The authors present a theoretical framework that describes the caregiving trajectory for a patient with cancer. Using this framework, the authors provide a clear delineation of the caregiving tasks during this period as well as the potential benefits and stresses to the caregiver.

Balducci and LaCoursiere provide information ranging from knowing what to expect at specific points in the dying process to whom to call when the patient dies. Education and research questions are outlined that specifically address this period in the illness trajectory. The chapter is important in highlighting the special responsibilities and needs of the caregiver during the terminal phase of the patient's illness.

Raveis In her discussion of the advances in cancer care, Raveis addresses the interesting conflict between the positive changes in medicine's ability to diagnose and treat cancer, and the negative impact these changes often have on family caregivers. On one hand, current developments in cancer research allow for earlier and more accurate detection, less invasive diagnostic procedures, less radical surgery, reduced side effects of treatment, broader availability of aggressive treatment to vulnerable populations, and increased survivorship. On the other hand, each of these developments can increase the level of burden on family caregivers. The duration of care and the demands of coping with treatment and disease-related side effects have increased. Lastly, caregivers have to make difficult treatment decisions and are often very stressed by the responsibilities of decision-making. As cancer care has shifted from being primarily hospital based to home and community based, caregiving has shifted as well, and costs to the caregiver are very high.

The author makes recommendations for future work in these various areas, with the goal of addressing needs of caregivers through various stages of the disease.

Cross-cutting Issues Impacting Caregivers and Caregiving

The final section of the book addresses a variety of issues that can have an impact on family caregivers. These range from spirituality in caregiving, to ethical and legal issues, and finally to legal and policy questions. The chapters provide information about the larger issues that caregivers must address beyond providing direct care to their loved ones.

Puchalski Spirituality is an important dimension in the lives of cancer patients and their caregivers, and this chapter provides an overview of the elements of spirituality that are relevant for these individuals. Pulchalski emphasizes that addressing the spiritual needs of the caregiver is as important as addressing the needs of the individual with cancer; however, addressing the spiritual needs of the caregiver is an area that has been overlooked in terms of education and research.

In this context, spirituality is clarified as not necessarily religious in nature, but rather it is a process that gives meaning and substance to one's life. Addressing spiritual needs can contribute to the care of the patient with cancer in several ways: (a) it helps the caregiver to acknowledge and potentially alleviate the suffering of the patient with cancer; (b) it is an area of knowledge that can assist the professional caregiver to support the patient with cancer and their family; and (c) it is an area of exploration that can help professional caregivers to understand their own spirituality.

Baldwin This chapter explores the economic aspects of cancer care and the financial burdens that family caregivers experience. National cancer care costs have risen significantly over the last decade, and changes in insurance coverage and management of care have placed a large financial burden on family caregivers. Cancer care requires expensive treatments in both hospital and community-based settings, and there are also significant demands related to home care, transportation, medications, nutritional needs, and lost wages of both the patient and the caregiver. Patients and their caregivers who are poor face additional burdens related to unemployment, diminished access to healthcare, inadequate education, substandard housing, and chronic malnutrition. These factors contribute to delay in seeking early care, thus affecting both the incidence and survival of this population.

Frank-Stromborg and Burns In their chapter, Frank-Stromborg and Burns provide an overview of key legal issues that the patients with cancer and their caregivers may need to address. These include: (a) the obligation for family members to provide care; (b) the legal issues that caregivers may need to address regarding decision-making; and (c) the complexities of state regulations and laws regarding living wills, durable power of attorney, and other documents that are relevant during treatment and end-of-life care. The authors provide a helpful summary of the most current regulations regarding Medicare and Medicaid, and reimbursement for various types of home care and end-of-life care. Also addressed in this chapter are legal implications of care and decision-making for individuals in lesbian, gay, or transsexual relationships.

Kaufman, O'Mara, and Ceccarelli Policy addressing the family caregiver's has received more attention at the federal level in recent years; however, the target of this activity has been caregivers in general, not specifically caregivers of cancer patients. Cancer patients often have specific needs that differ from the needs of the other populations requiring caregiving, such as Alzheimer's patients. In order to provide the types of cancer care advocated by the authors in this book, appropriate policies supporting cancer caregiving must be in place at the federal, state, and local levels. This chapter provides a summary of existing policies that support family caregivers and addresses the areas of deficiency. The authors conclude with recommendations for further work in political advocacy for cancer patients and their caregivers.

Smith and Paulk End-of-life decision-making can be difficult for everyone involved in caring for cancer patients, both professionals and family members. The purpose of this chapter is to help increase healthcare professionals' awareness of how ethical issues and decision-making can impact caregivers of patients with cancer. The chapter addresses both general ethical principles as well as issues that are specific to families.

The authors present several important areas of ethical care. These include: (a) an overview of the four foundational concepts of clinical ethics: respect for autonomy, nonmalfeasance, beneficence, and justice; (b) a discussion of the various levels of competence of an individual to make a decision regarding treatment and end-of-life options; and (c) a caution to healthcare professionals to be aware of cultural differences regarding decision-making.

Smith and Paulk also provide a comprehensive review of the barriers to ethical end-of-life care, addressing issues such as lack of advance planning on the part of individuals and their primary care providers; inadequate documentation of preferences through living wills and assignment of healthcare proxies; and decision-making at the end-of-life.

Summary

This book provides a comprehensive review of topics related to the care of patients with cancer, the needs of the caregivers, and issues related to different stages of the disease process. Broader issues such as legal implications, spiritual needs, ethical considerations, and policy implications are also explored. Each of the chapters provides an overview of the topic and makes recommendations for future work in the areas of practice, education, research, and policy and advocacy, making this book useful for a variety of readers. The format of the book allows the reader to explore specific areas of interest or read the entire text, which will provide an in-depth understanding of the issues that caregivers of patients with cancer face. It is the hope of the editors that readers of the book will find this information useful, especially when assisting caregivers of patients with cancer to provide optimal care not only to their family members, but also to themselves as they move through the course of the caregiving experience.

References

Administration on Aging. (n.d.). Resources: Common caregiving terms. Retrieved from http://www.aoa.gov/prof/aoaprog/caregiver/careprof/progguidance/resources/caregiving_terms.asp.

Blanchard, C., Albrecht, T., & Buckdeschel, J. (1997). The crisis of cancer: Psychological impact on family caregivers. *Oncology, 11*(2), 189–194.

Burton, L., Newsom, J., Schulz, R., Hirsch, C., & German, P. (1997). Preventive health behaviors among spousal caregivers. *Preventive Medicine, 26*, 162–169.

Cameron, J., Franche, R., Cheung, A., & Stewart, D. (2002). Lifestyle interference and emotional distress in family caregivers of advanced cancer patients. *Cancer, 94*(2), 521–527.

Cancer Statistics. (2012). Cancer facts and figures, 2012, CA. *A Cancer Journal for Clinicians, 62*(1), 10–29.

Carter, P. (2003). Family caregivers' sleep loss and depression over time. *Cancer Nursing, 26*(4), 253–259.

Carter, P., & Chang, B. (2000). Sleep and depression in cancer caregivers. *Cancer Nursing, 23*(6), 410–415.

Cawley, M., & Gerdts, E. (1988). Establishing a cancer caregivers program. An interdisciplinary approach. *Cancer Nursing, 11*(5), 267–273.

Conkling, V. (1989).Continuity of care issues for cancer patients and families. *Cancer, 64*(1 Suppl.), 290–294.

Crews, J. E., & Talley, R. C. (2011). Introduction: The multiple dimensions of caregiving and disability. In R. C. Talley (Series Ed.), & R. C. Talley & J. E. Crews (Vol. Eds.), *The multiple dimensions of caregiving and disability*. New York: Springer.

Ganz, P. (1990). Current issues in cancer rehabilitation. *Cancer, 65*(3 suppl.), 742–751.

Given, B., Wyatt, G., Given, C., Sherwood, P., Gift, A., DeVoss, D., et al. (2004). Burden and depression among caregivers of patients with cancer at the end-of-life. *Oncology Nursing Forum, 31*(6), 1105–1117.

Glajchen, M. (2004). The emerging role and needs of family caregivers in cancer care. *Journal of Supportive Oncology, 2*(2), 145–155.

Goldstein, M., Concato, J., Fried, T., Kasl, S., Johnson-Hurzeler, R., & Bradley, E. (2004). Factors associated with caregiver burden among caregivers of terminally ill patients with cancer. *Journal of Palliative Care, 20*(1), 38–43.

Grov, E., Dahl, A., Moum, T., & Fossa, S. (2005). Anxiety, depression, and quality of life in caregivers of patients with cancer in late palliative phase. *Annals of Onncology, 16*(7), 1185–1191. Retrieved from http://annonc.oxfordjournals.org/cgi/content/abstract/16/7/1185?etoc.

Grunfeld, E., Coyle, D., Whelan, T., Clinch, J., Reyno, L., Earle, C., et al. (2004). Family caregiver burden: Results of a longitudinal study of breast cancer patients and their principal caregivers. *Canadian Medical Association Journal, 170*(12), 1795–1801.

Haley, W., LaMonde, L., Han, B., Burton, A., & Schonwetter, R. (2003). Predictors of depression and life satisfaction among spousal caregivers in hospice: Application of a stress process model. *Journal of Palliative Medicine, 6*(2), 215–224.

Harding, R., & Higginson, I. (2003). What is the best way to help caregivers in cancer and palliative care? A systematic literature review of interventions and their effectiveness. *Palliative Medicine, 17*(1), 63–74.

Hayman, J., Langa, K., Kabeto, M., Katz, S., DeMonner, S., Chernew, M., et al. (2001). Estimating the cost of informal caregiving for elderly patients with cancer. *Journal of Clinical Oncology, 19*(13), 3219–3225.

Health Plan of New York & National Alliance for Caregiving. (n.d.). Care for the family caregiver: A place to start. Retrieved from http://www.caregiving.org/pubs/brochures/CFC.pdf.

Higginson, I., & Wasde, A. (1990). Palliative care: Views of patients and their families. *British Medical Journal, 301,* 277–281.

Hodges, J., Humphris, G., & Macfarlane, G. (2005). A meta-analytic investigation of the relationship between the psychological distress of cancer patients and their careers. *Social Science and Medicine, 60,* 1–12.

Horowitz, A. (1985). Family caregiving to the frail elderly. In C. Eisdorfer (Ed.), *Annual review of gerontology and geriatrics* (Vol. 5, pp. 194–246). New York: Springer.

Hudson, P. (2004). Positive aspects and challenges associated with caring for a dying relative at home. *International Journal of Palliative Nursing, 10*(2), 58–65.

Irwin, M., Hauger, R., Patterson, T., Semple, S., Ziegler, M. & Grant, I. (1997). Alzheimer caregiver stress: Basal natural killer cell activity, pituitary-adrenal cortical function and sympathetic tone. *Annals of Behavioral Medicine, 19*(2), 83–90.

Jensen, S., & Given, B. (1993). Fatigue affecting family caregivers of cancer patients. *Supportive Care in Cancer, 1,* 321–325.

Kiecolt-Glaser, J. K., Dura, J. R., Speicher, C. E., Trask, O. J., & Glaser, R. (1991). Spousal caregivers of dementia victims: Longitudinal changes in immunity and health. *Psychosomatic Medicine, 53,* 345–362.

King, A., Oka, R., & Young, D. (1994). Ambulatory blood pressure and heart rate response to the stress of work and caregiving in older women. *Journal of Gerongology, 49,* 239–245.

Koop, P., & Strang, V. (2003). The bereavement experience following home-based family caregiving for persons with advanced cancer. *Clinical Nursing Research, 12,* 127–144.

Kurtz, M., Given, B., Kurtz, J., & Given, C. (1994). The interaction of age, symptoms, and survival status on physical and mental health of patients with cancer and their families. *Cancer Supplement, 74*(7), 2071–2078.

Kurtz, M., Kurtz, J., Given, C., & Given, B. (2004). Depression and physical health among family caregivers of geriatric patients with cancer: A longitudinal view. *Medical Science Monitor, 10*(8), CR447–CR456.

Laizner, A., Yost, L., Barg, F., & McCorkle, R. (1993). Needs of family caregivers of persons with cancer: A review. *Seminars in Oncology Nursing, 9*(2), 114–120.

Lee, S., Colditz, G., Berkman, L., & Kawachi, I. (2003). Caregiving and risk of coronary heart disease in US women: A prospective study. *American Journal of Preventive Medicine, 24*(2), 113–119.

MacVicar, M., & Archbold, P. (1976). A framework for family assessment in chronic illness. *Nursing Forum, 15*(2), 180–194.

Metlife & National Alliance for Caregiving. (2012). 2006 MetLife foundation family caregiver awards program. Retrieved from http://www.raconline.org/funding details.php?funding id=2726.

Montazeri, A., McEwen, J., & Gillis, C. R. (1996). Quality of life in patients with ovarian cancer: Current state of research. *Supportive Care in Cancer, 4*(3), 169–179.

National Alliance for Caregiving & AARP (NAC/AARP). (2009). *Caregiving in the U.S.* Washington: National Alliance for Caregiving & AARP. Retrieved from http://www.caregiving.org/data/09finalreport.pdf.

National Family Caregiver Association (NFCA). (n.d.). What is family caregiving? Retrieved from http://www.thefamilycaregiver.org/what/what.cfm.

Nijboer, C., Triemstra, M., Tempelaar, R., Sanderman, R., & van den Bos, G. (1999). Determinants of caregiving experiences and mental health of partners of cancer patients. *Cancer, 86*(4), 577–588.

Northouse, L., Rosset, T., Phillips, L., Mood, D. Schafenacker, A.,& Kershaw, T. (2006). Research with families facing cancer: The challenge of accural and retention. *Research in Nursing and Health, 29*(3), 199–211.

Pasacreta, J., McCorkle, R. (2000). Cancer care: Impact of interventions on caregiver outcomes. *Annual Review of Nursing Research, 18,* 127–148.

Schulz, R., & Beach, S. (1999). Caregiving as risk factor for mortality. *Journal of the American Medical Association, 282,* 2215–2219.

Soothill, K., Morris, S., Harman, J., Francis, B., Thomas, C., & McIllmurray, M. (2001). Informal carers of cancer patients: What are their unmet psychosocial needs? *Health & Social Care in the Community, 9*(6), 464–475.

Strang, V. R., & Koop, P. M. (2003). Factors which influence coping: Home-based family caregiving of persons with advanced cancer. *Journal of Palliative Care, 19*(2), 107–114.

Vitaliano, P. P., Russo, J., & Bailey, S. L., Young, H. M., & McCann, B. S. (1993). Psychosocial factors associated with cardiovascular reactivity in older adults. *Psychosomatic Medicine, 55,* 164–177.

Vitaliano, P. P., Schulz, R., Kiecolt-Glaser, J., & Grant, I. (1977). Research on phsyiological and physical concomitants of caregiving: Where do we go from here? *Annals of Behavioral Medicine, 19*(2), 117–123.

Vitaliano, P. & Katon, W.(2006). Effects of stress on family caregivers: Recognition and management. *Psychiatric Times, 13,* 24–28.

Weisman, A., & Worden, J. W. (1976). The existential plight in cancer: Significance of the first 100 days. *International Journal of Psychiatric Medicine, 7*(1), 1–15.

Wellisch, D., Mosher, M., & Van Scoy, C. (1978). Management of family emotion stress: Family group therapy in a private oncology practice. *International Journal of Group Psychotherapy, 28*(2), 225–231.

Williamson, G., Shaffer, D., & Schulz, R. (1998). Activity restriction and prior relationship history as contributors to mental health outcomes among middle-aged and older spousal caregivers. *Health Psychology, 17*(2), 152–162.

Wingate, A., & Lackey, N. (1989). A description of the needs of noninstitutionalized cancer patients and their primary care givers. *Cancer Nursing, 12,* 216–225.

Yost, L., McCorkle, R., Buhler-Wilkerson, K., Schultz, D., & Lusk, E. (1993). Determinants of subsequent home health care nursing service use by hospitalized patients with cancer. *Cancer, 72*(11), 3304–3312.

Part I
Issues Effecting the Care Triad

Chapter 2
Diagnostic Issues: Family Dynamics and Caregiving for an Individual with Cancer

Diana J. Wilkie and Stuart J. Farber

Annually, nearly 1.6 million Americans will be diagnosed with cancer (Siegel et al. 2011). For the vast majority of these people, their cancer care is delivered in outpatient settings. Living with a new cancer diagnosis is a 24-hour experience, which means that family caregivers face responsibility for much of the care needed by persons diagnosed with cancer (Given et al. 1997). Caregivers' responsibilities are magnified by the many advances in cancer treatments, especially aggressive combination therapies that increase the complexity of patient needs over the trajectory of the cancer experience. The care needs also are exceptionally complex, for the people who will eventually die from their cancers.

This chapter addresses caregiving during the diagnostic phase of the cancer trajectory, a phase in which family dynamics set an important context for cancer caregiving throughout the other phases. Three models are presented to set a context for patient- and family-centered cancer care. A case example showcases the current status of caregiving during the diagnostic phase of cancer care. This case also highlights future directions for research and ways to implement conceptual frameworks. Such information can enhance the caregiving experience as patients and their caregivers begin to navigate the acceptable options for curative and palliative cancer care treatments.

Conceptual Models for Cancer Care

As the patient and family begin the cancer caregiving experience at the time of cancer diagnosis, three models are important to high quality cancer care: (1) the cancer trajectory; (2) cancer resource allocation; and (3) the roles of the professional

D. J. Wilkie (✉)
University of Illinois at Chicago, 845 South Damen Avenue (MC802),
Chicago, IL 60612-7350, USA
e-mail: diwilkie@uic.edu

S. J. Farber
School of Medicine, University of Washington,
Box 356390 Seattle, WA, USA
e-mail: sfarber@u.washington.edu

R. C. Talley et al. (eds.), *Cancer Caregiving in the United States,*
Caregiving: Research, Practice, Policy
DOI 10.1007/978-1-4614-3154-1_2, © Springer Science+Business Media, LLC 2012

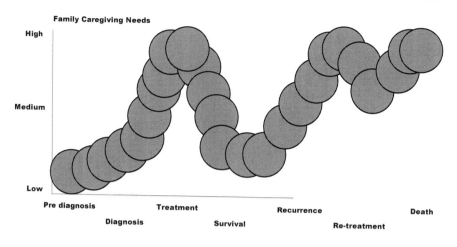

Phase of Cancer Care

Fig. 2.1 Cancer trajectory

caregivers, especially in sharing the bad news of a cancer diagnosis. Each model is briefly described and then discussed from the perspective of one patient and her family caregivers.

Cancer Trajectory

Cancer caregiving begins with the first sign or symptom of a tumor and continues over the entire cancer trajectory. After the patient notices and acknowledges the lump, hemoptysis, bloody stool or elevated PSA level for example, diagnostic procedures begin to determine if there is a malignancy and if so the type, stage, and other characteristics. This diagnostic phase of the cancer trajectory leads to the many other phases of cancer care including the treatment, survival with monitoring, recurrence, re-treatment, and palliative and terminal phases (Fig. 2.1). The diagnostic phase of the cancer trajectory helps to predict the course likely for each individual. At each phase, the patient requires professional and family caregiving.

Unfortunately, the patient and family caregivers without previous experiences with cancer do not know or anticipate the demands of caregiving over the cancer trajectory (Faulkner et al. 1994a; Waldrop 2006). Those with previous cancer experiences may approach the bad news with considerable anger (Faulkner et al. 1994b). Professional caregivers play an important role in exploring the family's prior experience with cancer and setting the stage for realistic hope (Kutner et al. 1999; Links and Kramer 1994; Trask et al. 2008). Those experiences are an important context for discussions about the patients' probable cancer trajectory and ways that cancer care resources should be tailored to meet the patient and family caregiver needs (Shields 1998; Trask et al. 2008).

Fig. 2.2 World Health Organization resource allocation model: current model of care for people diagnosed with cancer

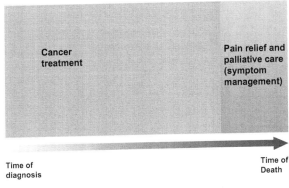

Fig. 2.3 World Health Organization: proposed resource allocation model for people diagnosed with cancer

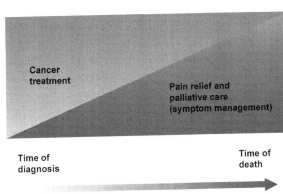

Cancer Resource Allocation

Over the cancer trajectory, most cancer resources have been traditionally allocated during the diagnostic and treatment phases. The current model of resource allocation emphasizes that most health care resources are focused on cancer treatment until it is clear that the cancer cannot be cured, when the focus of care changes to palliative management of pain and other symptoms (Fig. 2.2; World Health Organization [WHO] 1996).

Figure 2.3, however, shows an alternate simultaneous care model proposed by the WHO (1996). In this simultaneous care model, from the first sign of cancer in the diagnostic phase, cancer treatments and palliative care are implemented concurrently. Figure 2.3 shows that most of the cancer care resources are focused on cancer treatment at the diagnostic phase, however, some are focused on palliative care. Later in the cancer trajectory, the focus shifts to palliative care, however, antitumor treatments continue as appropriate to control symptoms and improve quality of life. The simultaneous care model is consistent with patient- and family-centered care at the diagnostic phase as well as throughout the cancer trajectory. Descriptive research findings support the feasibility and effectiveness of implementing the simultaneous care model on patient level variables in people diagnosed with advanced stage lung cancer (Pitorak et al. 2002, 2003). Although these findings are encouraging, little research is available to document the effect of implementing the simultaneous model in the early phases of cancer care, especially effects on caregivers (Bakitas et al. 2004, 2006, 2009a, b, 2010; Byock et al. 2006; Meyers et al. 2004; Temel et al. 2010).

Professional Caregiver Roles

Professional caregivers typically interact with patients and family caregivers in one of the three typical roles: consultant, collaborator, and guide (Farber et al. 2002). All of the roles require the use of communication skills and cancer expertise at the time of a cancer diagnosis, however, several traits help define each role. Understanding the relationship that professional caregivers share with the patient and their family caregivers helps to clarify the most effective role for a specific case and provides realistic hope about the future in the context of the cancer type and stage (Links and Kramer 1994; Shields 1998).

Consultant. The consultant caregiver provides expert, professional information about the cancer and treatment options to the patient, family, and other professional caregivers (Farber et al. 2002). The consultant role is based on the consultant's medical authority and expert cancer knowledge, the sharing of that knowledge with others for educational purposes, and referral to other members of the cancer care team in order to determine and support the diagnostic process and plan of care (Farber et al. 2002). The consultant presents information that helps the patient and family understand the cancer diagnosis, prognosis, and treatment. This information is often presented through dialogue (Faulkner et al. 1994a), however, it can also be written or available in forms such as videotapes (Cull et al. 1998) or audiotapes. The patient or family decides which cancer therapy plan best meets their goals and needs. If they are unable to make a decision, the consultant caregiver makes the decision based on the cancer facts, e.g., the cancer type, stage, and available therapies (Farber et al. 2002).

Collaborator. In the role of collaborator, professional caregivers exchange information with the patient and family to facilitate a common understanding of the cancer diagnosis and illness experience, and they all work together to choose the cancer treatment path (Farber et al. 2002). The collaborator role includes that of the consultant and also includes additional traits. Based on his original research findings, Farber (Wilkie et al. 2012) stated that the collaborator:

- "Acts as a coordinator, assuring all members of the team are providing patient and family care harmonious with the treatment plan.
- Serves as a facilitator, working with the patient/family and other team members to promote the care plan.
- Provides a therapeutic role by promoting healing through discussions and actions with the patient and family regarding medical, psychological, spiritual, and social issues related to the care plan.

- Is a team member, working within the care plan using and respecting other team members' skills."

Farber (Wilkie et al. 2012) suggest the following set of questions assist the collaborator to provide patient- and family-centered cancer care.

- "What have you been told about your condition?
- What do you feel is happening?
- What would you like to see happen?
- What are your other concerns?"

The patient's and family caregivers' responses to these questions help the collaborator to develop a patient- and family-centered plan of care that addresses the patient's goals and safety as well as the complexity of care needed to implement the cancer care treatment plan. The discussion should especially address the caregiving needs and whether the family caregivers can meet them safely. In addition, the dialogue helps the professional caregiver understand the resources available to meet these caregiving needs. Asking the patient and family about their illness experiences helps to identify and clarify the important issues for everyone, which typically include physical, emotional, and spiritual concerns (Shields 1998). With this broader understanding of the illness experience, the professional caregiver is able to facilitate the team members as they provide care. The collaborator uses relationships and personal self to create a therapeutic experience for the patient and family. Both the professional and personal connections of this role are important.

Guide. The guide role requires the professional caregiver to consult and collaborate with the patient and family, showing them the way to accomplish their goals by virtue of the guide's greater understanding of the medical context and how to achieve the patient's and family's needs within it (Farber et al. 2002). Farber (Wilkie et al. 2012) suggests that the guide role includes two additional traits:

- Advisor—acting to promote a cancer care treatment path that is most appropriate for the unique experience of the patient and family.
- Advocacy—assisting the patient and family in overcoming the barriers that impede the path of their cancer care.

The advocacy role of the guide goes beyond using professional skills to augment those of the patient and family. The guide also engages in direct supportive actions on their behalf.

There is danger in the guide role not present when the professional caregiver takes the role of the consultant or collaborator. The professional caregiver may be taking the patient where the professional caregiver wants him/her to go, not where the patient wants to go. Yet, without the professional caregiver's active involvement, the patient in need of guidance would find it extremely difficult to find a cancer care path that would achieve his/her treatment goals (Wilkie et al. 2012).

Compared to the consultant and collaborator roles, the guide develops deeper professional and personal connections. Unlike in the consultant role, the guide's efficacy is not solely based on professional knowledge. The guide invests enough of him/herself to be personally involved. Both the guide's professional and personal selves become essential elements in providing care to this patient and family. As a result, for the patient and family caregivers, no other professional caregiver can easily replace the guide. If the guide is working as part of a team, this impact is not overwhelming. There are other team members with whom to share the professional caregiving role when the guide is not available. However, if the guide works independently, this role can create significant tension and should be taken into account when such a role is considered. What does the guide do when he/she wants to be home with his/her family and the patient has a problem? When no one knows the patient and his family quite as well as the guide does, the patient's quality of care will decline steeply when the guide is not involved. Despite these potential tensions, the personal satisfaction of serving as a guide is high (Wilkie et al. 2012).

In summary, each of these three roles is important for professional caregivers to deliver high quality care at the time of a cancer diagnosis and initiation of a cancer treatment plan, be it for curative or palliative intent. None of the roles has a higher or lower value (Farber et al. 2002). Which role the professional caregiver plays will depend on many factors.

- What role does the patient and family wish?
- What role does the situation demand?
- What role does the professional caregiver feel comfortable playing?

Ultimately the role or roles the professional caregiver plays will be defined by the relationship shared with the patient and family and the personal and professional connections among all parties involved. Ideally, professional caregivers have the ability to play all three of these roles. However, rarely is the ideal a reality in clinical practice. Some professional caregivers are better or worse in each of these roles. It is important for each professional caregiver to understand the roles he/she is capable of performing and to recognize when the patient or family needs the support of a role with which he/she is uncomfortable. In such a case, another professional team member can be asked to provide this role, such as a nurse, consultant, mental health therapist, clergy member, physician, or the hospice team. The professional caregiver's understanding and facility with each of these roles is a dynamic process and will grow deeper over time. Most professional caregivers find that they continue to grow and develop in skill and understanding of these roles during their entire career (Balint and Shelton 1996; Emanuel and Emanuel 1992; Farber et al. 1999, 2002, 2003a).

Current Status

Stage of disease and the time that has passed since diagnosis are important variables in the family's responses to cancer (Woods et al. 1989). The diagnostic phase of cancer care is associated with high levels of stress for both the patient and the caregivers. During this time, they absorb the meaning of the cancer diagnosis and keep appointments with specialists for second opinions and specific recommendations regarding the cancer stage, searching for the treatment options most appropriate for the patient's cancer. The stress evolves not only from the emotional work of coping with the reality of the cancer diagnosis, but also from the enormity of the decisions patients and family members make about the acceptable treatment course (Albrecht et al. 2003). Patient- and family-centered cancer care during the diagnostic phase sets the stage for addressing the stress and forging effective relationships among the professional caregivers, patient, and family caregivers.

In order to provide high quality care to people with cancer and their families, professional caregivers must elicit, document, display, and assist in implementation of the patient's wishes for cancer care, including disease modifying treatments, palliative and end-of-life care (Morrison and Morris 1995). Helping patients to articulate their priorities sets the stage for family caregivers to participate most effectively in the cancer care treatment plan. Attending to the patient's wishes also requires the professional caregivers to recognize that family dynamics are central to this process (Grinyer and Thomas 2001; Lewis 1993; Lewis et al. 1993; Shields 1998; Stetz et al. 1994; Woods and Lewis 1995). Professional caregivers need to know that attending to the patient's wishes facilitates patient- and family-centered cancer care and it is not assisted suicide or euthanasia if the patient opts not to accept disease-modifying treatments.

The following case, Gypsy, exemplifies several important issues for patients, family caregivers, and professional caregivers during the diagnostic phase of cancer. As you read the case, identify the role her professional caregivers assumed, evaluate the model for the care that Gypsy and her family received, and make some conclusions about the family dynamics in this case. Gypsy's Cancer Diagnosis. (© 1994 D. J. Wilkie and D. B. Lawrence, modified with permission.)

Gypsy coughed bright red blood onto a tissue as she sat at the bedside of her husband, who was dying from chronic renal failure. Gypsy knew at the moment she saw the blood that she had lung cancer. After all, she had smoked one to two packs of cigarettes per day for 50 years, and her father died from lung cancer at age 42. She always knew she would get lung cancer. Still it wasn't easy when she heard the chest x-ray results at the same time that her husband was so near to death. It was difficult for her to undergo diagnostic staging scans only four days after he died and biopsy bronchoscopy two days before Christmas, two weeks after her first hemoptysis.

Gypsy learned the test results from her pulmonologist as she awoke in the recovery room without her family. She shared the news with her family as soon as she was able to see them. A few days later in his office, the pulmonologist sat with her and her family to discuss her options. He was gentle and kind as he told her that she had poorly differentiated nonsmall cell lung cancer. It was metastatic to the other lung, both kidneys, and possibly the cervical spine. He told her that surgery, chemotherapy, or radiation therapy would not cure her stage IV lung cancer. He promised he would control her symptoms and keep her comfortable. He also suggested that she see a medical oncologist and consider chemotherapy or radiation therapy as a means to control the hemoptysis. She agreed to the consultation.

The medical oncologist met with Gypsy and two of her three family members. He sat down next to Gypsy and talked with her about her lung cancer. As he talked, he drew pictures to show her and her family members what he was saying. He showed her where the tumors were in both of her lungs, both kidneys and her spine. He told her there were therapies that could be used to control her cancer but that none of them would cure her cancer. He talked about the advantages and disadvantages of each therapy and about not doing anything to treat her cancer but doing everything possible to keep her comfortable. Then he asked her which option she preferred.

Gypsy didn't hesitate, she told him that, as a 73-year-old woman, she didn't want to go through chemotherapy; she didn't want to lose her hair. She wanted to try radiation because it was likely to help the hemoptysis, which by now was very disturbing to her. She didn't want to cough and bleed to death.

Gypsy started radiation therapy to her lung, driven daily to treatments by her son. Her son and daughter also accompanied her when she saw her lawyer in order to deal with her husband's estate, revise her own will, and to specify her wishes in a living will. She created and signed a durable power of attorney and a durable power of attorney for health care in which she specified no home hospice; she did not want her son and daughter-in-law to take care of her, as they had done for her husband. Although his death was peaceful and her son and daughter-in-law valued the care-giving experience, Gypsy did not want them providing the level of personal, intimate care to her that they had willingly provided to her husband; she could accept that care from strangers, but not family. Gypsy discussed her wishes with her son, daughter, daughter-in-law and her physicians. She told her family that she had purchased cremation services for herself at the same time as she had taken care of her husband's final arrangements.[1]

Gypsy's case demonstrates several important aspects of patient- and family-centered decision-making at the time of diagnosis. Facilitating patient-centered decision-making requires the cancer care team, which consists of the patient, family caregivers, and professional caregivers, to reach consensus about the treatment goals. This consensus is necessary despite the uncertainty and barriers to understanding and accepting the cancer diagnosis, prognosis and the patient's wishes (Farber et al. 2003b; Shields 1998).

In Gypsy's situation, both physicians gave her the bad news in a humane way that helped her and her family caregivers come to a common understanding of the meaning of her medical diagnosis and prognosis (Buckman 1992; Shields 1998). All family members were identified by name and family role and accommodated in the small examination rooms (Buckman 1992). These practices are important to create a welcoming environment for the family caregivers and integrate them into the cancer care team (Speice et al. 2000). Professional caregivers understood which family members were authorized to receive Gypsy's health information subject to the Health Insurance Portability and Accountability Act (HIPAA) of 1996 (HHS 2003), and Gypsy signed appropriate permission documents to provide for ongoing communication between professional and her family caregivers. Research findings suggest that an audiotape recording of the discussion could have helped family members who were not present to reach a common understanding (Bruera et al. 1999).

Providing alternates to the office visit as a means of communicating with the physician, such as telephone and e-mail, encourages caregivers to be active team members (Speice et al. 2000). These methods allow the caregivers to be extra ears, ask questions, recall details, take notes, and gather and share important information, especially about symptoms (Speice et al. 2000). Together, the physician, Gypsy and her family reached a consensus about her treatment goals, the critical first step in patient- and family-centered decision-making at the time of a cancer diagnosis. This outcome was facilitated by the physician eliciting both Gypsy's and her family caregivers' understandings of the illness and expectations about the diagnosis and prognosis (Farber et al. 2002; Speice et al. 2000).

---

[1] From *How can I be dying, I feel so good? Gypsy's escape from lung cancer* (1994), by D. J. Wilkie and D. B. Lawrence, *Washington State Cancer Pain Initiative News, 2*(1), 1, 6–7. Copyright 1994 by D. J. Wilkie & D. B. Lawrence. Modified with permission.

Gypsy's prognosis was less uncertain than many people must cope with when their cancers are diagnosed. Her physicians clearly stated that they could not cure her cancer, however, they promised they would do everything possible to promote her comfort and emphasized that radiation therapy was integral to her long-term comfort. This focus was consistent with the simultaneous care model (Fig. 2.3; WHO 1996). Cancers diagnosed at earlier stages require considerable skill and expertise for the health care provider to address the many uncertainties experienced by the patient and family caregivers regarding the prognosis, especially if one or more family members are health professionals (Frogge et al. 1998).

Gypsy clearly articulated her wishes, and by doing so demonstrated her understanding and acceptance of the diagnosis and prognosis. She also communicated her values and priorities. Her family did not challenge her wishes because they recognized and respected her need for control. Had Gypsy's family focused on different wishes, such as prolonging her life to lengthen the time between the deaths of both parents, reaching consensus would have been more difficult.

All of Gypsy's family members knew her diagnosis and prognosis, which facilitated communication among team members. Family dynamics regarding those who know the diagnosis and those who do not can lead to difficulties for the entire cancer care team. Speice et al. (2000) cite several strategies that professional caregivers reported were useful in minimizing such difficulties:

- "Ask in advance how much information the patient wants the family to know
- Have interactions with the patient and family together, as much as possible
- Provide the same information to the patient and family
- Remind the family that the patient is the first priority
- Ask the family how they would feel if information was kept from them."

Farber (Wilkie et al. 2012) recommends that patient- and family-centered communication guide the team to a culturally appropriate way of disclosing the cancer diagnosis to the patient, family or both. For example if a Chinese-American woman's son requests that she not be told her diagnosis, several questions can guide the team to a culturally appropriate and family-centered response:

- Ask the patient, "Do you have any concerns about your health?" Allow her to say what she understands.
- Next ask, "Do you have any questions about your health?" Respond to her reply or if she gives an uncertain answer try another tack.
- Ask, "Do you want me to talk to you about your health or would you rather I talk with your children?" She may reply that she wants you to talk to her children.
- Then ask, "Who do you want to make decisions about your health?" It is likely that she will say her children, however, especially her son should make all decisions about her treatment.
- Then ask her children to meet in a place where the discussion of diagnosis, prognosis and treatments can continue in privacy and without interruption.

Using the questions in this example, the professional caregiving team will be able to honor the family's request to withhold disclosure of the diagnosis because it is culturally appropriate and based on the patient's wishes. These simple questions provide the team with the guidance they need to minimize difficulties encountered when the patient does or does not wish to know his/her diagnosis and prognosis or to make treatment decisions. Similar questions can guide the professional care team in determining which family members the patient wishes to be told and how much and how they should be told (Faulkner et al. 1994a; Speice et al. 2000). This type of patient- and family-centered communication can be very helpful with most families and is critically important for families with dysfunctional family dynamics (Faulkner et al. 1994b; Speice et al. 2000).

As the treatment plan is being developed, professional caregivers need to negotiate a common point of view about the initial management path while maintaining flexibility. The patient and caregivers benefit when the professional caregivers provide a context for the care that will be needed and specify who will provide the care, the family caregivers or the professionals. Professional caregivers should expect disequilibrium and help to restore balance in the family system while constructing a new future for the patient and family. In doing so, Farber (Wilkie et al. 2012) suggests the professionals should allow exploration of possible futures, and be mindfully "present" to the patient and family by asking open-ended questions such as:

- "What do you think will happen in the coming weeks?"
- "What role does spirituality play in your life?"
- "What is important to you in your life?"

Exploring responses to these questions guides the professional caregiver to gain insight about the patient's and caregivers' values and priorities. Farber (Wilkie et al. 2012) also stresses the importance of reminding them that the actual future is often experienced through an extremely unpredictable and circuitous path, as documented by his research with patients, family members, and providers (Farber et al. 2003b).

Application of Three Conceptual Models in Current Cancer Care

During the diagnostic phase of Gypsy's lung cancer experience, the pulmonologist acted solely in the consultant role. He used his expert skills and knowledge to diagnose her cancer and referred her to the medical oncologist for staging procedures and treatment options.

Her oncologist also played the consultant role when he used his professional knowledge to verbally describe and then illustrate the news about her cancer diagnosis. Although this role did not require a deep personal connection, her physician was caring and competent, which was important to Gypsy and her family members. Once Gypsy understood the knowledge provided by the professional caregiver, she decided what the diagnosis and prognosis meant to her and decided on the appropriate treatment, which was to accept the referral to the radiation oncologist. The family caregivers were a part of this process and supported her decisions, and Gypsy and her family made meaning of her disease through their interaction with her physicians.

"therapeutic alliance" among these three entities with the purpose of working toward a cancer cure or minimizing its side effects. This approach emphasizes establishing relationships that encourage mutual respect, strong communication and information sharing, and negotiation and problem-solving among the members of the alliance.

Integration of caregivers into the treatment team has implications for practice, research, and education, and the authors discuss these recommendations in detail. The overall value of the chapter is in providing an overarching framework for understanding and collaboratively addressing caregivers' needs.

Issues in Providing Care

This section addresses the broad array of issues that caregivers face in providing care to cancer patients. These include educational needs, short-and long-term care needs, end-of-life issues, and the impact of cancer treatment's changing status on the caregiver.

Glajchen In her chapter, Glajchen reviews the current status of education, training, and support programs for caregivers of patients with cancer. These topics are examined from the perspective of both efficacy, i.e., whether controlled trials show a treatment effect, and effectiveness, whether the treatment transfers to real world populations. Caregiver issues include unmet needs, the impact of caregiving on quality of life, and cultural and ethnic influences on caregivers. Interventions include strategies to increase knowledge, reduce anxiety and depression, provide medical care, offer comfort through hospice and palliative care, and increase confidence through problem-solving.

Glajchen notes that few effective strategies to address the needs of cancer caregivers have been documented, and many have limitations. Educational interventions have been developed in many settings, however, there is little outcome data to support them. Due to the variability in program type and setting as well as lack of standardization, it has been difficult to compare interventions. Hospice services can reduce anxiety and improve the quality of life and psychological status; however, outcomes of counseling and support interventions vary depending on the needs of the individual.

Bergamini and Hendrickson Several unique contributions to the discussion of caregivers of individuals with cancer are offered in this chapter. First, the authors present a discussion of the needs of caregivers at different points in the care trajectory of patients with cancer. Second, they offer a conceptual model for evaluating caregiver burden and quality of life effects. The authors suggest that the burdens of caregiving are inversely related to caregiver's quality of life. The model is then applied to the discussion of various aspects of caregiving and their implications for the patient and caregiver.

Finally, Bergamini and Hendrickson discuss the needs of caregivers of children with cancer and the needs of youth caregivers. Caregivers of children with cancer

The plan of care she selected was consistent with the WHO simultaneous care model (Fig. 2.3; WHO 1996), in which radiation therapy was planned to control her symptoms despite a diagnosis of advanced stage lung cancer. At the diagnostic phase of her cancer care, Gypsy's pulmonologist and oncologist both promised attentive, aggressive comfort care and implemented a plan of care to initiate control of her symptoms. The rest of Gypsy's cancer experience can be found on the Toolkit for Nurturing Excellence at the End-of-Life Transition and is available from http://www.tneel.uic.edu/.

Implications

Gypsy's case shows how the simultaneous care model, which is implemented by professional caregivers who enact a role consistent with the patient's preferences, can facilitate patient- and family-centered cancer care, beginning at the diagnostic phase of cancer. These conceptual models have important implications for clinical practice, research, and policy.

Practice. Similar to Gypsy's case, many professional caregivers play the consultant role as they interact with patients and family caregivers during the cancer diagnosis phase and perhaps throughout the entire cancer trajectory. However, not all patients are like Gypsy and her family. In some cases, the needs of the patient and family caregivers differ and could be met better by the professional caregiver assuming either the collaborator or guide roles (Davison et al. 2002).

Unfortunately, patient preferences and family dynamics as well as their needs infrequently direct professional caregivers in their implementation of the three roles. Although there are psychometrically valid and reliable measurements of patient preferences for control in the cancer treatment decision-making process, it is not clear if or how the three typical preferences (keep control, share control, and give away control; Degner et al. 1997) correspond to the professional caregiver roles for other phases of the cancer care process. Few tools have been validated as clinically useful measures of family dynamics in cancer care (Real del et al. 1998). Patient and family caregiver needs related to psychological and physical symptoms have been identified as common in patients and family caregivers living with the new cancer diagnosis (Darrow et al. 1998; Kristjanson and Ashcroft 1994; Wallberg et al. 2000; Wingate and Lackey 1989). Uncovering these preferences and needs currently requires skilled clinical interviews because screening tools appropriate for use in clinical settings are lacking.

The simultaneous model of cancer care is becoming more commonly implemented in clinical practice (Bakitas et al. 2009, 2010; Meyers et al. 2004; Pitorak et al. 2002, 2003; Temel et al. 2010). There is a critical need for additional emphasis on providing concurrent treatment of the cancer as well as palliative care appropriate to the patient's symptoms (Byock et al. 2006). The diagnostic phase of cancer provides a golden opportunity to initiate patient- and family-centered care that recognizes their current and potential needs across the entire cancer trajectory (Albrecht et al. 2003).

Table 2.1 Examples of cancer education materials for caregivers at the cancer diagnosis

Type of education material	Organization	Source: web site, phone number, other
General material for patients and professionals on each type of cancer	National Cancer Institute	http://cancersymptoms.org/
Comprehensive material for patients, family, friends, professionals. Some materials are available in Spanish and specific for people of Asian and Pacific Islander heritage	American Cancer Society	http://www.cancer.org (1-800-ACS-2345)
Comprehensive clearinghouse for web sites related to topics of interest to people living with cancer	Ortho Biotech Products, L.P.	http://www.cancer.com/
Material for patients and caregivers: – For managing ten common symptoms related to cancer treatments – Resources for recently diagnosed patients	Oncology Nursing Society	http://cancersymptoms.org/, http://www.ons.org/patientEd/ CancerDiagnosis.shtml
Flow Chart for professionals to communicate with patients and family	Palliative Medicine	(Faulkner et al. 1994a, b)
Material for physicians on breaking bad news and communicating with patients and caregivers	Education in Palliative and End of Life Care	http://www.epec.net/EPEC/ webpages/index.cfm
Material for health professionals on breaking bad news and communicating with people about health concerns	Toolkit for Nurturing Excellence at End of Life	http://www.tneel.uic.edu/

Education and Training. Currently, professional caregivers are predominately trained to use the consultant role, and they have insufficient flexibility in using the collaborator and guide roles. Communication difficulties can occur when the professional caregiver is unable to shift roles or lacks patient- and family-centered communication skills. These communication difficulties also can inflame family dynamics. Unless other members of the caregiving team assume responsibility for patient- and family-centered communications during the diagnostic phase of cancer care, gaps can occur in the caregiving process. Professional caregivers need to work as a team to deliver patient- and family-centered cancer care, however, they often lack the skills required for effective interdisciplinary work.

Education materials about cancer diagnosis and treatments designed for lay and professional caregivers are available from a number of organizations. These materials are readily available by calling or from web sites, a few of which are presented in Table 2.1.

Research. Little available research addresses effects of the simultaneous cancer care model for all people diagnosed with cancer. Like in Gypsy's case, it is more likely to occur in a cancer diagnosed at a stage clearly known for its high mortality within a relatively short time such as stage IIB or stage IV nonsmall cell lung cancer (Pitorak et al. 2003; Temel et al. 2010). Research in caregiving during the diagnostic phase of cancer is further impeded by a lack of clinically useful measurement tools that assist professional caregivers in selecting the role most appropriate for patient and family caregivers at various points in the cancer trajectory.

Policy. Current reimbursements for cancer care support the services of the physician, the captain of the professional caregiver team. This reimbursement plan negates the reality that multidisciplinary team is critical to effective patient- and family-centered care, not only at the diagnostic phase of cancer care but also throughout the entire cancer care trajectory.

Future Needs and Directions

Improving cancer care during the diagnostic phase requires a paradigm shift for clinical practice. Additional research and policy changes are important to implementing a model of simultaneous care that addresses patient and family preferences for caregiving roles.

Practice

Time-efficient screening tools are desperately needed in order to increase professional caregivers' insights into patient preferences, family dynamics, and the professional caregiver role most appropriate for the patient and his/her family caregivers. Given the explosion of informatics, computer-based tools can be used to capture, share, interpret, and implement patient wishes with consideration of family dynamics (Davison et al. 2002; Wilkie et al. 2003). Use of these tools can facilitate more efficient and effective cancer care, beginning at the diagnostic phase.

Education and Training

Professional caregivers need to be trained to use all roles as indicated by the patient's wishes and family dynamics. Improved communication skills are critical to patient- and family-centered cancer care.

Research

Refinement is needed for the existing patient preference tools (Degner et al. 1997) to also address family caregiver preferences. Development and testing of tools that identify preferences for professional caregiver roles and evaluate family dynamics at the diagnostic phase of cancer should be a priority for the National Institutes of Health (e.g., National Cancer Institute [NCI], National Institute on Aging), the American Cancer Society, and other cancer or family-oriented research organizations.

Policy

Continuity of cancer care from diagnosis throughout the cancer trajectory requires a multidisciplinary team effort and should be reimbursed accordingly. Indicators of success for NCI-funded comprehensive cancer programs should include measures of patient- and family-centered care throughout all phases of the cancer trajectory.

Conclusion

In conclusion, as showcased by Gypsy's story of her lung cancer diagnosis, a number of conceptual models inform patient- and family-centered cancer care at the diagnosis phase of cancer care. Professional caregivers should consider not only the phase of the cancer care, e.g., diagnosis, but also how to incorporate cancer treatments simultaneously with palliative care therapies. Additionally, the role assumed by the professional caregiver, e.g., consultant, collaborator, or guide, should fit the patient preferences and family dynamics. Clinical practice needs are tangled with education, research and policy changes that support a team approach to cancer care. The cancer care team must include professional caregivers, patients, and family caregivers all working toward patient-centered and family-focused care in order to overcome current deficits in cancer caregiving.

References

Albrecht, T. L., Ruckdeschel, J. C., Riddle, D. L., Blanchard, C. G., Penner, L. A., Coovert, M. D., et al. (2003). Communication and consumer decision making about cancer clinical trials. *Patient Education and Counseling, 50*(1), 39–42.

Bakitas, M., Bishop, M. F., Caron, P., & Stephens, L. (2010). Developing successful models of cancer palliative care services. *Seminars in Oncology Nursing, 26*(4), 266–284.

Bakitas, M., Lyons, K. D., Hegel, M. T., Balan, S., Barnett, K. N., Brokaw, F. C., et al. (2009). The project ENABLE II randomized controlled trial to improve palliative care for rural patients with advanced cancer: baseline findings, methodological challenges, and solutions. *Palliative & Supportive Care, 7*(1), 75–86.

Bakitas, M., Lyons, K. D., Hegel, M. T., Balan, S., Brokaw, F. C., Seville, J., et al. (2009). Effects of a palliative care intervention on clinical outcomes in patients with advanced cancer: the Project ENABLE II randomized controlled trial. *Journal of the American Medical Association, 302*(7), 741–749.

Bakitas, M., Stevens, M., Ahles, T., Kirn, M., Skalla, K., Kane, N., et al. (2004). Project ENABLE: a palliative care demonstration project for advanced cancer patients in three settings. *Journal of Palliative Medicine, 7*(2), 363–372.

Bakitas, M. A., Lyons, K. D., Dixon, J., & Ahles, T. A. (2006). Palliative care program effectiveness research: developing rigor in sampling design, conduct, and reporting. *Journal of Pain & Symptom Management, 31*(3), 270–284.

Balint, J., & Shelton, W. (1996). Regaining the initiative. Forging a new model of the patient-physician relationship. *Journal of the American Medical Association, 275*(11), 887–891.

Bruera, E., Pituskin, E., Calder, K., Neumann, C. M., & Hanson, J. (1999). The addition of an audiocassette recording of a consultation to written recommendations for patients with advanced cancer: A randomized, controlled trial. *Cancer, 86*(11), 2420–2425.

Buckman, R. (1992). *How to break bad news.* Baltimore: Johns Hopkins University Press.

Byock, I., Twohig, J. S., Merriman, M., & Collins, K. (2006). Promoting excellence in end-of-life care: A report on innovative models of palliative care. *Journal of Palliative Medicine, 9*(1), 137–151.

Cull, A., Miller, H., Porterfield, T., Mackay, J., Anderson, E. D., Steel, C. M., et al. (1998). The use of videotaped information in cancer genetic counselling: a randomized evaluation study. *British Journal of Cancer, 77*(5), 830–837.

Darrow, S. L., Speyer, J., Marcus, A. C., Ter Maat, J., & Krome, D. (1998). Coping with cancer: the impact of the Cancer Information Service on patients and significant others. Part 6. *Journal of Health Communications, 3 Suppl,* 86–96.

Davison, B. J., Gleave, M. E., Goldenberg, S. L., Degner, L. F., Hoffart, D., & Berkowitz, J. (2002). Assessing information and decision preferences of men with prostate cancer and their partners. *Cancer Nursing, 25*(1), 42–49.

Degner, L. F., Sloan, J. A., & Venkatesh, P. (1997). The control preferences scale. *Canadian Journal of Nursing Research, 29*(3), 21–43.

DHHS. (2003). Summary of the HIPAA Privacy Rule. Retrieved August 29, 2011, from http://www.hhs.gov/ocr/privacy/hipaa/understanding/index.html.

Emanuel, E. J., & Emanuel, L. L. (1992). Four models of the physician-patient relationship. *Journal of the American Medical Association, 267*(16), 2221–2226.

Farber, S. J., Egnew, T. R., & Herman-Bertsch, J. L. (1999). Issues in end-of-life care: Family practice faculty perceptions. *Journal of Family Practice, 48*(7), 525–530.

Farber, S. J., Egnew, T. R., & Herman-Bertsch, J. L. (2002). Defining effective clinician roles in end-of-life care. *Journal of Family Practice, 51*(2), 153–158.

Farber, S. J., Egnew, T. R., Herman-Bertsch, J. L., Taylor, T. R., & Guldin, G. E. (2003a). Issues in end-of-life care: patient, caregiver, and clinician perceptions. *J Palliat Med, 6*(1), 19–31.

Farber, S. J., Egnew, T. R., Herman-Bertsch, J. L., Taylor, T. R., & Guldin, G. E. (2003b). Issues in end-of-life care: patient, caregiver, and clinician perceptions. *Journal of Palliative Medicine, 6*(1), 19–31.

Farber, S. J., Egnew, T. R., Herman-Bertsch, J. L., Taylor, T. R., & Guldin, G. E. (2003). Issues in end-of-life care: Patient, caregiver, and clinician perceptions. *Journal of Palliative Medicine, 6*(1), 19–31.

Faulkner, A., Maguire, P., & Regnard, C. (1994a). Breaking bad news—A flow diagram. *Palliatiative Medicine, 8*(2), 145–151.

Faulkner, A., Maguire, P., & Regnard, C. (1994b). Dealing with anger in a patient or relative: A flow diagram. *Palliatiative Medicine, 8*(1), 51–57.

Frogge, M. H., Vance, R. B., Meyer, M., & Chong, F. A. (1998). Multidisciplinary rounds: patient-family-staff dynamics: when the patient/family are colleagues. *Cancer Practice, 6*(5), 258–261.

Given, B. A., Given, C. W., Helms, E., Stommel, M., & DeVoss, D. N. (1997). Determinants of family care giver reaction. New and recurrent cancer. *Cancer Practice, 5*(1), 17–24.

Grinyer, A., & Thomas, C. (2001). Young adults with cancer: the effect of the illness on parents and families. *International Journal of Palliative Nursing, 7*(4), 162–164, 166–170.

Kristjanson, L. J., & Ashcroft, T. (1994). The family's cancer journey: a literature review. *Cancer Nursing, 17*(1), 1–17.

Kutner, J. S., Steiner, J. F., Corbett, K. K., Jahnigen, D. W., & Barton, P. L. (1999). Information needs in terminal illness. *Social Science & Medicine, 48*(10), 1341–1352.

Lewis, F. M. (1993). Psychosocial transitions and the family's work in adjusting to cancer. *Seminars in Oncology Nursing, 9*(2), 127–129.

Lewis, F. M., Hammond, M. A., & Woods, N. F. (1993). The family's functioning with newly diagnosed breast cancer in the mother: the development of an explanatory model. *Journal of Behavioral Medicine, 16*(4), 351–370.

Links, M., & Kramer, J. (1994). Breaking bad news: Realistic versus unrealistic hopes. *Support Care Cancer, 2*(2), 91–93.

Meyers, F. J., Linder, J., Beckett, L., Christensen, S., Blais, J., & Gandara, D. R. (2004). Simultaneous care: a model approach to the perceived conflict between investigational therapy and palliative care. *Journal of Pain & Symptom Management, 28*(6), 548–556.

Morrison, R. S., & Morris, J. (1995). When there is no cure: Palliative care for the dying patient. *Geriatrics, 50*(7), 45–51.

Pitorak, E. F., Beckham Armour, M., & Sivec, H. D. (2002, July). *Project safe conduct integrates palliative goals into comprehensive cancer care: An interview with Elizabeth Ford Pitorak and Meri Armour.* Retrieved from http://www2.edc.org/lastacts/archives/archivesJuly02/featureinn.asp.

Pitorak, E. F., Beckham Armour, M., & Sivec, H. D. (2003). Project safe conduct integrates palliative goals into comprehensive cancer care. *Journal of Palliative Medicine, 6*(4), 645–655.

Real del, S., Stiefel, F., Leyvraz, S., Bauer, J., Gehring, T. M., & Guex, P. (1998). The Family System Test (FAST): A pilot study in families with a young adult member with cancer. *Support Care Cancer, 6*(4), 416–420.

Shields, C. E. (1998). Giving patients bad news. *Primary Care, 25*(2), 381–390.

Siegel, R., Ward, E., Brawley, O., & Jemal, A. (2011). Cancer statistics, 2011: the impact of eliminating socioeconomic and racial disparities on premature cancer deaths. *CA: A Cancer Journal for Clinicians, 61*(4), 212–236.

Speice, J., Harkness, J., Laneri, H., Frankel, R., Roter, D., Kornblith, A. B., et al. (2000). Involving family members in cancer care: Focus group considerations of patients and oncological providers. *Psycho-Oncology, 9*(2), 101–112.

Stetz, K. M., Lewis, F. M., & Houck, G. M. (1994). Family goals as indicants of adaptation during chronic illness. *Public Health Nursing, 11*(6), 385–391.

Temel, J. S., Greer, J. A., Muzikansky, A., Gallagher, E. R., Admane, S., Jackson, V. A., et al. (2010). Early palliative care for patients with metastatic non-small-cell lung cancer. *New England Journal of Medicine, 363*(8), 733–742.

Trask, P. C., Blank, T. O., & Jacobsen, P. B. (2008). Future Perspectives on the Treatment Issues Associated With Cancer and Aging. *Cancer, 113*(12, Supplement), 3514–3518.

Waldrop, D. P. (2006). At the eleventh hour: psychosocial dynamics in short hospice stays. *Gerontologist, 46*(1), 106–114.

Wallberg, B., Michelson, H., Nystedt, M., Bolund, C., Degner, L. F., & Wilking, N. (2000). Information needs and preferences for participation in treatment decisions among Swedish breast cancer patients. *Acta Oncology, 39*(4), 467–476.

Wilkie, D. J., Brown, M. A., Corless, I., Farber, S., Judge, K., Shannon, S., et al. (2012). Toolkit for Nurturing Excellence at the End-of-Life Transition for Nurse Educators (TNEEL-NE) CD ROM [CD-ROM, Version 2.0]. Seattle, WA: TNEEL Investigators.

Wilkie, D. J., Judge, M. K., Berry, D. L., Dell, J., Zong, S., & Gilespie, R. (2003). Usability of a computerized PAINReportIt in the general public with pain and people with cancer pain. *Journal of Pain & Symptom Management, 25*(3), 213–224.

Wingate, A. L., & Lackey, N. R. (1989). A description of the needs of noninstitutionalized cancer patients and their primary care givers. *Cancer Nursing, 12*(4), 216–225.

Woods, N. F., & Lewis, F. M. (1995). Women with chronic illness: their views of their families' adaptation. *Health Care Women International, 16*(2), 135–148.

Woods, N. F., Lewis, F. M., & Ellison, E. S. (1989). Living with cancer. Family experiences. *Cancer Nursing, 12*(1), 28–33.

World Health Organization (WHO). (Ed.). (1996). *Cancer pain relief: With a guide to opioid availability* (2nd ed.). Geneva: World Health Organization.

Chapter 3
The Emotional Responses of Family Caregivers: Living with Cancer and Helping Families Cope

Ruth McCorkle and Barbara Given

Although individuals and families have been living with cancer and its consequences for years, it was not until the National Cancer Act was signed in the early 1970s that cancer became recognized as a major public health problem. Initially, research and clinical resources focused primarily on finding novel discoveries to try to cure different types of cancers and developing comprehensive cancer centers to house clinical and basic scientific efforts. As more and novel cancer treatments became available that prolonged life expectancy, cancer was increasingly associated with chronicity, remissions, and exacerbations; thus, its emotional impact on patients and families became increasingly evident. Gradually a body of literature evolved that documented the impact of cancer on patients and demonstrated that the diagnosis was a time of crisis (Krouse and Krouse 1982; Northouse et al. 2000; McCorkle and Benoliel 1983; Weisman and Worden 1976). Simultaneously, there were scientific developments that documented that families also experienced a crisis associated with a cancer diagnosis, its subsequent treatment, and in most cases premature death. (Benoliel and McCorkle 1978; Giaquinta 1977; Hampe 1975; Given et al. 2004; MacVicar and Archbold 1976; Vachon 1982; Wellisch et al. 1978).

Recent years have seen an escalating trend toward early discharge of hospitalized patients and a shift of high utilization of ambulatory care services. As a result, increasing numbers of family caregivers are caring for cancer patients at home (Cawley and Gerdts 1988; Conkling 1989; McCorkle and Given 1991; McCorkle et al. 1993). This demand on families is not new, although the caregiver role has changed dramatically from promoting convalescence to providing high technology care and psychological support in the home. Members of the patient's family are of vital importance in meeting the patient's physical and psychosocial needs and accomplishing

R. McCorkle (✉)
School of Nursing, Yale University, 100 Church Street South, New Haven,
CT 06536-0740, USA
e-mail: Ruth.McCorkle@yale.edu

B. Given
School of Nursing, Michigan State University, B515-C West Fee Hall, East Lansing,
MI 48824-1315, USA
e-mail: Barb.Given@hc.msu.edu

R. C. Talley et al. (eds.), *Cancer Caregiving in the United States*,
Caregiving: Research, Practice, Policy,
DOI 10.1007/978-1-4614-3154-1_3, © Springer Science+Business Media, LLC 2012

treatment goals (Ganz 1990; Mor et al. 1987). The burden of caring for patients with a diagnosis of cancer however, may adversely affect families who lack adequate resources or who are insufficiently prepared for this new complex role. There is mounting evidence that changes in family roles and the burden placed on family caregivers may have negative effects on the psychological stability of both cancer patients and their caregivers (Given et al. 2004; McCorkle et al. 1993), particularly on the caregivers' emotional status and their ability to cope with increasing demands.

Family caregivers are now, due to the pressures from the health care system, expected to play a major role in assisting with the management of the disease, treatment, and treatment-related side effects. Cancer and its treatment may alter family identity, roles, communication patterns, employment, and daily functioning. These changes can occur over an extended period of time as family members deal with unfamiliar situations and demands as cancer treatment changes and continues, as the disease progresses, or as patients recover and survive.

Family caregivers indicate they feel ill prepared, have insufficient knowledge, and receive little assistance from the formal healthcare system to acquire the knowledge and skills they need to provide care. Family caregivers may not know how to take on the caregiving role, may be unfamiliar with what care they must provide, and may not utilize available resources (Given and Given 1992; Oberst et al. 1989). The impact of caregiving on cancer patients can be critical to the health and emotional well-being of the caregiver (Given et al. 1993; McCorkle et al. 1993; Northouse 1988; Oberst et al. 1989; Sales 1991; Schulz and Beach 1999; Sherwood et al. 2005; Weitzner et al. 1997b), and caregivers often neglect their own healthcare needs in order to assist their loved ones.

Family caregiving has been conceptualized as the provision of unpaid aid or assistance by one or more family members to another family member related to a healthcare problem (beyond that required as part of normal, everyday life). Caregiving may not always be distinguished from aid and assistance given as a part of the normal family relationship, so it may be difficult for family members to label. Some of the difficulty in defining the family caregiver role exists in the history and nature of the relationship between the caregiver and the care receiver, as well as the ambiguous and evolving demands of care that change and evolve due to both the nature of the disease trajectory as well as the complexity of the cancer treatment.

The purpose of this chapter is to provide a comprehensive synthesis of the literature on family caregivers' emotional responses to the role of caregiver and the identification of strategies for coping with cancer and its impact. For the review, a combination of computerized and manual searches was used and supplemented by the personal library collection of the authors. As both the interdisciplinary and nursing intervention studies were of interest, diverse databases were searched using the following key words: caregiver, caregiving, family, cancer, emotional distress, mood, depression, interventions, quality of life, and coping. Initially the search sought articles from 1976, and a large number of articles on family and caregiving were found, however, the majority of these articles was descriptive in nature and documented the need for caregiver interventions. Articles were retrieved through computerized databases, (MEDLINE®, CINAHL®, PsychINFO, and HealthSTAR®). For the final review, data-based studies that described emotional responses of family caregivers and interventions aimed at helping caregivers cope with their caregiving role and their emotional responses were selected. Although the original intent was to limit the review to studies that associated interventions with emotional outcomes, a lack of well-delimited outcome variables along with few rigorous intervention trials were revealed as major gaps in the literature.

Caregiver Emotional Responses

Descriptive studies have provided evidence that family members of patients with cancer experience distress due to their caregiving roles, and this distress continues over time (Given et al. 1990b, 1993; Northouse et al. 2000; Northouse and Peters-Golden 1993; Oberst and Scott 1988; Raveis et al. 1998). Recognition of the emotional burden that the diagnosis and treatment of cancer places on family caregivers has appeared in cancer literature since the early 1980s. See Table 3.1 for a summary of descriptive studies.

Caregiving emotional distress may be related to direct care tasks, complex medical procedures, disruption of daily routines, role overload, or the need to provide emotional support. A number of review articles describe the emotional impact of cancer on family caregivers (Cooley and Moriarty 1997; Kristjanson and Ashcroft 1994; Laizner et al. 1993; Northouse et al. 1995, 2000), including the presence of increased symptoms of depression, anxiety, psychosomatic symptoms, restrictions of roles and activities, strain in marital relationships, and poorer physical health among family caregivers. Various dimensions of caregiver reactions have been identified by previous researchers (Given et al. 1992; Stetz 1987, 1989). Depression and anxiety have most often been examined as indicators or symptoms of caregiver distress. Descriptive studies have documented that caregivers experience anxiety and depression, as well as a sense of helplessness and fear (Nijboer et al. 2001; Northouse et al. 1995; Oberst et al. 1989; Sherwood et al. 2005; Siegel et al. 1991; Weitzner et al. 1997b). Researchers report only about 25–30% of cancer caregivers are depressed or emotionally distressed.

Overall, caregiving is more stressful for women (both wives and daughters) than for men (both husbands and sons; Baider et al. 1996; Nijboer et al. 2001; Northouse et al. 1995, 2000; Raveis et al. 1998; Sales et al. 1992). In addition, wives, husbands, daughters, and sons appear to approach the practice of caregiving in different ways, which may affect caregivers' emotional outcomes (Gerstel and Gallagher 1993; Raveis et al. 1998). In married couples, husbands caring for wives with cancer focus on caregiving tasks while continuing their own activities and interests, such as gardening and yard work; they do not expect care needs to interfere with these activities. Wife caregivers, however, give priority to their husbands' needs and choices (Miller 1990) and may consider their own needs secondary. Wives focus attention on the interpersonal aspects of caregiving—such as how their relationships with their husbands are changing—and find changes to be uncomfortable. The differences

Table 3.1 Summary of Caregiver Descriptive Studies

Author	Conceptual Framework	Design	Sample	Measures	Results
Cameron et al. (2002)	Life style interference and illness intensive	Descriptive	54 Caregivers of patients with advanced cancer. 25 Women. 38 Spouses. Mean age 60.	Caregiver assistance scale. Caregiver impact scale. Profile of mood states.	Education and lifestyle interference correlates with emotional distress. More distress when limited in their valued activities and interests. No gender differences.
Carey et al. (1991)	Cognitive appraisal, stress and coping model	Descriptive, convenience, cross sectional	49 family caregivers of patients getting chemotherapy. 25 men, 25 women. Convenience, cross sectional	Hardiness, caregiver burden, caregiver health	Burden, hardiness, and caregiver health predicted 50% of negative caregiver appraisal. Less hardiness, more burden. Negative appraisal and age explained mood disturbance.
Fang and Manne (2001) health psychology	Psychological distress	Descriptive longitudinal (6 mo.)	197 cancer patients and spouses. Solid tumors 32% local rest late stage. Mean age 56 (SDII) spouse 108 men, 89 women	Psychological distress of mental health inventory. Spaniers dyadic adjustment. CARES for patient.	Higher levels of patients functional measurement associated with poor marital quality it only related to distress at wave I. Patient distress mediated impact of functional impairment on spouse distress, at all times.
Given et al. (1993) health psychology	Social stress and coping	Cross sectional sample	196 convenience community breast solid tumors	CESD, CRA, symptom distress, OARS. Life orientation test	Caregiver optimism proved to be a significant predictor of mental health and reactions to caring.
Haley et al. (2001)	No framework	Descriptive	40 dementia and 40 lung cancer spouse. Convenience sample of terminal patients	ADL, CESD memory and behavior check lest life satisfaction. MOS - health perception physical function.	Caregiver showed depression lower life satisfaction and poorer physical health than non caregivers cancer caregivers more hours of care. 57% wives and 29% husbands at clinical depression

Table 3.1 (continued)

Author	Conceptual Framework	Design	Sample	Measures	Results
Kristjanson et al. (1996)	Family model fulfillment theory	Descriptive longitudinal	89 with advanced cancer	Fulfillment, family functioning, family health index	Patients quality of life correlated with family health. Families more stressed than normative population
Nijboer et al. (2001)	Social and psychological resources	Descriptive longitudinal over 6 months	148 dyads with colorectal cancer	CESD, care tasks. Social support. List interactions. Mastery extraversion and neuroticism. CRA	Effect of social and psychological resources on caregiver. Experiences small. No effect on depression. Caregiver with low daily support and those with low mastery perceived caregiver in negative way and were more depressed.
Nijboer et al. (2000) the gerontologist	No framework	Longitudinal 6 months	N=148. Colorectal. 64% female caregiver X age 63. SDCII	CRA. CESD. Co-morbidity. Rotterdam symptom checklist	Women, younger caregiver and those with higher SES experienced caregiver more negatively. Suggest that caregiver distress is multi-dimensional
Nijboer et al. (1999)	Nijboer's framework based on Given's. Cognitive stress theory	Longitudinal descriptive	148 dyads of newly diagnosed colorectal disease. 54 men, 54 women caregivers. Mean age 63	Marital scale CESD. Rotterdam symptom list. Activity restriction. CRA	Low burden. Depression mean 9 (SD8). Those with stoma more burden and more depression. Patient dependency correlated with depression of caregiver.
Northouse et al. (1995)	Stress and coping uncertainty	Descriptive	81 women with a first recurrent breast cancer, and husbands	Social support question, adjustment (PAIS), uncertainty, symptom distress, hopelessness	Symptom distress and hopelessness accounted for the most distress and husbands adjustment. Wife and husbands adjustment scores were related.

Table 3.1 (continued)

Author	Conceptual Framework	Design	Sample	Measures	Results
Northouse et al. (1998)	Cognitive appraisal model of stress	Descriptive longitudinal	Breast. 58 couple's malignant breast. 73 benign. Cognitive appraisal model of stress	Smilktstein stress. Dyadic adjustment. Family apgar. Mishel uncertainty. Beck hopeless. BSI, BA IS	Male and female adjustment corresponded.
Northouse et al. (2000)	Stress and coping	Longitudinal descriptive	131 couples. 58 with a breast cancer diagnosis and 73 with a benign diagnosis	Partners adjustment scores (PAIS)	Strongest predictor of husband adjustment was hopelessness and own baseline level. Husband and wife adjustment affected each other. Individual variables explained 32% husband's distress and 57% role problems
Northouse et al. (2000)	Cognitive appraisal model of stress.	Descriptive	56 couples colon cancer patients. Average age 61. 91% Caucasian.	PAIS, hopelessness, BSI	Emotional distress over time correlation between patients spouse adjustment marital satisfaction predicted spouses adjustment
Oberst and Scott (1988)	Descriptive, stress and coping	Longitudinal	40 patients and their spouses. Non terminal, treated surgically	State anxiety, brief symptom index, vulnerability index	Patient and spouse distress similar. Spouse less distressed to 10 days at home. High vulnerability at 90 and 190 days with clinical depression
Oberst et al. (1991)	Cognitive appraisal stress and coping	Cross sectional	72 patients with radiation. 35 women, 37 men	Self care burden POMS	Symptom distress predicted burden

Table 3.1 (continued)

Author	Conceptual Framework	Design	Sample	Measures	Results
Raveis et al. (1998)	No framework listed	Descriptive	164 cancer outpatients age 60-90 and their adult caregivers	Constraints of caregiving, CESD, caregiver burden	Predictors of depression were constants of caregiving and caregiver burden. No patient characteristics were productive, health limiting condition. Sense of filial obligation and greater caregiver burden correlated with CESD
Raveis et al. (1999)	No framework listed	Descriptive Panel study	164 patients with adult daughters mean age 39 (SD 8). 90% white. Recent diagnosis	STAIS scores. Constraints of caregiving. Caregiver burden appraisal of care situation	Health limiting condition greater sense of filial obligation. Increased caregiver burden. Correlated with caregiver burden anxiety. Overload with caregiver responsibilities correlated with anxiety. More tasks actually lowered anxiety
Siegel et al. (1991) annals of oncology.	No conceptual model.	Convenience sample	295 spousal caregiver. Solid tumors 96%. Caucasian 64%. Wives mean age 60	Burden. Disease burden. Reduced activity days. Intensity of burden	Wives experienced more burden. Wives more time burden. Extent of patient disease more burden. Number of days restricted more burden. Number of symptoms associated with burden
Stommel et al. (1990)	No framework	Longitudinal descriptive	307 caregivers of patients with solid Tumors	CRA Caregiver involvement. Informal support/ formal support. Service utilize financial. CESD	Patient health, nor caregiver process linked to burden. Caregiver depression dominates caregiver perceptions burden but depression independent of current care situations. Depression independent of variations in care processes

Table 3.1 (continued)

Author	Conceptual Framework	Design	Sample	Measures	Results
Given et al. (2004)	Family caregiving model	Prospective Longitudinal	152 caregivers of patients on chemotherapy who died	CRA Caregiver involvement. CESD patient symptoms.	Caregivers 45-54 highest depression. Caregivers 35-44 sense of abandonment. Younger caregivers description in lives
Sherwood et al. (2005)	Family caregiving model	Inception cohort of caregivers	488 caregivers of patients over 65	Cognitive scale. Neuropsychiatric scale. ADL, IADL. Recency of care demands. CRA. CESD	Care recipients mental health, functional status and recency of care demands predicted caregiver burden. Burden predicted depressive symptoms
Coristine et al. (2003)	No framework	Focus groups of caregiver	30 caregivers following death		Non-spouses had the most roles to manage and they had the most difficulty with care. Some caregivers could not continue care. Unable to satisfy patient wishes
Grunfeld et al. (2004)	No framework	Longitudinal study	89 caregivers of women with advanced breast cancer	Kainofsky SF36. HAD. Zarit Burden. Family care	Caregivers became more depressed as they moved from palliative to terminal care, had higher burden. Burden predicted anxiety and depression.
Kurtz et al. (2004)	Family caregiving model	Inception cohort of caregivers longitudinal	491 cancer patient caregiver dyads	SF36. Physical Functioning. CRA. CESD	Caregiving affected work Caregiver perceptions of burden played central role on depression and physical health contextually patient symptoms, patient depression, comorbidity, cancer site and living arrangement

between wives and husbands have been attributed to normative roles. Women are also more emotionally distressed by the caregiving role and care demands.

Nijboer et al. (1999) studied colorectal cancer patients and their partners. Caregiver experiences were assessed by the Caregiver Reaction Assessment (CRA) scale, which contains four negative subscales (disrupted schedule, impact on finances, lack of family support, and impact on health) and one positive subscale (self-esteem). The mental health of caregivers was assessed in terms of depression and quality of life. The researchers concluded that although caregiving may lead to depression, especially in those experiencing loss of physical strength, caregivers may sustain their quality of life through increased self-esteem from caregiving.

Providing emotional support can be as—or more—emotionally burdensome than providing direct care (Carey et al. 1991). Changes or restrictions in work roles and career opportunities, increased financial costs and demands, and strain in marital relationships all lead to increased burden (Bradley et al. 2004; Grunfeld et al. 2004; Stommel et al. 1995; Weitzner et al. 1997a). Raveis et al. (1998) found that care-providing daughters who had an existing health condition themselves reported limitations in their ability to care and reported higher levels of depression.

These accounts present persuasive documentation that caring for a person with cancer is a stressful experience and can have major emotional and physical consequences for caregivers. In their review of caregiver research, Sales et al. (1992) concluded that a significant number of cancer caregivers exhibited emotional distress and physical symptoms. Predictors of emotional distress included a number of illness-related variables, including more advanced stages of cancer, disability and complex care needs (Sherwood et al. 2005).

In general, the descriptive literature on caregivers of cancer patients highlights: (1) the increasing number of complex tasks assumed by cancer caregivers; (2) the high proportion of unmet emotional and physical caregiver needs; (3) the subjective nature of the caregiving experience which encompasses both positive and negative elements; and (4) the conceptualization of caregiver burden as directly linked to negative caregiving reactions.

Characteristics of Caregivers at Risk for Emotional Distress

There are a number of factors related to increased caregiver emotional distress and should be considered when planning interventions. These include, however, are not limited to gender, age, socioeconomic status, living arrangements, family role, developmental stage, and clinical variables associated with the patient.

Gender has been shown to be differentially related to caregiver distress. Levels of depression among caregivers are highest for wives, followed by daughters, then other female caregivers, sons, and finally husband caregivers (Stommel et al. 1990). Spousal caregivers appear to be at particular risk for caregiver distress, because they typically provide the most extensive and comprehensive care, maintain their role longer, tolerate greater levels of disability among family members than adult children and other nonspousal caregivers, experience more lifestyle adjustment, and exhibit lower levels of well-being (Given et al. 2004; Nijboer et al. 2000; Northouse et al. 2000; Siegel et al. 1991).

Age contributes to caregiver distress (Nijboer et al. 2000). Intergenerational caregivers are often middle-aged (adult caregivers) of parents, and are more likely to suffer role conflicts due to multiple and competing role demands, whereas intragenerational caregivers suffer from caregiver role entrenchment. Elderly spouse caregivers may have fewer defined roles to perform than adult children caregivers and may respond to demands of cancer care by isolating themselves from social and family roles to become completely focused on providing care. Older and aging families living with cancer may have other problems related to care tasks, such as decreased physical abilities resulting from the caregiver's own frailty and comorbid conditions such as diabetes and cardiovascular disease, social isolation, and diminished family resources. Caregivers of younger patients may report more distress from care than those caring for older patients (Given et al. 1993; Schumacher et al. 1993). Older caregivers may have more established patterns of decision making that may ease the decision-making process related to cancer (Coristine et al. 2003).

Cancer care is most burdensome for patients and caregivers with low incomes and limited financial resources if there are substantial out-of-pocket costs. Unemployed or low-income caregivers may experience more emotional distress because they have fewer resources and less capacity to respond to distress. Davis-Ali et al. (1993) concluded that higher-income families may not concern themselves with the financial hardships of cancer care because they are able to purchase or seek resources. Income and overall financial concerns cause distress for caregivers during long periods of caregiving (Clipp and George 1992), as resources become depleted.

Living arrangements may need to be altered, either temporarily or permanently, to manage the care of cancer patients. The patient may move into the caregiver's home to facilitate care, or family members may move into the home of the patient to provide care. Secondary caregivers are much more involved in parental care than spousal care situations. When a patient is widowed, single, or divorced, more caregivers are involved. Studies show that caregivers who live with the person with cancer are more depressed than those who live in separate households (Stommel and Kingry 1991).

Current and previous role relationships between patients and their family caregivers need to be considered. Family caregiving is a stressful normative expectation with the feelings of obligation and attachment, and individuals often assume caregiving responsibilities to show that they are committed to supporting the family (Cicirelli 1992). Both recipient and caregiver bring a history of interactions that may enhance or complicate the care process. Therefore, it is important to consider not only the influence of family relationships but also the quality of relationships in terms of impact on the evolving care recipient–caregiver relationship (Nijboer et al. 1999; Northouse et al. 2005).

Family developmental stage may differentially influence caregiver's emotional responses and availability because roles often conflict, compete with, and are disrupted by care demands (Kristjanson and Ashcroft 1994). If caregiving is required "off time" in younger families, care challenges are even more burdensome and emotionally stressful because not only are they unexpected, however, the needed support may also not be available. Kristjanson and Ashcroft described how emotional distress may be greater during a transition from one developmental stage to another, and it is during transitions that most family dysfunction is likely to occur. Spouses reported decreases in family functioning and social support combined with increases in emotional distress over time. Families with better spousal communication may experience less disruption, role conflict, and role strain over time (Nijboer et al. 2001; Northouse et al. 1995, 1998, 2000; Kurtz et al. 2004).

Patient-related Factors for Caregivers Emotional Distress

There are a number of factors associated with the clinical characteristics of the patient that may influence the caregiver's emotional responses. For example, a relationship between a caregiver's emotional distress and actual care demands is assumed to exist, however, has not been systematically examined. Nor has the amount of time or hours per day devoted to cancer care, the inability to control timing of care, the intimacy of care required, and the amount of physical care provided been systematically examined. The severity of illness and complexity of treatment that make care necessary are integral to determining the risk for negative caregiver reactions and emotional distress. The stage of cancer; length of illness; phase in treatment trajectory; symptom experience; impact of cancer and treatment on functional, psychological, and mobility status; and patient role changes will influence the cancer care demands of families and thus, the level of concurrent emotional distress (Given et al. 1993; Kurtz et al. 2004; Morita et al. 2002; Sherwood et al. 2004).

Severity and duration of patient illness, symptoms, and physical decline are thought to be related to caregiver emotional distress. Oberst and James (1985) and Oberst and Scott (1988) have documented emotional reactions of family caregivers in the early phase of diagnosis, treatment, and threat of illness. Constancy in adjustment—that is, change in patient status, or either improvement or deterioration—may influence the caregiver's emotional responses over time. Caregiver emotional distress may continue even after patient status improves (Given et al. 1993; McCorkle et al. 1993; Northouse and Peters-Golden 1993) or varies with treatment type, phase, and stage of disease. In the terminal stages, families may be overwhelmed with the demands of not only the illness, but also poor prognosis and threat of approaching death. Patient reactions to illness appear to influence family member reactions, and at times family member emotional distress equals or exceeds that of the patient (Carey et al. 1991; Given et al. 1990b).

Several small-scale studies have shown that recurrent disease may be associated with caregiver emotional distress (Given and Given 1992; Northouse et al. 1995). However, Schumacher et al. (1993) found that depression among caregivers of patients with recurrent disease was significantly related to caregiver gender, perceived adequacy of social support, and coping efficacy rather than recurrent disease per se.

Patient symptom distress may also lead to caregiver emotional distress, which may be manifested as anger, anxiety, frustration, or depression. This distress affects the demands on family caregivers' ability to provide care, or even to care for themselves. Care for difficult symptoms, such as pain management, influences the level of caregiver strain (Kurtz et al. 2004; Miaskowski et al. 1997; Musci and Dodd 1990). Research on the effects of patient functional status on caregiver distress have been mixed. Severity of functional impairment (e.g., activities of daily living, cognitive and social functioning) and severity of symptoms have been found significantly related to caregiver emotional distress (Clipp and George 1992; Given et al. 1993; Kurtz et al. 2004; Oberst et al. 1989). Impaired patient cognitive function produces higher caregiver distress than impaired physical functioning. Family caregivers may adapt to the demands that impaired physical functioning places upon them, however, caring for patients with cognitive deficits produces high and sustained levels of caregiver emotional distress (Carey et al. 1991).

Interventions to Help Caregivers Cope

There are a number of interventions that have been suggested to assist family caregivers of cancer patients. The difficulty, however, is that most do not meet the methodological rigor needed to have confidence in findings that are available. The literature includes a number of studies describing strategies to help caregivers cope with living with cancer and its consequences. The interventions include a range of educational, psychoeducational, support, and skills-building strategies targeted at the patient and family caregiver as a dyad and to family caregivers alone. The value of providing information to cancer caregivers has been reported consistently in the research literature (Wilson and Morse 1991; Zahlis and Shands 1991). Reported in the literature with equally consistent frequency however, is the difficulty that caregivers have in obtaining information from healthcare professionals, particularly physicians and nurses (Dyck and Wright 1988; Wilson and Moore 1991; Zahlis and Shands 1991). Despite the fact that it is often difficult to obtain, caregivers report that information is a critical element in helping them to cope with the patient's illness (Gotay 1984; Northouse 1989).

In addition to providing information about the physical aspects of the illness, caregivers need to learn more about the emotional aspects of illness and recovery (Northouse and Peters-Golden 1993). According to Oberst and Scott (1988), caregivers need to be informed about what to expect regarding the emotional aspects of the illness for both themselves and the patient. In this manner, caregivers can be proactively reassured that their own and the patient's psychological distress is to be expected and not a sign of poor coping.

The times when caregivers appear to be in the greatest need of information are at the time of diagnosis (Northouse 1989), during the hospital period, especially at the time of surgery (Northouse 1989; Northouse and Swain 1987), at the start of new treatments (Wilson and Moore 1991) and at the time of recurrence. Despite the documented importance of providing information to caregivers, only a few intervention programs have been reported that demonstrated how and what information should be provided. Outcomes associated with educational interventions were not clearly described nor were consistent variables and measures used to describe relevant outcomes. This makes replication of studies difficult at best. It undermines the importance of conducting research in an effort to bolster caregiver supports and makes it difficult to build on past work to meet caregiver needs.

Heinrich and Schag (1985) developed the "Stress and Activity Management" (SAM) intervention for cancer patients and their spouses and consisted of structured, small group meetings that met weekly for 2 hours over a 6-week period. Groups were designed to: educate patients and spouses about cancer and its impact; teach specific skills that could be used to manage stress and daily problems such as relaxation techniques, physical and recreational activities; and promote problem solving. Among the 92 patients who met eligibility criteria, 51 participated in the study along with 25 of their spouses. Twenty-six patients and 12 spouses were randomized to the treatment group and 25 patients and 13 spouses to the control group. The primary outcome variables included psychological adjustment, depression and anxiety, which improved for both treatment and control groups, supporting the notion that natural improvement in psychological status will occur over time. The SAM patients and spouses reported high satisfaction with the intervention, although due to the self-selected nature of the treatment and control groups, it is likely that the control subjects would have also been satisfied. Support for the unique and positive impact of the SAM treatment intervention came from the improvement in scores on the Cancer Information Test, indicating that the program increased participant's knowledge about cancer and coping. This finding is noteworthy because most patients and spouses had been living with cancer for about 2 years and demonstrated minimal knowledge about their illness. SAM spouses in particular were more satisfied with the education and support they received than the control spouses who received the usual care and were not routinely included in physician office visits. Despite the small number of subjects studied and the self-selected nature of the sample, this study is noteworthy in several respects including: a well-described replicable intervention, randomization, and clear delineation of outcome variables. Barg et al. (1998) implemented a 6-hour psychoeducational Caregiver Cancer Education Program (CCEP) that addressed symptom management, psychosocial support, and resource identification. A convenience sample of 150 caregivers attended sessions. The majority of caregivers were female and cared for patients over 50 years of age. Sixty-one percent of the caregivers assumed the caregiver role less than 6 months previously. Twenty-two percent provided less than 5 hours of care per week, while 32% provided 6–20 hours per week. Thirty-eight percent of the caregivers reported their health suffered due to caregiving and 20% reported being very stressed. The majority of patients received assistance, and 70% reported that their families were not working well together. Forty-six percent reported inadequate financial resources. Thirty-five percent were emotionally overwhelmed with caregiver roles; 61% reported all of their activities centered on caregiving, requiring them to adjust their schedules and relinquish other activities. Psychosocial issues, such as watching the patient becoming more ill and not knowing what to do, were reported as the most difficult issues they faced. Many caregivers were ambivalent in the role, however, saw it as an important task. The methodological limitations include convenience sample, lack of clinical data on patients and shortness of follow-up intervals.

In a randomized control design, Blanchard et al. (1997a) implemented a coping with cancer (CWC) intervention for spouses of cancer patients. Thirty spouses were randomized to the CWC group and 36 to usual services. The intervention was a problem-solving approach to reduce or manage problems underlying caregiver distress. An experienced oncology social worker conducted six 1-hour individual counseling sessions. Measures included a battery of standardized measures. Assessments occurred at baseline, after completing the 6-week intervention, and again at 6 months. Mean caregiver age was 55 years in the control group and 50 years in the experimental group. The average length of caregiving time was 21 months for the intervention group and 31 months for the control group. Number of hours of care provided per week was 2.7 for the experimental and 3.1 for the control group. The two most common cancer diagnoses were breast, followed by lung. Results revealed a significant intervention main effect of time on spouse psychosocial well-being and on coping. Univariate follow-up revealed significantly reduced depression in both groups as well as reduction in avoidance coping in both the groups. Qualitatively, spouses and patients reported that the intervention helped to improve their communication. Methodological limitations of this study include small sample size, time since inception of caregiving, lack of variation in age of caregivers, and lack of discussion of patient's clinical data.

Houts et al. (1996) described a prescriptive problem-solving model for how care should be managed at home and for the kind of information and training family caregivers should receive. The Prepared Family Caregiver model, which is summarized in the acronym COPE (Creativity, Optimism Planning, and Expert information), teaches caregivers how to develop and implement plans that address both medical and psychosocial problems and are coordinated with care plans of health professionals. The model is based on extensive research regarding unmet emotional and physical needs of caregivers and problem solving training and therapy. According to the authors, the program empowers family members and patients to cope with illness and can help to moderate caregiver emotional stress, although outcomes used in the research design to document the program's effectiveness remain inadequately described.

Jepson et al. (1999) examined changes in the psychosocial status of caregivers ($N = 161$) of postsurgical patients with cancer. In a longitudinal, randomized trial, these investigators analyzed how caregiver distress was affected by whether caregivers had physical problems of their own and whether patients received a home-care intervention. Half of the patients were randomly assigned to receive a standardized home-care nursing intervention in which 32% were referred to home care; the other half received a standardized intervention over a 4-week period consisting of three home visits and six phone calls from an oncology clinical nurse specialist. The intervention focused on assessing and monitoring problems, helping with symptom management, teaching self-care, and coordinating resources. Data were collected at the time of the patients' discharge and approximately 3 and 6 months later. Overall, psychosocial status improved from baseline to 3 months and was about the same at 6 months. Among caregivers with physical problems, the psychosocial status of those in the treatment group declined compared to those in the control groups in the 3 months after discharge; an opposite pattern was observed during the following 3 months. Results indicated that caregivers who have physical problems of their own are at risk for psychological morbidity, which may have a delayed effect. This delay may reflect the replacement of initial optimism with discouragement as caregivers face the reality of long-term illness. This research suggests that it may be important for clinicians to assess who is responsible for providing care to their patients at home and whether caregivers have health problems of their own that might interfere with their abilities to take on this role. In the event, caregivers report health problems, referrals for supplemental care are essential. These findings warrant additional investigation.

Bultz et al. (2000) found that partners of breast cancer patients provided support at a time when their own coping abilities were taxed by the challenge of cancer. Among 118 consecutive patients approached, 36 patients and their partners participated in a randomized controlled trial of a brief psychoeducational group intervention for partners only. Patients whose partners received the intervention at 3 months reported less mood disturbance, greater confidant support, and increased marital satisfaction.

Support, Counseling and Psychotherapy

The sources of support available to cancer patients are many and varied ranging from one-on-one interaction to a myriad of formal support groups and networks. Sources of support for family caregivers have lagged far behind those provided for patients (Northouse and Peters-Golden 1993). Spouses in particular report little support from health professionals, often due to limited contact with physicians and nurses in hospital and outpatient settings (Northouse 1988; Northouse and Northouse 1987).

There is a dearth of information regarding the effectiveness of supportive and counseling interventions with cancer caregivers. This is despite the implications from studies of educational interventions that many seem to be inadequate.

Goldberg and Wool (1985) conducted a 12-session intervention of social support counseling over 6 months with spouses and adult children of newly diagnosed lung cancer patients in treatment, using a randomized control group design. Fifty-three caregivers were assigned to the counseling intervention or to usual treatment. Caregivers and patients were assessed at initial treatment, prior to implementing the intervention, and again at 8 and 16 weeks. The support functions of the intervention were: to help maintain the social support system, to promote the patient's sense of autonomy, to be an advocate in the care system, to encourage communication between patient and family, and to facilitate mutual expressions of feelings. No changes were found on the measures of psychosocial or physical functioning for the caregiver. The interventionists were social workers and psychologists. The investigators attributed the lack of findings to the characteristics of the subjects who participated. The caregivers were doing well and thus had limited or no distress. They recommended screening caregivers so interventions can be targeted to those who need them.

Blanchard et al. (1997a) reported on the effect of a six-session intervention with spouses of cancer patients. They used a problem solving intervention to help spouses solve individually identified problems. Results at 6 month follow up showed no significant impact associated with the intervention, even for those spouses who were most distressed. Interestingly, patients of spouses who received the intervention showed significant decline in depression. It could not be determined whether this was related to altered communication between spouses and patients following the intervention or relief on the part of patients that spouses were receiving help. Findings suggested the importance of studying the spouse/patient dyad as opposed to each person individually.

Pfefferbaum et al. (1977) described a comprehensive program for breast cancer patients and their families that followed families pre and postoperatively and impacted positively on coping outcomes. In this program, a mental health professional worked with the surgical team to provide counseling to patients and family members who were identified ahead of time as being in need of emotional assistance. The researchers concluded that this notion of identifying caregivers who are at high risk for problems in specific areas and tailoring interventions to their special needs seems to be an important direction for future research.

If caregivers are unable to satisfactorily deal with the multiple demands and have overwhelming feelings and affect associated with them, the potential exists for deterioration of the caregivers' emotional and physical health (Axelsson and Sjoden 1998; Hull 1992). Institutional and home hospice services have been used to help patients and caregivers deal with the insults to physical and emotional well-being that are imposed by terminal illness. They have also incorporated caregivers into patients' care by educating them and supporting their caring efforts. In this sense, recent studies have shown an increase in hospice supported home care with an emphasis on supporting the primary caregiver role (Schachter 1992).

> As is the case with other caregiver intervention research, efforts to describe and standardize interventions need to be undertaken so that interventions can be successfully replicated across studies. In addition, outcomes must be clearly described and measured in several areas including physical health, emotional health, utilization of costly health care services and functional productivity. (Schachter 1992, p. 63)

Research Implications

Among the small number of studies in this area, many used small convenience samples that lacked randomization. Although convenience samples are often used in caregiver research, their use makes it difficult to generalize results. Small sample sizes may not reveal hypothesized relationships because statistical power is low. Future studies should attempt to employ strategies to maximize sample size, such as multi-site studies, longitudinal randomized clinical trials, and secondary analyses of large data sets. Many studies included in this chapter used a cross-sectional design. The use of longitudinal designs is preferred and would greatly enhance our understanding of caregiver emotional responses to interventions over time, including the potential preventive nature of caregiver interventions over time and the optimal timing of interventions. Recruitment and retention of diversity of caregivers in longitudinal studies is an important area needing further attention. Diversity needs to be ethnic, racial and cultural to examine common and varied needs. Difficulties retaining subjects in family research has been outlined (Cooley and Moriarty 1997; Moriarty 1990). Creative strategies for recruiting and retaining caregivers who are experiencing the unique emotional stresses associated with caring for a loved one with cancer are needed.

Attrition was noted as a problem in the longitudinal studies that were described. The use of statistical techniques to determine whether a remaining sample differs from the initial sample is important in terms of assessing the internal validity of the study (Cook and Campbell 1979). Given et al. (1990a) proposed strategies to minimize attrition in research with family caregivers. Data collectors need to be prepared to deal with high subjective distress. Ongoing communication by the researchers with the subjects, continuity of subject contact with consistent data collectors and creation of a positive interpersonal relationship between research team and subjects are essential to minimize subject attrition.

Many studies revealed selection bias, often to well-adjusted caregivers who were accepting of support, able to obtain respite care for participation purposes, and usually were willing to avail themselves to a group style intervention. Efforts to recruit the most vulnerable caregivers, such as those who are homebound or have chronic medical conditions themselves, must be developed and described.

Other areas for future research include the impact of ethnic differences and nontraditional family styles on caregiver needs and intervention response. A family's social and ethnic background may influence relationships with and perceptions of health care professionals, access to care issues and roles in caring for the patient. To date, little attention has been paid to social and cultural issues in cancer caregiver research.

Another notable gap in the cancer caregiver research relates to variation in family structure. Most research is done from the perspective of the traditional marriage dyad or a two parent family structure (Kristjanson and Ashcroft 1994). There are many other types of families that may have needs different from those of traditional couples and may warrant the development and testing of innovative interventions strategies. For example, remarried and blended families, gay and lesbian couples with and without children, and unmarried partners may have unique needs and properties that require definition. Errors in the development of interventions may occur if research findings generated from other family forms are applied inappropriately. Further research to address these gaps is needed.

A lack of well-delimited outcome variables was revealed as a major gap in the literature. Outcomes, or the results of care, are frequently viewed as indicators of the quality of service provided. Globally, outcomes can be categorized into those related to the quality and need for services, the cost of care and access to care issues. In this age of soaring health care costs and diminishing nonessential services, the documentation of outcomes associated with interventions, especially those geared toward vulnerable caregivers is paramount. In addition to outcomes, common measures are needed to assess needs, burdens, and caregiver health.

Overall, nurse and nonnurse researchers have developed interventions targeted at caregivers of cancer patients. In general, nurses tend to develop interventions that are geared toward increasing the proficiency of caregivers to address the physical and psychosocial needs of the patient. Nonnurse researchers tend to develop a greater abundance of individual and group psychological interventions directed specifically at the caregiver. Since research examining the efficacy of caregiver interventions is clearly in its infancy, the field would be greatly enhanced with an emphasis on interdisciplinary efforts that capitalize on each discipline's theoretical orientation and clinical strengths. Interventions in those experiencing high levels of distress also need to be tested at different points in the cancer trajectory to determine, for example, if interventions are most effective at certain points in the illness, whether interventions can be preventive across illness stages or whether different types of caregiver interventions need to be implemented at different stages of the cancer. Multimodal interventions that combine more than one type, such as problem solving and support or education and support are needed.

Policy Implications

Current trends in health care focus on cutting costs in acute care settings resulting in a shift of care from the hospital to the home. Despite what may seem to some to be societal cost savings and enhanced efficiency of the health care system, the locus of the financial, physical and emotional burden of cancer care is often shifted to family caregivers who may incur emotional, economic, and physical consequences. Intervention initiatives underscore the need for caregiver advocacy in these changing times.

Advocacy groups are needed to champion the needs of family caregivers, especially for high risk caregivers who have no voice. The passage of the Family Leave Bill in 1993 is noteworthy, however, it is extremely limited. Efforts are needed to secure both federal and state financial support for family caregivers. Mental health services are needed for individual and family counseling, including adequate coverage and reimbursement for both in-patient and out-patient services. Community health centers need to organize local support groups for adults as well as school age children. Respite programs that provide relief need to be expanded along with comprehensive mental health services. There need to be state tax credits to allow families full advantage of essential services such as respite. These measures are critical so that programs to assist caregivers can be adopted through policy initiatives as changes in the health care system continue to evolve. Families are an important resource in person power to provide needed care to patients to prevent them from using more costly services and long-term care resources before they are needed.

Clinical Implications

Despite the fact that a cancer diagnosis causes major changes in family roles and functioning in addition to increased responsibility for caregivers, data supporting the effectiveness of caregiver interventions are limited at best. A seminal review by Blanchard et al. (1997b) reported that between 20 and 30% of partners suffered from psychological impairment and mood disturbance as a result of a spouse's cancer. The review goes on to describe factors that may predict high levels of caregiver emotional distress. The authors highlighted the need to explore the mediating role of suggested risk factors on specific outcome variables such as family functioning and emotional distress and suggested that interventions be targeted to high-risk individuals. Factors suggested to effect distress levels in caregivers are summarized below:

- *Disease stage.* Advanced disease is often accompanied by higher distress.
- *Patient's emotional adjustment.* This is correlated with caregiver adjustment.
- *Gender.* Female family members are more distressed than males.
- *Age.* This is inversely related to emotional distress.
- *Socioeconomic status and other life stressors.* Lower SES and more life stressors correlated with higher distress.
- *Personality traits.* Caregiver optimism may predict caregiver reactions.
- *Coping and social support.* Previous history of caregiver depression predicts more distress. Perceived coping efficacy may mediate effect between caregiver strain and depression. Social support may mediate relationship between functioning and caregiver depression.
- *Caregiver health.* Caregivers' previous health predicts their adjustment.
- *Marital adjustment.* Good communication correlated with the ability to meet demands.
- *Family functioning.* Lower distress found in spouses and children if families are not rigid or chaotic.

While additional work is needed with regard to the identification of factors that predict those at highest risk for distress, clinicians need to become knowledgeable about the factors we know influence caregiving. Once caregivers who are at risk for emotional distress are identified, they can be referred to services to address their needs.

Educational Implications

Given the levels of emotional distress documented in the literature cited previously, there is a tremendous need to better prepare health professionals to be attentive to the emotional needs of the caregiver. Physicians and other professionals have to be taught during their training programs about the value of the family care role. With this training, they are more likely to apply it to their ongoing practice settings. Professionals need to understand how to assess the dynamics within a family to understand when challenges and conflicts might occur, and to recognize caregivers who are at risk for high levels of emotional distress. Primary care clinicians for their health care needs will see most of these caregivers; it is these professionals that must be targeted for ongoing educational training, including continuing education credits. Professionals need to be taught how to assess caregivers' capacity to provide care in light of the patients' actual and anticipated needs. Caregiving training programs are available, however, effective home care will be enhanced when professionals assess the needs of their patients along with the capacity of the family caregivers to provide the care. Professionals need to have the knowledge and skills to facilitate caregiver role acquisition and determine when emotional distress extends beyond expected levels and warrants treatment. Family caregivers need to be included in the patient's plan of care and kept informed about what to expect. Once professionals grasp that family caregivers can play a critical role in enhancing patient clinical outcomes, they may be willing to assess the caregiver's health and emotional capacity to provide care as a partner in the process. By forming partnerships with family caregivers, professionals can achieve the clinical outcomes they desire for the patient.

References

Axelsson, B., & Sjoden, P. (1998). Quality of life of cancer patients and their spouses in palliative home care. *Palliative Medicine, 12,* 29–39.

Baider, L., Kaufman, B., Peretz, T., Manor, O., Ever-Hadani, P., & De Nour, A. K. (1996). Mutuality of fate: Adaptation and psychological distress in cancer patients and their partners. In L. Baider, C. Cooper, & A. Kaplan De-Nour (Eds.), *Cancer and the family* (pp. 187–224). New York: Wiley.

Barg, F. K., Pasacreta, J. V., Nuamah, I. F., Robinson, K, D., Angeletti, K., Yasko, J. M., et al. (1998). A description of a psychoeducational intervention for family caregivers of cancer patients. *Journal of Family Nursing, 4*(4), 394–413.

Benoliel, J. Q., & McCorkle, R. (1978). A holistic approach to terminal illness. *Cancer Nursing, 1,* 143–149.

Blanchard, C. G., Toseland, R. W., & McCallion, P. (1997a). The effects of a problem solving intervention with spouses of cancer patients. *Journal Psychosocial Oncology, 14,* 1–21.

Blanchard, C., Albrecht, T., & Ruckdeschel, J. (1997b). The crisis of cancer: Psychological impact of family caregivers. *Oncology, 11,* 189–194.

Bradley, C. J, Given, B., Given, C., & Kozachik, S. (2004). Physical, economic, and social issues confronting patients and families. In C. Yarbo, M. Frogge, & M. Goodman (Eds.), *Cancer nursing: Principles and practice* (6th ed.). Boston: Jones and Bartlett.

Bultz, B., Speca, M., Brasher, P., Geggie, P., & Page, S. (2000). A randomized controlled trial of a brief psychoeducational support group for partners of early stage breast cancer patients. *Psycho-Oncology, 9*(4), 303–313.

Carey, P., Oberst, M., McCubbin, M., & Hughes, S. (1991). Appraisal and caregiving burden in family members caring for patients receiving chemotherapy. *Oncology Nursing Forum, 18*(8), 1341–1348.

Cawley, M. M., & Gerdts, E. K. (1988). Establishing a cancer caregivers program: An interdisciplinary approach. *Cancer Nursing, 11,* 267–273.

Cicirelli, V. G. (1992). *Family caregiving: Autonomous and paternalistic decision making.* Newbury Park: Sage.

Clipp, E., & George, L. (1992). Patients with cancer and their spouse caregivers. *Cancer, 69,* 1074–1079.

Conkling, V. K. (1989). Continuity of cares issues for cancer patients and families. *Cancer, 64,* 290–294.

Cook, T. D., & Campbell, D. T. (1979). *Quasi-experimentation: Design and analysis issues for field settings.* Chicago: Rand-McNally.

Cooley, M. E., & Moriarty, H. J. (1997). An analysis of empirical studies examining the impact of the cancer diagnosis and treatment of an adult on family functioning. *Journal of Family Nursing, 3*(4), 318–347.

Coristine, M., Crooks, D., Grunfeld, E., Stonebridge, C., & Christie, A. (2003). Caregiving for women with advanced breast cancer. *Psycho-Oncology, 12,* 709–719.

Davis-Ali, S. H., Chesler, M. A., & Chesney, B. K. (1993). Recognizing cancer as a family disease: Worries and support reported by patients and spouses. *Social Work in Health Care, 19*(2), 45–65.

Dyck, S., & Wright, K. (1988). Family perceptions: The role of the nurse throughout an adults' cancer experience. *Oncology Nursing Forum, 12,* 53–56.

Fang, C. Y., & Manne, S. L. (2001). Functional impairment, martial quality, and patient psychological distress as predictors of psychological distress among cancer patients' spouses. *Health Psychology, 20*(6), 452–457.

Ganz, P. A. (1990). Current issues in cancer rehabilitation. *Cancer, 65,* 742–751.

Gerstel, N., & Gallagher, S. (1993). Kin keeping and distress: Gender, recipients of care, and work-family conflict. *Journal of Marriage and Family, 55,* 598–607.

Giaquinta, B. (1977, October). Helping families face the crisis of cancer. *American Journal of Nursing, 77,* 1585.

Given, B., & Given, C. (1992). Patient and family caregiver reaction to new and recurrent breast cancer. *Journal of the American Medical Women's Association, 47*(5), 201–212.

Given, B. A., Keilman, L. J., Collins, C., & Given, C. W. (1990a). Strategies to minimize attrition in longitudinal studies. *Nursing Research, 39,* 184–186.

Given, B., Stommel, M., Collins, C., King, S., & Given, C. (1990b). Responses of elderly spouse caregivers. *Research in Nursing and Health, 13,* 73–85.

Given, C., Given, B., Stommel, M., Collins, C., King, S., & Franklin, S. (1992). The Caregiver Reaction Assessment (CRA) for caregivers of persons with chronic physical and mental impairments. *Research in Nursing and Health, 15,* 271–283.

Given, C., Stommel, M., Given, B., Osuch, J., Kurtz, M., & Kurtz, J. (1993). The influence of the cancer patient's symptoms, functional states on patient's depression and family caregiver's reaction and depression. *Health Psychology, 12*(4), 277–285.

Given, B., Wyatt, G., Given, C., Sherwood, P., Gift, A., DeVoss, D., et al. (2004). Burden and depression among caregivers of patients with cancer at the end of life. *Oncology Nursing Forum, 31*(6), 1105–1115.

Goldberg, R. J., & Wool, M. S. (1985). Psychotherapy for the spouses of lung cancer patients: Assessment of an intervention. *Psychotherapy Psychosomatic, 43,* 141–150.

Gotay, C. C. (1984). The experience of cancer during early and advanced stages: The views of patients and their mates. *Social Science and Medicine, 18,* 605–613.

Grunfeld, E., Coyle, D., Whelan, T., Clinch, J., Reyno, L., Earle, C., et al. (2004). Family caregiver burden: Results of a longitudinal study of breast cancer patients and their principal caregivers. *Canadian Medical Association Journal, 170*(12), 1795–1801.

Haley, W., LaMonde, L., Han, B., Narramore, S., & Schonwetter, R. (2001). Family caregiving in hospice: Effects on psychological and health functioning among spousal caregivers of hospice patients with lung cancer of dementia. *Hospice Journal, 15*(4), 1–17.

Hampe, S. (1975). Needs of the grieving spouse in a hospital setting. *Nursing Research, 24,* 113–119.

Heinrich, R. L., & Schag, C. (1985). Stress activity management: Group treatment for cancer patients and spouses. *Journal of Consulting and Clinical Psychology, 43,* 439–446.

Houts, P. S., Nezu, A. M., Nezu, C. M., & Bucher, J. A. (1996). The prepared family caregiver: A problem-solving approach to family caregiver education. *Patient Education & Counseling, 27*(1), 63–73.

Hull, M. M. (1992). Coping strategies of family caregivers in hospice home care. *Oncology Nursing Forum, 19,* 1179–1187.

Jepson, C., McCorkle, R., Adler, D., Nuamah, I., & Lusk, E. (1999). Effects of home care on caregivers' psychosocial status. *Image: Journal of Nursing Scholarship, 31*(2), 115–120.

Kristjanson, L., & Ashcroft, T. (1994). The family's cancer journey: A literature review. *Cancer Nursing, 17,* 1–17.

Kristjanson, L., Sloan, J., Dudgeon, D., & Adaskin, E. (1996). Family members' perception of palliative cancer care: Predictors of family functioning and family members' health. *Journal of Palliative Care, 12*(4), 10–20.

Krouse, H., & Krouse, J. (1982). Cancer as crisis: The critical elements of adjustment. *Nursing Research, 31,* 96–101.

Kurtz, M., Kurtz, J., Given, C., & Given, B. (2004). Depression and physical health among family caregivers of geriatric patients with cancer: A longitudinal view. *Medical Science Monitor, 10*(8), CR447–CR456.

Laizner, A., Shedga, L., Bard, F., & McCorkle, R. (1993). Needs of family caregivers of persons with cancer: A review. *Seminars in Oncology Nursing, 9*(2), 114–120.

MacVicar, M., & Archbold, P. (1976). A framework for family assessment in chronic illness. *Nursing Forum, 15*(2), 180–194.

McCorkle, R., & Benoliel, J. Q. (1983). Symptom distress, current concerns and mood disturbance after diagnosis of life threatening disease. *Social Science and Medicine, 17,* 431–438.

McCorkle, R., & Given, B. (1991). Meeting the challenge of caring for chronically ill adults. In P. Chin (Ed.), *Health policy: Who cares?* (pp. 2–7). Kansas City: American Academy of Nursing.

McCorkle, R., Yost, L.S., Jepson, C., Malone, D., Baird, S., & Lusk, E. (1993). A cancer experience: Relationship of patient psychosocial responses to caregiver burden over time. *Psycho-Oncology, 2,* 21–32.

Miaskowski, C., Kragness, L., Dibble, S., & Wallhagen, M. (1997). Differences in mood states, health status, and caregiver strain between family caregivers of oncology outpatients with and without cancer-related pain. *Journal of Pain and Symptom Management, 13*(3), 138–147.

Miller, B. (1990). Gender differences in spouse management of the caregiving role. In E. K. Abel & M. K. Nelson (Eds.), *Circles of care: Work and identity in women's lives* (pp. 92–104). Albany: State University of New York Press.

Mor, V., Guadagnoli, E., & Wool, M. (1987). An examination of the concrete service needs of advanced cancer patients. *Journal of Psychosocial Oncology, 5,* 1–17.

Moriarty, H. J. (1990). Key issues in the family research process: Strategies for nurse researchers. *Advances in Nursing Science, 12,* 1–14.

Morita, T., Chihara, S., & Kashiwagi, T. (2002). Family satisfaction with inpatient palliative care in Japan. *Palliative Medicine, 16*(3), 185–193.

Musci, E. C., & Dodd, M. J. (1990). Predicting self-care with the patients and family members after the states and family functioning. *Oncology Nursing Forum, 17*(3), 393–400.

Nijboer, C., Triemstra, M., Tempelaar, R., Sanderman, R., & van den Bos, G. (1999). Determinants of caregiving experiences and mental health of partners of cancer patients. *Cancer, 86*(4), 577–588.

Nijboer, C., Triemstra, M., Tempelaar, R., Mulder, M., Sanderman, R., & van den Bos, G. (2000). Patterns of caregiver experiences among partners of cancer patients. *Gerontologist, 40*(6), 738–746.

Nijboer, C., Tempelaar, R., Triemstra, M., van den Bos, G., & Sanderman, R. (2001). The role of social and psychological resources in caregivers of cancer patients. *Cancer, 89*(5), 1029–1039.

Northouse, L. L. (1988). Social Support in patients' and husbands' adjustment to breast cancer. *Nursing Research, 37,* 91–95.

Northouse, L. (1989). A longitudinal study of the adjustment of patients and husbands to breast cancer. *Oncology Nursing Forum, 16,* 511–516.

Northouse, L., & Peters-Golden, H. (1993). Cancer and the family: Strategies to assist spouses. *Seminars in Oncology Nursing, 9,* 74–82.

Northouse, L. L., & Swain, M. A. (1987). Adjustment of patients and husbands to the initial impact of breast cancer. *Nursing Research, 36,* 221–225.

Northouse, L., Dorris, G., & Charron-Moore, C. (1995). Factors affecting couples' adjustment to recurrent breast cancer. *Social Science and Medicine, 41*(1), 69–76.

Northouse, L., Templin, T., Mood, D., & Oberst, M. (1998). Couples' adjustments to breast cancer and benign breast disease: A longitudinal analysis. *Psycho-Oncology, 7,* 37–48.

Northouse, L., Mood, D., Templin, T., Mellon, S., & George, T. (2000). Couples' patterns of adjustment to colon cancer. *Social Science and Medicine, 50,* 271–284.

Northouse, L., Kershaw, T., Mood, D., & Schafenacker, A. (2005). Effects of a family intervention on the quality of life of women with recurrent breast cancer and their family caregivers. *Psycho-Oncology, 14,* 478–491.

Northouse, P. G., & Northouse, L. L. (1987). Communication and cancer: Issues confronting patients, health professionals, and family members. *Journal of Psychosocial Oncology, 5,* 17–46.

Oberst, M., & James, R. (1985). Going home: Patient and spouse adjustments following cancer surgery. *Topics in Clinical Nursing, 7,* 46–57.

Oberst, M., & Scott, D. (1988). Post-discharge distress in surgically treated cancer patients and their spouses. *Research in Nursing and Health, 11,* 223–233.

Oberst, M. T., Thomas, S., Gass, K. A., & Ward, S. E. (1989). Caregiving demands and appraisal of stress among family caregivers. *Cancer Nursing, 12,* 209–215.

Oberst, M., Huges, S., Chang. A., & McCubbin, M. (1991). Self care burden, stress appraisal, and mood among persons receiving radiotherapy. *Cancer Nursing, 14*(2), 71–75.

Pfefferbaum, B., Pasnan, R. O., & Jamison, K. (1977). A comprehensive program for psychosocial care for mastectomy patients. *International Journal of Psychiatry Medicine, 8,* 53–71.

Raveis, V., Karus, D., & Siegel, K. (1998). Correlates of depressive symptomatology among adult daughter caregiver of a patient with cancer. *Cancer, 83*(8), 1652–1663.

Raveis, V., Karus, D., & Pretter, S. (1999). Correlates of anxiety among adult daughter caregivers to a parent with cancer. Journal of *Psychosocial Oncology, 17*(3/4), 1–26.

Sales, E. (1991). Psychosocial impact of the phase of cancer on the family: An updated review. *Journal of Psychosocial Oncology, 9,* 1–18.

Sales, E., Schulz, R., & Beigel, D. (1992). Predictors of strain in families of cancer patients: A review of the literature. *Journal of Psychosocial Oncology, 10,* 1–26.

Schachter, S. (1992). Quality of life for families in the management of homecare patients with advanced cancer. *Journal of Palliative Care, 8,* 61–66.

Schulz, R., & Beach, S. R. (1999). Caregiving as a risk factor for mortality: The caregiver health effects study. *Journal of the American Medical Association, 282*(23), 2215–2219.

Schumacher, K., Dodd, M., & Paul, S. (1993). The stress process in family caregivers of persons receiving chemotherapy. *Research in Nursing and Health, 16,* 395–404.

Sherwood, P., Given, B., Given, C., Schiffman, R., Murman, D., & Lovely, M. (2004). Caregivers of persons with a brain tumor: A conceptual model. *Nursing Inquiry, 11*(1), 43–53.

Sherwood, P., Given, C., Given, B., & von Eye, A. (2005). Caregiver burden and depression: Analysis of common caregiver outcomes. *Journal of Aging and Health, 17*(2), 125–147.

Siegel, K., Raveis, V., Mor, V., & Houts, P. (1991). The relationship of spousal caregiver burden to patient disease and treatment-related conditions. *Annals of Oncology, 2*(7), 511–516.

Stetz, K. M. (1987). Caregiving demands during advanced cancer: The spouse's needs. *Cancer Nursing, 10,* 260–268.

Stetz, K. M. (1989). The relationship among background characteristics, purpose in life and caregiving demands on perceived health of spouse caregivers. *Scholarly Inquiry for Nursing Practice, 3,* 133–153.

Stommel, M., & Kingry, M. (1991). Support patterns for spouse-caregivers of cancer patients. The effect of the presence of minor children. *Cancer Nursing, 14*(4), 200–205.

Stommel, M., Given, C. W., & Given, B. (1990). Depression as an overriding variable explaining caregiver burdens. *Journal of Aging and Health, 2*(1), 81–102.

Stommel, M., Given, B. A., Given, C. W., & Collins, C. E. (1995). The impact of frequency of care activities on the division of labor between primary caregivers and other care providers. *Research on Aging, 17*(4), 412–433.

Vachon, M. L. S. (1982). Grief and bereavement: The family's experience before and after death. In I. Gentles (Ed.), *Care for the dying and the bereaved.* Toronto: Angelican Book Centre.

Weisman, A., & Worden, J. (1976). The existential plight in cancer: Significance of the first 100 days. *International Journal of Psychiatry in Medicine, 7,* 1–15.

Weitzner, M., Meyers, C., Stuebing, K., & Saleeba, A. (1997a). Relationship between quality of life and mood in long-term survivors of breast cancer treated with mastectomy. *Supportive Care in Cancer, 5*(3), 241–248.

Weitzner, M., Moody, L., & McMillan, S. (1997b). Symptom management issues in hospice care. *American Journal of Hospice and Palliative Care, 14*(4), 190–195.

Wellisch, D., Mosher, M. B., & VanScoy, C. (1978). Management of family emotional stress: Family group therapy in a private oncology practice. *International Journal Group Psychotherapy, 28*(2), 225–231.

Wilson, S., & Moore, J. M. (1991). Living with a wife undergoing chemotherapy. *Image, 23,* 78–84.

Zahlis, E., & Shands, M. E. (1991). Breast cancer: Demands of one illness on the patient's partner. *Journal of Psychosocial Oncology, 9,* 75–93.

Chapter 4
The Impact of Health Disparities on Cancer Caregivers

Carol D. Goodheart

The daily routine of giving care to a person ill with cancer is difficult under the best of circumstances. In the dynamic ebb and flow of need and care, crisis and chronicity, the on-going strain exacts a toll, even for people who take pride and satisfaction in being able to provide care. Difficulties are magnified when the climate for caregiving is worsened by such factors as poverty, discrimination, substandard access to services and treatment, language or cultural barriers.

Health disparities are defined by the working group of the National Institutes of Health (NIH) as "differences in the incidence, prevalence, mortality, and burden of cancer and related adverse health conditions that exist among specific populations in the United States. These population groups may be characterized by gender, age, ethnicity, education, income, social class, disability, geographic location, sexual orientation" (National Cancer Institute [NCI] 2005, p. 2). This chapter addresses the current status and future directions for cancer care research, practice and services, education and training, and public policy, as they pertain to increasing resilience and reducing the caregiving hardships created by health disparities.

Background

The changing demographics and distribution of income in the United States paint a revealing picture of the challenges for the future of cancer care and the concomitant effects on caregivers. Demographics are shifting rapidly in the twenty-first century. Today, more than 7 out of 10 people in the population are White Americans. By 2050, close to half of all Americans will be persons of color (U.S. Census Bureau 2004). The pattern of income distribution for the country is becoming increasingly skewed as the gap widens between the wealthiest 25% and the poorest 25% of the population. The Federal Reserve reports a 70% increase between 1998 and 2001 in the wealth difference between the richest 10% and the poorest 20% of families;

C. D. Goodheart (✉)
114 Commons Way, Princeton, NJ 08540, USA
e-mail: carol@drcarolgoodheart.com

R. C. Talley et al. (eds.), *Cancer Caregiving in the United States,*
Caregiving: Research, Practice, Policy,
DOI 10.1007/978-1-4614-3154-1_4, © Springer Science+Business Media, LLC 2012

the gap between ethnic minorities and Whites escalated by 21% in the same brief period of time (Hagenbaugh 2003). This type of disparity results in a worsening of overall health status because less of the general population has access to healthcare (Wilkinson 1992).

Consider the following examples of cancer occurrence, mortality, and health insurance, in which each number in an aggregate statistic has a human face and one or more significantly affected caregivers behind it:

- African Americans have the highest cancer incidence and death rates of any group in the United States; their death rate is 30% greater than Whites (NCI 2005). These figures represent the largest total health disparity among all groups and occur for multiple reasons, including poverty and a historic pattern of discrimination and differences in medical care.
- Hispanics/Latinos represent about 12% of the population, however, they make up 25% of the nation's uninsured. By 2050, they will represent almost a quarter of the country's population (U.S. Census Bureau 2004). The strain on the health care system and on families will increase proportionately if the nation does not have adequate and culturally appropriate care and caregiving support services.
- Asian Americans have an incidence rate for liver cancer that is more than three times the rate for Whites; their stomach cancer rate is more than twice as high (NCI 2005). More research is needed to understand fully the reasons for these differences.
- Poor White Appalachian Kentucky women have a cervical cancer rate that is almost twice as high as the incidence rate reported for White American women overall (Institute of Medicine 1999). Concerted education and screening efforts are needed to respond to this trend.

These examples imply differences not only for people with cancer, but also for those who take care of them and the communities in which they live. However, it is not helpful to make blind assumptions about the health status of a particular ethnic or cultural group. Former Surgeon General David Satcher illustrates this reminder well: "Asian-Americans are often viewed as a 'model' ethnic minority because of their low unemployment and disease rates. Asian-American/Pacific Islander women age 65 and older, however, have the highest death rate from suicide of all women in their age group, four times higher than the rate among elderly black women and twice the rate of white women" (Satcher 2001, pp. 131–132).

Broad categorizations may mask considerable individual differences. People are heterogeneous both within and between groups. It is necessary to avoid cultural stereotyping and to consider such factors as acculturation status and ethnic identity, including the reality that many people have multiple ethnic identities. There exists a useful distinction between generalizations and stereotypes (Galanti 1997): A generalization is a starting point, indicating common trends, however, further inquiry is needed to discover if the statement is appropriate to a particular individual. A stereotype is an ending point, one in which no further attempts are made to discover if a person fits the statement.

Caregiving situations and resources differ for: a poor Mexican agricultural worker family that travels hundreds, or even thousands of miles within the United States each year (alternatively, the family may be separated during the harvest seasons and reunited in Mexico for only a small portion of the year, depending on the feasibility of border crossings), a working-class Cuban American gay man in Miami, a wealthy Argentinean American heterosexual couple in Chicago, and a Puerto Rican American single middle-class working mother with two children in New York City. Although all are classified as Hispanic/Latino and may have commonalities such as language and religion, they have diverse personal circumstances, identities, immigration/citizenship status, levels of acculturation, and cultural backgrounds. Not all of them will face the same degree of disparity in access to health care and support services.

Race is a social construct associated with power, status, and access to opportunity. Institutional racism and overt discrimination in the United States have been ameliorated somewhat by better public policies and social norms for social equality, however, disparities remain widespread in health care systems.

Current Status

Guided by the caution not to over-generalize and fall into cultural stereotyping, it is useful to understand the underlying contributing factors that produce cancer disparities and affect families directly. The reduction of health disparities in the United States will depend upon applying the current knowledge to health policies for the future. There are several issues to consider as one evaluates the status of cancer caregiving.

First, cancer caregiving is becoming more difficult in general, because medical treatments are aggressive in the attempt to save lives. There are many side effects produced by surgery, chemotherapy, and radiation that create physical and emotional sequelae. Many of the treatments are done on an outpatient basis, and hospital stays are short. This leads to hardship for care recipients and family caregivers, who must cope with debilitating symptoms and frightening procedures at home. Also, even when the treatments end and the result is remission or cure, some survivors need on-going care.

Second, although the focus of this chapter is on family caregivers, it is important to note that there are actually several classes of caregivers relevant to a full consideration of health disparities: professionals (e.g., physicians, nurses, psychologists, social workers), paid nonprofessionals (e.g., aides, community workers), and informal caregivers (e.g., family members are most typical, however, sometimes the daily primary caretaker is a friend or neighbor). Each group faces particular demands. For example, the preponderance of hospital and nursing home aides are women, are underpaid, under-trained, and/or under-supported for the complexities of the job, and are often from ethnic minority cultures themselves, which may not match the cultures of the individuals with cancer under their care.

Third, the literature on cancer caregivers in the context of health disparities is quite limited. It is necessary to draw upon several related streams of research and to extrapolate from them in order to gain a clearer understanding for cancer care.

The resources used in this chapter include information on cancer, disparities, cross-cultural issues, and caregiving for other diseases and conditions such as Alzheimer's disease and disabilities.

Research

Research reports on ethnic minority family caregivers reveal both positive and negative consequences associated with the role. Sociocultural status may increase the risk of being in harm's way for members of some groups, however, cultural heritage may provide well-developed protective and coping resources to counterbalance some of the risk.

Work

Many caregivers reduce the number of hours they work each week to provide care. A study of caregivers for frail elders finds the burden of reduced employment is more likely to be experienced by families of African Americans and Hispanic/Latinos than the families of Whites (Covinsky et al. 2001). This finding may be a reflection of socioeconomic status, cultural values, or a combination of the two.

Health

African American caregivers are at greater risk to become ill themselves, and they are less likely than Whites to have formal support as their care recipients' conditions deteriorate (Williams and Dilworth-Anderson 2002). Although caregiving places similar restrictions on both Black and White families, the variable associated with physical health is race, not caregiving (Haley et al. 1995).

Resilience

African American caregivers show more resilience than Whites on measures of depression and life satisfaction. However, they are still vulnerable to increases in physical symptoms over time (Haley et al. 1995; Roth et al. 2001).

Learning

When given a culturally sensitive psychoeducational program on caregiving, Hispanic/Latina caregivers respond very positively. They increase their knowledge;

they increase their awareness of community-based services, and they increase their willingness to attend support groups (Morano and Bravo 2002).

Religion

Hispanic/Latinas and African Americans turn increasingly to religion after they become caregivers. White caregivers do not show this change (Navaie-Waliser et al. 2001).

Resourcefulness

African American caregivers have higher resourcefulness scores than Whites, and a more benign appraisal of disruptive behavior in their sick elderly care recipients. Despite this, coping efforts for both groups are similar (Gonzalez 1997).

Hospice Use

Many ethnic minority groups underutilize hospice services for end of life care. A study of a large metropolitan facility in Virginia found the hospice provided end of life care service at the following rates: 30% of Caucasians, 20% of Asians, 19% of Hispanic/Latinos, and 18% of African Americans (O'Mara and Arenella 2001). Barriers to hospice access were identified in a national study (Gordon 1996). The admission criteria impeded access for African Americans, especially the primary caregiver requirement, whereas problems with language, reimbursement, and severity of illness impeded access for Hispanic/Latinos, who were the most underserved group. Apart from the existence of barriers, there may be cultural preferences for end of life care among some groups, which could account for a portion of the underutilization patterns.

Disparities in Cancer Caregiving

In looking at a different subset of the research literature, some of the factors that make cancer caretaking harder may be identified.

Unequal Cancer Treatment Perhaps the most striking factor is unequal cancer treatment. There are significant racial and ethnic differences for the implementation of cancer diagnostic tests, treatments, and analgesics (Institute of Medicine 1999, 2003).

Of great significance for caregivers, how does one care for someone in daily cancer pain? Pain management is inadequate for nearly everyone. However, it is more difficult for women, those in rural areas, the elderly, and people of color to manage. The treatment of pain for African Americans is inadequate compared to that for Whites. African Americans have a 63% greater likelihood of having untreated cancer pain than Whites. Patients treated in centers primarily serving African American or Hispanic/Latino populations have a 77% probability of being undermedicated for pain, and physicians underestimate the severity of cancer pain in African Americans. African American women with breast cancer are less likely than Whites to receive radiation and African American men with prostate cancer are less likely than Whites to receive the newer surgical treatments. Further, African American men are twice as likely as Whites not to receive any treatment at all for prostate cancer. These findings provide disturbing evidence of unequal burden (Institute of Medicine 1999, 2003).

Gender Disparity Women comprise three out of four caregivers for dying cancer patients, however, when they are terminally ill are less likely than men to receive family care and must rely on paid assistance (Emanuel et al. 1999). However, paid home health care is being reduced across the country in the national effort to lower health care costs. Some studies show a more equitable distribution of caregiving between the sexes, but overall, women spend 50% more time than men do as caregivers (U.S. Department of Health and Human Services 1998a). Women are overburdened both as caregivers and as those in need of care. The implications of gender disparity in cancer care are compounded when one takes into account caregiver ethnicity research findings on the percentage of individuals caring for parents: 19% of Whites, 28% of African Americans, 34% of Hispanic/Latino Americans, and 42% of Asian Americans (AARP 2001). The intersection of gender and ethnicity research highlights the disproportionate role burden on ethnic minority women caregivers.

Stress, Depression and Anxiety The risks for stress, depression, and anxiety increase with the problems accompanying cancer. Often, ethnic minority and socioeconomically disadvantaged people are at additional risk for depression and anxiety. Racism and discrimination are stressful events adversely affecting both physical and mental health; in addition, clinical environments that are incompatible with the cultures of the people served are a deterrent to obtaining appropriate care (U.S. Department of Health and Human Services 2001). Schultz et al. (2001) used a stress process framework to explore the implications of race-based housing segregation and economic divestment on the lives and health (including depression) of women caring for children in urban environments. The women reported the following life stressors, which were significantly associated with symptoms of depression: financial and safety worries, contact with the police, and unfair treatment concerns. It seems reasonable to hypothesize that if one adds the stress of caring for a child, adult partner, or aging parent with cancer, this can only increase the risk for anxiety and depression.

Thwarted Prevention Efforts Tobacco products are advertised, displayed, and promoted disproportionately to ethnic minority communities, most noticeably in Hispanic/Latino and Asian neighborhoods. Lung cancer is the leading cause of cancer deaths for Hispanic/Latinos (U.S. Department of Health and Human Services 1998b).

Other Centers for Disease Control and Prevention data show an increase in smoking prevalence among Hispanic/Latino high school students from 1991 (25.3%) to 1997 (34%), and a plateau at that high prevalence rate since then (Kann et al. 2000). The rate for lung cancer occurrence among Southeast Asians in the United States is 18% higher than the rate for White Americans (Coultas et al. 1994). An evaluation of Proposition 99-funded efforts to prevent and control tobacco use in California (Elder et al. 1993) found the highest number of tobacco displays in Asian neighborhoods (6.4 per store), compared to Hispanic/Latino (4.6 per store) and African American stores (3.7). The lowest number of displays was found in White neighborhoods. Ethnic minority communities are not benefiting to the same extent as White communities in the national public health campaign to eradicate smoking and greatly reduce the incidence of lung cancer. Although tobacco promotion is reviewed here, it is important to note that alcohol consumption and the associated health risks show a similar pattern of thwarted prevention efforts.

Unmet Psychosocial Needs Caregivers have more concerns about managing daily life, emotions, and social identity than do the cancer sufferers themselves (Soothill et al. 2001). This reflects the comparative neglect of caregivers. Perhaps not surprisingly, 43% of caregivers report significant unmet needs, which makes functioning in the role of caregiver more difficult (Soothill et al. 2001).

Practice and Services

Cancer health disparities and hardships in caregiving are strongly linked to the barriers to care. The process of understanding and removing these barriers will go a long way toward increasing the comfort of family caregivers and improving access and utility of services.

Financial Resources Poverty, small incomes combined with long work hours, and lack of health insurance constitute a daunting barrier to cancer care and to the needed services for caregivers. Too often, health care quality and access in the United States are governed by the ability to pay for consultation, treatment, education about the disease, and support services. Disparities are associated with socioeconomic differences and "tend to diminish significantly, and in a few cases, disappear altogether when socioeconomic factors are controlled" (Institute of Medicine 2003, p. 5).

Language The United States is made up of people who speak many languages, each of which expresses a distinctive culture. Almost 18% of US residents speak a language other than English at home, including 10.7% Spanish, 3.8% Indo-European, and 2.7% Asian languages (U.S. Census Bureau 2003). Currently, there are insufficient translators and written materials for many ethnic minority groups, which would aid in caregiving. Translation is often unavailable in some settings. When available, it may be carried out by children, teens, adult relatives, as well as by maintenance workers in some institutions. This could create an awkward or taboo interpersonal situation, one in which the translator's relationship, development, or language skill is not appropriate to the task. The best translators are "cultural brokers" (Fadiman 1997), who are equals, rather than inferiors, to the health care professional. The best-written materials are conceptual translations, not literal ones.

Some effort has been made to address language needs. The NCI offers material in Spanish via its website (www.cancer.gov) and will mail *Cancer Fact Sheets* in Spanish. Families can also call 1-800-4CANCER, the Cancer Information Service of NCI; translators are available upon request. If one is not immediately available, arrangements can be made for a call by appointment. Information specialists at the American Cancer Society (ACS) provide most of their basic documents in Spanish and answer cancer questions from callers speaking any language (ACS 2003). ACS also has some materials in other languages, e.g., the materials for the Asian *Tell A Friend* screening program are written in Chinese (Mandarin), Korean, Vietnamese, and two Filipino languages—Ilokano and Tagalog (www.cancer.org). Increasingly, language and culture-specific resources are available on cancer facts, care, and options. However, if translators are not available to discuss care in practice settings too, the results are likely to be poor communication, disparities in service, and errors.

Cultural Unfamiliarity and Differences The culture of biomedicine is a strange and exotic culture for members of many ethnic minority cultures. Biomedical and ethnic minority cultures may hold very different views and beliefs about health and sickness, dietary needs, dying, polite communication, authority, family/gender/caregiver roles, folk medicine practices, social customs, and the relationship among mind, body, and spirit. Because of these potential differences, misunderstanding and discouragement on both sides of the cultural divide are quite common.

Anne Fadiman's award winning book, *The Spirit Catches You and You Fall Down* (1997), gives a rich illustration of the clash between conscientious and humane medical professionals and the loving caregiving refugee parents and family of a Hmong child. Geri-Ann Galanti's text, *Caring for Patients from Different Cultures* (1997), is an example-filled resource that discusses many cultural group norms and practices. Familiarity with resources such as these books is recommended for health care professionals who want to become more culturally competent in their work with patients and families.

Time Pressure During Medical Consultations Typically, visits with physicians are brief for everyone, and this brevity creates frustration for physicians, patients, and family members. Many people wish they had more time to ask questions and to clarify or expand upon the discussion. Time pressure increases if there are additional demands in the room, such as a need for translation, a need to ascertain if one's message is being understood, or a need to negotiate differences in approaching a problem and arrive at a mutually agreeable compromise. When the pressure flusters a caregiver, she or he is less likely to hear and give important information related to cancer options and care. The same may be said for patients, physicians, nurses, and any other allied health professionals present during consultations.

Limited Access to Support Services When caregivers do not have such basics as transportation, respite from caregiving and work responsibilities, or language facility, they cannot avail themselves of informational, psychoeducational, advocacy, or support services. A good number of cancer treatment centers now have grants and programs to facilitate participation and support for caregivers, although more are needed.

Health Professionals' Attitudes and Knowledge   Even among well-intentioned health care professionals, little time is spent on learning cross-cultural medicine, nursing, psychology, or social work. Increasing numbers of programs are being offered to health care professionals on diversity issues and guidelines for best practices, although there remains a long road ahead until widespread cultural competence is reached.

Education and Training

A survey of physicians in Los Angeles found that although 71% believe language and culture are important for care delivery, more than half of them had no cultural competency training (Cho and Solis 2001). A national survey of physicians, conducted by the Kaiser Family Foundation, found a majority of physicians aware of racial disparities in health treatment, however, not believing it to be a widespread problem. Conversely, 77% of African American physicians disagreed, believing race and ethnicity do have an impact on how people are treated (Kaiser Family Foundation 2002, March).

Despite these statistics, cultural competency training is on the rise. Many health care professionals grasp the importance of language and cultural differences in providing cancer care and experience the impact of this in their practices. Cross-cultural education has evolved from cultural sensitivity models to cultural competence models, which are skill based and designed to be less subjective. The growing awareness of the fundamental inequities related to health disparities has provided an impetus for the expansion of this educational focus. In line with these advances, accreditation standards and guidelines have formalized the curriculum requirements for multicultural education in training programs for physicians, nurses, and psychologists. A lag in multicultural education and training remains for the time being. However, it may be expected to decrease over time with advances in training opportunities.

Public Policy

In recent years, there has been a growing recognition of health disparities and beginning steps are underway to alter the circumstances. Little is directed yet toward caregivers, however, they may benefit indirectly from changes in policy that have an impact on their care recipients. In 2000, the NCI established the Center to Reduce Cancer Health Disparities. Under the auspices of the center, a network of 18 institutions creates and implements cancer control, prevention, research, and training programs in ethnic minority and underserved communities. Another initiative located at NCI is the Comprehensive Minority Biomedical Branch, whose mission is to increase the participation of ethnic minority scientists and institutions in cancer research, benefiting ethnic minority communities over time. Also in 2000, the Minority Health and Health Disparities Act was passed and signed into law. It authorized funding for the National Center on Minority Health and Health Disparities at the NIH ; authorized the Agency for Healthcare Research and Quality to conduct and support activities, research to measure health disparities, and identify causes and remedies; and authorized the Health Resources and Services Administration to support research and demonstration projects to train health professionals on reducing health care disparities.

Combining both Federal and State resources, the National Breast and Cervical Cancer Early Detection Program is a model screening program for underserved poor and ethnic minority women in all 50 states. This is a state Department of Health administered program, with matching funds and support provided through the Centers for Disease Control and Prevention. In addition, combining local community and agency collaboration, the ACS has established a partnership, the Minority Outreach & Education Coalition, to provide cancer education programs to underserved residents.

The progress has been exemplary, however, the public policy trend is not all positive. There are concerns about the stability of funding for cancer screening, registry, prevention, and education programs, based on burgeoning federal and state budget deficits and rising health care costs.

Future Directions

The primary goal for future research, practice, education, and policy is the eradication of cancer health disparities. Equal care is the path toward equal outcome. To the extent that cancer health disparities can be reduced, the burden on caregivers will be reduced proportionately.

Research

There is a need for more research that is specifically targeted to investigate cancer family caregivers. A great deal is more known about the caregivers of people with other conditions, such as Alzheimer's disease. Much of the recent comparison work on caregiving has been done with African American and Hispanic/Latino groups. As this body of literature grows, it will be useful to study caregivers from other cultural groups as well. Particularly within biopsychosocial and family systems theoretical frameworks, there is ample room to expand the knowledge base and test interventions for underserved and understudied cancer caregivers. The area of cancer caregiver research remains open for creative investigation by researchers in all salient health fields.

Practice and Services

In order to improve cancer health care practices and services, it will be necessary to improve communication and outreach efforts to family caregivers. Based on current experiences, future efforts are likely to be most successful if they are tailored to the specific needs of ethnic minority groups and accommodate differences in language fluency, dietary practices, gender sensitivity, cultural and religious beliefs, and the special concerns of a growing population of the aged. Within this context:

- More psychoeducational services for caretakers are needed to teach disease information, coping skills, self-care and patient-care, how to access services, and how to make the use of group support systems (both formal and informal).
- More practical services are needed to insure that caregivers have reliable modes of transportation, communication, respite, and medical backup available to them.
- More bilingual-bicultural staff is needed in cancer care centers to lessen the barriers created by language differences.
- More community health workers, who are recruited, trained, and retained locally, are needed. Community health workers are the cultural brokers who translate language and culture, identify needs, screen for problems, and refer and mediate between the family and the health care system. They are often the bridge between health care systems and ethnic minority communities.

Implementation of these needed services will require additional resources from insurers, hospitals, agencies, and the government.

Innovative programs for caregivers may be adapted for differing populations. For example, the Stanford Assistance Program (Stanford University School of Medicine) offers an outstanding multicultural interventions program for dementia caregivers. The model for ethnicity and caregiving takes into account explanatory and cultural beliefs about disease and caregiving, attitudes toward caregiving, assessment issues, implications for caregivers, and implications for service utilization and the development of effective interventions. The program might be adapted to cancer caregivers by modifications such as removing the material focused on disruptive behavior in dementia and adding appropriate material on pain, side effects, and symptom relief in cancer (D. Gallagher-Thompson 2003, personal communication; Gallagher-Thompson et al. 2003). At a national meeting of the Cancer Patient Education Network, Ana Marchena, a Health Education Specialist at Memorial Sloan Kettering Cancer Center, presented a program on establishing a program for caregivers of cancer patients. This cancer caregiver program could be modified for diverse cultural groups.

In the future, the Internet and combinations of Internet, telecommunications, and face-to-face contact may be used increasingly as a source of information and support. Of course, many caregivers affected by health disparities due to language barriers or poverty do not have ready access to the new "infomatics." Public libraries provide free public access to computers with Internet availability, as do some hospitals in conjunction with the American Cancer Society.

The Computer Retrieval of Information on Scientific Projects (CRISP; crisp.cit.nih.gov), which is a database of federally-funded biomedical research, summarizes projects in progress that may develop into promising intervention programs for caregiving members of ethnic minority populations. Two such examples are *Web-Based Support for Informal Caregivers in Cancer* (Gustafson 2006) and *Tele-Care for Caregivers of the Terminally Ill* (Rubert 2000). It seems likely that technology-based options will supplement, but not supplant, the resources needed for human contact, support, and respite.

Education and Training

The education and training system serves as the mechanism to translate the evolving knowledge base into better practices that serve the public well-being. The goal is full integration of multicultural competence training, including an understanding of the psychological and physical impact of bias and stereotyping, into all core professional education programs for health professionals: physicians, nurses, psychologists, social workers, occupational therapists, physical therapists, and dieticians. Professionals must understand that bias exists and has an impact on health care delivery, however, learning new multicultural skills can mitigate it. As health care professionals and educators learn and grow, the health care educational system will both teach and reflect these changes.

The full implementation of training will take time. For now, in addition to core training programs for those entering the professions, multicultural competence training may be disseminated through continuing education courses and institutional in-service programs. It has been shown that training for professionals in cultural competence has a direct influence on the quality of service patients and family caregivers receive.

Public Policy

The major public research and intervention policy initiatives begun over the past decade, and discussed earlier in the chapter, will need continued growth and sustainable funding if they are to come to fruition. New initiatives are needed to offer basic protections for caregivers. For example, Ezekiel Emanuel, MD, a director of the Commmonwealth-Cummings Project on the End of Life, suggests that the vital services provided by family caregivers be recognized by the introduction of tax credits (ACS 2000).

As health care reform cycles to the forefront of economic and political debates again, it will be important to consider how best to maintain the policy gains of the past 15 years related to cancer caregiving and health disparities. Further legislative and legal means may be needed to block insurance discrimination, to allow for continuity of care in government-backed health plans such as Medicare and Medicaid, and to maintain adequate resources to enforce civil rights laws (Institute of Medicine 1999).

Summary

The impact of health disparities on cancer caregivers is discussed in terms of the current status of cancer care research, practice, education, and policy. Future directions for these four areas are explored with an eye toward improving both health care conditions and the quality of life for caregivers from diverse cultural groups.

There is less direct research and intervention literature on caregivers for individuals with cancer is available than on other populations, perhaps because the cancer population is less homogeneous and the disease course more widely variable. Cancer occurs across the life span—in children and adolescents, adults in the prime of life, and the elderly. Cancer may run a fast course from diagnosis to death, or it may result in long-term remission or cure. Cancer treatments may extend life considerably, but leave the person with significant disabilities. Cancer family caregivers may be children, adolescents, adults, or elderly themselves. Although this heterogeneity makes research and intervention for cancer caregivers more difficult, the need is imperative. The hallmark of a healthy society is fair and equitable treatment for all. If the United States is to meet the challenge of eliminating health disparities, we must insure that services for cancer care and cancer caregiving are responsive to the needs of all members of our diverse society.

References

American Association for Retired Persons (AARP). (2001, June). *In the middle: A report on multicultural boomers coping with family and aging issues.* Washington: AARP.

American Cancer Society (ACS). (2000, February 10). Study finds women fill most caregiving needs. *ACS News Today.* Retrieved from http://www.cancer.org/docroot/NWS/content/NWS_2_ 1x_Study_Finds_Women_Fill_Most_Caregiving_Needs.asp.

American Cancer Society (ACS). (2003). *Cancer information services.* Retrieved from http:// www.cancer.org/AboutUs/HowWeHelpYou/HelpingYouGetWell/cancer-information-services.

Cho, J., & Solis, B. M. (2001). *Healthy families culture and linguistics resources survey: A physician perspective on their diverse member population.* Los Angeles: LA Care Health Plan.

Coultas, D. B., Gong, H., Jr., Grad, R., Handler, A., McCurdy, S. A., & Player, R. (1994). Respiratory diseases in minorities of the United States. *American Journal of Respiratory and Critical Care Medicine, 149,* S93–S131.

Covinsky, K. E., Eng, C., Lui, L. Y., Sands, L. P., Sehgal, A. R., Walter, L. C., Wieland, D., Eleazer, G. P., Yaffe, K. et al. (2001). Reduced employment in caregivers of frail elders: Impact of ethnicity, patient clinical characteristics, and caregiver characteristics. *Journal of Gerontology, 56*(11), M707–M713.

Elder, J. P., Edwards, C., & Conway, T. L. (1993). *Independent evaluation of Proposition 99-funded efforts to prevent and control tobacco use in California.* Sacramento: California Department of Health.

Emanuel, E. J., Fairclough, D. L., Slutsman, J., Alpert, H., Baldwin, D., & Emanuel, L. L. (1999). Assistance from family members, friends, paid care givers, and volunteers in the care of terminally ill patients. *New England Journal of Medicine, 341*(13), 956–963.

Fadiman, A. (1997). *The spirit catches you and you fall down.* New York: Farrar, Straus and Giroux.

Galanti, G. A. (1997). *Caring for patients from different cultures: Case studies from American hospitals* (2nd ed.). Philadelphia: University of Pennsylvania Press.

Gallagher-Thompson, D., Hargrave, R., Hinton, L., Arean, P., Iwamasa, G., & Zeiss, L. (2003). Interventions for a multicultural society. In D. Coon, D. Gallagher-Thompson, & L. Thompson (Eds.), *Innovative interventions to reduce dementia caregiver distress: A clinical guide* (pp. 50–73). New York: Springer.

Gonzalez, E. W. (1997). Resourcefulness, appraisals, and coping efforts of family caregivers. *Issues in Mental Health Nursing, 18*(3), 209–227.

Gordon, A. K. (1996). Hospice and minorities: A national study of organizational access and practice. *Hospice Journal, 11*(1), 49–70.

Gustafson, D. H. (2006). *Web- Based Support for Informal Caregivers in Cancer.* Retrieved from http://search.engrant.com/project/ZWheNy/web-based_support_for_informal_caregivers_in_cancer.

Hagenbaugh, B. (2003, January 23). Nation's wealth disparity widens. *USA Today*, p. 1.

Haley, W. E., West, C. A. C., Wadley, V. G., & Ford, G. R. (1995). Psychological, social, and health impact of caregiving: A comparison of Black and White dementia family caregivers and noncaregivers. *Psychology and Aging, 10*(4), 540–552.

Institute of Medicine (IOM). (1999). Executive Summary. In M. A. Haynes & B. D. Smedley (Eds.), *The unequal burden of cancer: An assessment of NIH research and programs for ethnic minorities and the medically underserved (pp 1–15).* Washington: National Academy Press (http://www.nap.edu/openbook.php?record_id=6377&page=16).

Institute of Medicine (IOM). (2003). Summary. In B. D. Smedley, A. Stith, & A. R. Nelson (Eds.), *Unequal treatment: Confronting racial and ethnic disparities in health care (pp. 1–28).* Washington: National Academies Press (http://www.nap.edu/openbook.php?record_id=10260&page=R1).

Kaiser Family Foundation. (2002, March). *National survey of physicians Part I: Doctors on disparity in medical care.* Retrieved from http://www.kff.org/content/2002/20020321a/.

Kann, L., Kinchen, S. A., Williams, B. I., Ross, J. G., Lowry, R., Grunbaum, J. A. et al. (2000). *Youth Risk Behavior Surveillance—United States, 1999.* Retrieved from http://www.cdc.gov/mmwr/preview/mmwrhtml/ss4905a1.htm.

Morano, C. L., & Bravo, M. (2002). A psychoeducational model for Hispanic Alzheimer's disease caregivers. *Gerontologist, 42,* 122–126.

National Cancer Institute. (2005). *Cancer health disparities: Fact sheet.* Retrieved from http://www.cancer.gov/cancertopics/factsheet/disparities/cancer-health-disparities.

Navaie-Waliser, M., Feldman, P. H., Gould, D. A., Levine, C., Kuerbis, A. N., & Donelan, K. (2001). The experiences and challenges of informal caregivers: Common themes and differences among Whites, Blacks, and Hispanics. *Gerontologist, 41,* 733–741.

O'Mara, A. M., & Arenella, C. (2001). Minority representation, prevalence of symptoms, and utilization of services in a large metropolitan hospice. *Journal of Pain and Symptom Management, 21*(4), 290–297.

Roth, D. L., Haley, W. E., Owen, J. E., Clay, O. J., & Goode, K. T. (2001). Appraisal, coping, and social support as mediators of well-being in Black and White family caregivers of patients with Alzheimer's disease. *Psychology and Aging, 16*(3), 427–436.

Rubert, M. P. (2000). *Tele-Care for Caregivers of the Terminally Ill.* Retrieved from http://search.engrant.com/project/93hsFY/tele-care_for_caregivers_of_the_terminally_ill

Satcher, D. (2001). American women and health disparities. *Journal of the American Medical Women's Association, 56*(4), 131–133.

Schultz, A., Parker, E., Israel, B., & Fisher, T. (2001). Social context, stressors, and disparities in women's health. *Journal of the American Medical Women's Association, 56,* 143–149.

Soothill, K., Morris, S. M., Harmon, J. C., Francis, B., Thomas, C., & McIllmurray, M. B. (2001). Informal Carers of Cancer Patients: What are their unmet psychosocial needs? *Health and Social Care in the Community, 9*(6), 464–475.

U.S. Census Bureau. (2003). *Census 2000, Summary File 3, Table PCT10. Detailed List of Languages Spoken at Home for the Population 5 Years and Over by State:* 2000 Internet release date: February 25, 2003. Retrieved from http://www.census.gov/population/cen2000/phct20/tab05.pdf

U.S. Census Bureau. (2004). *National interim projections consistent with Census 2000 (released March, 2004), Summary table 1a, Projected population of the U.S. by race and Hispanic origin: 2000–2050.* Retrieved from http://www.census.gov/population/www/projections/popproj.html.

U.S. Department of Health and Human Services. (1998a). *Informal caregiving: Compassion in action.* Washington: U.S. Department of Health and Human Services, Office of the Assistant Secretary for Planning, Evaluation, and Administration on Aging.

U.S. Department of Health and Human Services. (1998b). *Tobacco use among US racial/ethnic minority groups—African Americans, American Indians and Alaska Natives, Asian Americans and Pacific Islanders, and Hispanics: A report of the Surgeon General.* Atlanta: U.S. Department of Health and Human Services, Centers for Disease Control and Prevention.

U.S. Department of Health and Human Services. (2001). *Mental health: Culture, race, and ethnicity—Executive summary—A supplement to mental health: A report of the Surgeon General.* Rockville: U.S. Department of Health and Human Services, Public Health Service, Office of the Surgeon General.

Wilkinson, R. G. (1992). Income distribution and life expectancy. *British Medical Journal, 304,* 165–168.

Williams, S. W., & Dilworth-Anderson, P. (2002). Systems of social support in families who care for dependent African American elders. *Gerontologist, 42,* 224–236.

Chapter 5
Education, Training, and Support Programs for Caregivers of Individuals with Cancer

Myra Glajchen

More than 52 million adults currently provide care to relatives in the United States (Family Caregiver Alliance 2011; Schulz and Beach 1999). These family caregivers become active members of the healthcare team with little or no preparation in disease management, sometimes under sudden and extreme circumstances. As this has occurred, the demanding role of caring for patients has fallen to untrained, inexperienced family members. Involvement of family caregivers is essential for the optimal treatment of the cancer-pain patient, especially in assuring treatment compliance, continuity of care, and social support (Warner 1992). In response, the medical community has sought to develop education, support, and training programs to guide family members caring for patients with cancer.

Developing effective interventions that fulfill caregivers' physical and emotional needs is a demanding process. In order to design effective caregiver interventions, clinicians, researchers, and educators must have a clear understanding of the role caregivers assume and the needs they have as a result of these demanding roles. Research conducted over the past 20 years has given us a good understanding of caregivers' roles and their needs. As a result, several types of interventions have been developed with the goal of addressing these needs. In general, four types of interventions can be identified: (1) educational or informational; (2) counseling or psychotherapy; (3) hospice or palliative home care; and (4) problem-solving or skill-building. The intended outcomes of these programs for caregivers include increasing knowledge and confidence, reducing anxiety and depression, providing medical and psychosocial services, and improving skills. However, whether current interventions result in the intended outcomes is unclear.

The purpose of this chapter is to provide the reader with an understanding of the current status of education, training, and support programs for caregivers of patients with cancer. The chapter begins with a review of caregivers' roles, needs, and the impact of caregiving. Next, a description is provided of each type of intervention and its intended outcome, followed by a review of literature regarding whether existing

M. Glajchen (✉)
Institute for Education and Research in Pain and Palliative Care, Beth Israel Medical Center,
First Avenue at 16th Street, NY 10003, New York, USA
e-mail: mglajchen@chpnet.org

R. C. Talley et al. (eds.), *Cancer Caregiving in the United States,*
Caregiving: Research, Practice, Policy,
DOI 10.1007/978-1-4614-3154-1_5, © Springer Science+Business Media, LLC 2012

interventions have demonstrated effectiveness and efficacy in meeting caregivers' needs. Programs of education, training, and support were included for review if they were designed for the caregivers of cancer patients and had been published in the peer-reviewed literature. Pasacreta and McCorkle (2000) evaluated the literature on the impact of interventions on caregiver outcomes. This chapter summarizes and augmentes their findings with literature and new developments published subsequent to their review.

Both program efficacy and effectiveness are described to illuminate the association between program and outcome. Efficacy refers to whether controlled trials show a treatment effect, while effectiveness refers to whether the treatment transfers well to real-world populations. Randomized controlled trials measure efficacy and provide enhanced internal validity; however, they may have limited generalizability to real-world settings. On the other hand, effectiveness approaches offer enhanced external validity, and are generalizable. However, they are typically less-controlled than efficacy studies, thereby limiting the assumptions that can be made about causality. Both efficacy and effectiveness studies are included in this review. The chapter concludes with recommendations for future research and challenges confronting the field of caregiving as a whole. The multifaceted role of persons caring for patients with cancer, especially advanced cancer, is a demanding role that poses significant challenges. As care of the cancer patient has shifted from the hospital to the home, the role of family caregiver has been transformed into a complex, multifaceted role that a caregiver may be ill-prepared to assume. To fully understand the role of the caregiver caring for someone with cancer, it is useful to first describe the cancer continuum. This term has been used since the mid-1970s to describe the various transition points that comprise the disease trajectory in cancer. These milestones include cancer prevention, detection, diagnosis, treatment, survivorship, end-of-life, and death (National Cancer Institute 2005). The role of the caregiver in cancer will shift along with the needs of the person with cancer. In addition, for the caregiver whose loved one dies, bereavement must be added as the last transition point along the continuum.

For purposes of the discussion, a caregiver will be defined as a relative or friend who provides unpaid help to people with cancer as they are unable to do things for themselves because of the illness or related disability. This kind of help can include household chores, finances, personal or medical needs (Levine 2004). The prevalence of caregiving in cancer is not currently known. However, we do know that an estimated 1.3 million people are diagnosed with cancer in the United States each year, and that many of these people are living longer with the disease (National Cancer Institute 2005). From this, we can infer that many of the nations' caregivers are taking care of their loved ones with cancer. Caregivers of cancer patients are expected to function broadly, providing direct care, assistance with activities of daily living, case management, emotional support, companionship, and medication supervision (Levine 2004). Caregivers assume such tasks for a variety of reasons, including a sense of familial obligation and loyalty, altruism in the face of their loved one's suffering, as well as more practical reasons such as lack of paid help and lack of insurance coverage for services (Family Caregiver Alliance 2011). Caregivers of people with cancer may assist specifically by providing meals, providing transportation, completing insurance forms, and providing such personal care as toileting and dressing. Caregivers may be expected to provide patients with emotional support, conversation, and other forms of distraction.

Generally speaking, patients with cancer experience side-effects and symptoms as a result of advancing disease and such treatment as chemotherapy, radiation therapy and surgery. As many people with cancer experiences pain at some point along the disease trajectory, caregivers are likely to be called upon to help manage cancer-related pain. An overview of the caregiver's role in cancer pain management can serve as a prototype for any type of symptom management during the course of cancer diagnosis and treatment.

The prevalence of pain in patients with cancer is now widely known. Thirty to 45% of cancer patients experience pain at diagnosis and in the early stages of the illness, while an average of 75% of patients with advanced cancer have pain (Agency for Health Care Policy and Research [AHCPR] 1994). Cancer pain management is therefore a major focus of the caregivers' role. First, caregivers function as nurse's aides when they are required to assess and report the patient's pain and manage the pain management regimen. Caregivers must attempt to determine the source, nature, and amount of pain. They must keep records and control the technical aspects of pain management. Caregivers frequently dispense pain medication or remind the patient to take a scheduled dose, which requires decision-making about which type of medication to give, when, and in what dosage (Ferrell et al. 1995). It generally falls to the caregiver to fill and refill pain prescriptions, which presupposes such skills as proficiency with insurance reimbursement, the ability to follow medical instructions, and the ability to anticipate the need for refills ahead of time (Glajchen 2003). With increasingly high-tech home care and pain management protocols, family caregivers are frequently expected to help manage patient-controlled analgesia pumps, epidural catheters, and home infusions. The technical aspects of these interventions can be terrifying for even the most sophisticated of caregivers. In addition to managing the patient's pain regimen, the caregiver is expected to identify and report treatment side effects or new symptoms.

Cancer patients may face an array of side-effects and symptoms as they move along the disease trajectory. Fatigue, drowsiness, and sleep problems have been reported in 51–68% of cancer patients; nausea, vomiting, anorexia, and cachexia have been reported in 10–40% of patients; while reports of anxiety, mood disorder, and depression are well-documented in 25–50% of cancer patients (National Cancer Institute 2005; Hickock et al. 2005). Management of these complicated side-effects frequently falls to the caregiver in the outpatient setting.

Finally, caregivers may be expected to function as legal and medical assistants for patients with cancer. Patients face an overwhelming array of decision-making during the course of diagnosis and treatment. Decisions about treatment options, role changes, and finances are generally made by the patient-family unit (Vachon 1998; Warner 1992). Caregivers are expected to manage home care professionals; manage medical emergencies; facilitate transitions (e.g., home to hospital to hospice or long-term care facility); obtain medical, financial, and legal advice; and prepare for the death and funeral.

In summary, caregivers of cancer patients have multifaceted role expectations and needs, which they may be ill-prepared to assume. In addition, caregivers have their own emotional responses to the patients' diagnosis and prognosis, and may require coaching and emotional support separate and apart from the patient (Given et al. 2001; Kozachik et al. 2001). Despite the high prevalence of family caregiving, the healthcare system does little to address caregivers' needs and concerns: They are automatically assumed capable of performing complex medical care tasks at home, their symptom management and coping skills are seldom appraised, and their own physical health is rarely considered (Northouse et al. 2002). Moreover, in this era of high patient volume and brief patient appointments, caregivers may be acknowledged only briefly during the decision-making and discharge planning portions of patients' medical visits (Glajchen 2003).

Unmet Needs of Caregivers

Extensive research has been performed to identify the needs of caregivers, and to characterize their unmet needs. Shelby et al. (2002) reported their findings from a comprehensive literature review regarding those needs most often reported by cancer patients and their caregivers. They found that 60–90% of patients and their caregivers reported a need for assistance in at least one area. The most frequently reported needs related to personal adjustment to illness (38–70%), psychosocial support (30–60%), transportation (31–58%), financial assistance (50–52%), home care (10–42%), and medical information (3–29%). Although most of the literature has focused on adult caregivers of adult cancer patients, there is a growing body of literature on grandparents, young adults, and children as caregivers (Hunt et al. 2005; Lewis et al. 2005; Sands et al. 2005).

Caregivers of cancer patients frequently report unmet needs in physical, psychosocial, economic and instrumental, or concrete, domains. In their review, Shelby et al. (2002) found that 18–30% of patients and caregivers reported that assistance for at least one need was unmet. Findings from recent landmark studies also convey a picture of rising expectations and unmet needs for caregivers carrying out a variety of medical tasks at home (Emanuel et al. 2000; Schulz and Beach 1999; United Hospital Fund 2000). For example, Emanuel and his team interviewed terminally ill adults and their caregivers to determine how their needs for assistance were being met. Unmet needs were reported by 87% of patients, who required help with transportation (62%), homemaking services (55%), nursing care (29%), and personal care (26%). Most patients relied completely on family and friends to provide this assistance; only 15% relied on paid assistance (Emanuel et al. 2000). For caregivers of cancer patients, such care may translate into 20 or more hours of care a week, the equivalent of an unpaid part-time job (United Hospital Fund 2000).

Impact of Caregiving on Quality of Life

Caregivers of cancer patients have described the experience as impacting many domains of life, including medical, psychosocial, and economic. In general, caregiving is associated with high levels of chronic stress and emotional strain, especially in the context of an illness such as cancer. For example, caregivers of patients with cancer-related pain report even higher levels of depression, tension, and mood disturbance than caregivers of pain-free patients (Miaskowski et al. 1997). From a physical and practical perspective, caregiving has been described as relentless. While such physical impact is often obvious to the healthcare professional, the emotional toll of caregiving cannot be overlooked. In this realm, caregivers describe stress and strain that can parallel or surpass that of the patient. One prospective population-based cohort study found that caregiver strain increased mortality risk by 63% within 5 years. Specifically, after adjusting for sociodemographic factors, and underlying caregiver disease, older spousal caregivers who were providing care and experiencing caregiver strain had mortality risks that were 63% higher than noncaregiving controls (Schulz and Beach 1999).

The cancer patient's stage of illness and goals of care have been shown to impact the burden of caregiving. Caregivers of patients receiving palliative care have been shown to have significantly lower quality of life and physical health scores than caregivers of patients in active, curative treatment (Weitzner et al. 1999). The physical and emotional demands of caregiving reach their peak as the disease progresses to the terminal phase. In addition to assuming many of the patients' prior domestic responsibilities, family caregivers may have to forego social activities and work duties that result in job insecurity and isolation. Caregivers providing end-of-life care have been shown to experience increased emotional distress, regardless of the amount of care provided, when limited in their ability to participate in valued activities and interests (Cameron et al. 2002).

Not only has caregiver burden been identified as an issue during the patient's life, inefficient psychological symptom control for patients during the last months of a cancer patient's life may predispose the surviving partner to long-term psychological morbidity (Bass et al. 1991; Valdimarsdóttir et al. 2002). Bass et al. (1991) evaluated the influence of caregiving and bereavement support on adjusting to an older relative's death. They found that caregivers' perceptions of the support provided to the patient before death had a significant impact on their subsequent bereavement adjustment. In fact, the caregiver's perception of the patients' care was more important for surviving spouses' and children's adjustment than support given directly to these family members during bereavement.

The Influence of Culture and Ethnicity on Caregiving in Cancer

Studies show that Hispanic and African-American patients and caregivers underutilize community health resources, including counseling and support groups, home care, residential care, and hospice services. The reasons for this underutilization are many. One important reason is that strong ties may prevent minority caregivers from seeking help outside of the family unit (Cox and Monk 1996). In a study comparing African-American, Caucasian, and Hispanic caregivers, Guarnaccia and Parra (1996) found that 65% of Hispanic patients and 60% of African-American patients lived with the caregiver. The minority families relied more on informal caregiving from friends and relatives and had larger social support networks than the Caucasian families. However, this increased the sense of obligation to provide care for older family members which is associated with more caregiving hours, greater resignation about caregiving, higher caregiver strain, and a larger reduction in household income than that reported by Caucasian caregivers (Cox and Monk 1996; Guarnaccia and Parra 1996). A study by Covinsky et al. (2001) analyzed reports of employment loss due to caregiving. Results showed that African-American and Hispanic caregivers were more likely than Caucasian caregivers to reduce their work hours to care for the patient. In addition, minority caregivers were reluctant to use formal nursing home services for their loved one. The decision to reduce work hours rather than place their relative in a nursing home was associated with increased psychological, social, and financial burden.

Accepting the burden of caregiving may lead to depression. Caregivers who have no outside help are more depressed than those who receive help from secondary informal caregivers or formal resources. Despite reporting stress, many Hispanic and African-American caregivers do not seek outside help even when they are aware of support groups and other resources. The barrier to care may be a reluctance to share familial problems with outsiders. However, minority caregivers respond better to direct recruitment efforts through personal contacts and face-to-face interviews, strategies that are often too labor-intensive for typical caregiver programs.

Similarly, underuse of hospice services has been reported in both the African-American and Hispanic communities. For African-Americans, barriers to hospice use include lack of availability, lack of community awareness, lack of trust in social service providers, and misperceptions of the role of hospice services. Since African-Americans rely heavily on closely knit groups of friends and family, they are less inclined to welcome strangers, such as hospice workers, into their networks (Gordon 1995). In addition, a prerequisite to hospice care is the presence of a primary caregiver in the home. Since African-American family members often have to work, no one is at home to care for the patient, and the patient may thus be barred from hospice care. Members of the African-American community may also be uncomfortable with the concept of palliative care, which seems to encourage the patient to give up and stop fighting (Gordon 1995). These cross-cultural issues are important in assessing caregivers' needs and in designing clinical and educational programs to meet those needs (Glajchen 2004).

Caregiver Intervention Strategies

Despite the fact that caregiver burden and distress have been studied since the early 1980s, few documented, effective intervention strategies have been developed to support persons caring for patients with cancer. The lack of definition and standardization in type of caregiver intervention, method of service delivery, and outcome variables present major challenges in their evaluation and replication.

The overall goal of interventions delivered to caregivers should be to promote the caregiver's physical and emotional well-being so that the caregiver can more effectively attend to the needs of the patient with advanced cancer (Given et al. 2001). The goals of interventions developed for caregivers have focused on increasing knowledge through education and information; reducing anxiety and depression through counseling and psychotherapy; providing medical care and emotional comfort through palliative and hospice home care; and increasing confidence through problem-solving and skill-building.

Goals of Information or Educational Interventions

Education is an effective tool for helping cancer patients and their families understand the disease process, pain, other symptoms and treatment options (Glajchen et al. 1995). Clinicians generally agree upon the value of providing information to caregivers. Information tailored to the caregiver's situation provides them with guidance for implementing care. More importantly, adequate information may help reduce the stress of caregiving and the associated feelings of inadequacy and helplessness arising from ambiguity (Given et al. 2001). Information about the disease trajectory, the anticipated course, and the range of emotions experienced by families helps normalize the experience and enhances the sense of control so often missing in cancer.

Despite this widespread agreement, however, one of the most common frustrations cited by caregivers is the difficulty they experience in obtaining information from healthcare providers, especially physicians and nurses. The most important periods along the disease trajectory for caregivers to receive information appears to be at the time of diagnosis, during the period of hospitalization, at the initiation of new treatment, at the time of recurrence, and during the end-of-life phase (McCorkle and Pasacreta 2001). However, owing to the chronic nature of cancer, and the range of tasks that need to be mastered at different points, caregivers' information needs change over time (Wong et al. 2002).

Caregivers want factual information about cancer, its treatment, related symptoms and side effects. They need specific details about what to do and how the particular cancer is likely to behave. Caregivers want to be involved in treatment planning, however, they also want to be acknowledged for their expertise, their own needs, and their hard work (United Hospital Fund 2000). Unfortunately for caregivers, studies have shown that doctor-patient communication is low in patient-caregiver centeredness, medical issues tend to dominate, and systems obstacles such as lack of time and fragmentation in care further hinder information exchange (Wong et al. 2002).

In a recent survey of the information and education needs of cancer outpatients and their caregivers, the priority areas listed were management of pain, weakness and fatigue, followed by the types of services available to facilitate patient care at home (Wong et al. 2002). In the area of pain management, caregivers need to understand pharmacologic issues and medication instructions. Specifically, caregivers have been shown to need instruction about which medications to use for pain relief, when to give the medication, how to assess the efficacy of pain control, how to monitor for side effects, and how to identify negative results or ineffectiveness (Ferrell et al. 1995).

The role of family caregivers in fostering or hindering treatment compliance should not be underestimated. Caregivers' knowledge and attitudes about such symptoms as pain and fatigue management may influence the patient. If caregivers harbor fears of addiction, overdosing, or indirectly causing discomfort through side effects, they may guard the medication supply, limit its use, and undermedicate the patient (Juarez and Ferrell 1996). Caregivers need training in the management of side effects, as these can cause patients to abandon their treatment protocols for cancer. Educating caregivers about anticipated side effects and strategies for their amelioration is, therefore, essential.

Caregivers have been shown to benefit from education in nonpharmacologic strategies for reducing such symptoms as pain, fatigue, depression, and anxiety, including such techniques as massage, the use of heat and cold compresses, energy conservation, rest and restoration strategies, relaxation and distraction. Caregivers have responded favorably to training in the use of relaxation techniques, as such skills promote confidence and reduce helplessness. Similarly, skills in positioning with pillows, mobilizing the patient, and assisting with ambulation in an effort to promote pain relief and reduce fatigue can be taught (Ferrell et al. 1995). Caregivers report that they learn these skills through trial and error, and would like more assistance from the formal healthcare system (Given et al. 2001).

Especially important in cancer is the need to educate caregivers about alternative health practices that can exacerbate unwanted symptoms and undermine treatment effectiveness. Toxic side effects such as irreversible neuropathy, bleeding, and electrolyte imbalance can result from alternative medical approaches to cancer treatment (Montbriand 1994). Desperate families may make erroneous decisions based upon misinformation in the media and on the Internet. Caregivers must be educated on the importance of reporting all alternative health practices to a healthcare provider.

Importantly, caregivers must be educated about the support services that are available to them. Several studies have shown that patients and caregivers underutilize available resources owing to perceived lack of access, lack of information or emotional exhaustion.

Are Informational or Educational Interventions Effective?

Although several descriptive investigations have reported the value of educational programs for caregivers, a paucity of outcome data exists. In their review, Pasacreta and McCorkle (2000) identified several studies designed to evaluate the effectiveness of an educational intervention program. Two of the studies (Carmody et al. 1991; Grahn and Danielson 1996) loosely supported the usefulness of educational intervention programs for caregivers; however, each of the studies had important methodological flaws, especially in delineating outcome variables. Therefore, limited information could be gathered from these studies other than the implication that the programs were beneficial for the caregivers.

A handful of the studies reviewed by Pasacreta and McCorkle (2000) were designed to evaluate an educational intervention titled "I Can Cope," developed by Johnson et al. or some variation of this program (Johnson 1982; Diekmann 1988; Reele 1994). The "I Can Cope" program was designed to teach patients about cancer, its treatment, and physical and psychological management techniques. However, caregivers often attended the program and some variations of the program were developed specifically for them (Johnson and Norby 1981). The findings from the studies were mixed. Participants in one of the studies reported increased knowledge, reduced anxiety, and an improved sense of purpose in their lives (Johnson 1982). In another study, nonattendance was a problem, which the researchers attributed to the group format and the fear associated with cancer (Diekmann 1988). Participants in the third study reported the group experience to be a positive one, although the program did not appear to improve quality of life or coping skills (Reele 1994).

Robinson et al. (1998) developed a 6-hour psychoeducational program that focused on communication, symptom management and community resources for caregivers of cancer patients. Participants were evaluated at baseline and again eight weeks later. However, although caregivers reported feeling less overwhelmed after the series, the outcomes and specific measures were not reported by the authors, making replication impossible. In addition, recruitment difficulties further hampered program evaluation.

A successful educational intervention program reported in the literature was developed by Ferrell et al. (1995). These researchers reported on a successful educational intervention used with 50 family caregivers of elderly cancer patients. Caregivers were educated in pain assessment, pharmacologic interventions, and nonpharmacologic interventions. Caregivers participating in this program reported improved knowledge and quality of life.

Edgar et al. (2002) reported their experience of a pilot study conducted to evaluate an Internet intervention for cancer patients and their family members. Participants received a one-on-one teaching session with a medical librarian where they learned to find information specific to their needs. Follow-up interviews found that the sessions were well received and participants reported positive well-being, in large part due to the intervention. Other types of intervention are less well described in the literature. They are: coaching patients and families to ask questions; booklets, pamphlets, fact sheets, and information cards; touch screen information systems; webcasts; and computerized information systems (Wong et al. 2002).

Although many more educational programs are provided in a variety of settings across the country, it is difficult to review or compare them for several reasons. First, some of the most innovative programs are developed at the local level, in small social service agencies that lack the capability for outcome measurement or publication. Second, in the context of real practice, caregiver programs may be offered in such disparate settings as the hospital, church, area agency on aging, social service agency or cancer advocacy group, further complicating replication and comparison. Third, the lack of standardization in format and approach can leave the reader wondering about such issues as the needs assessment, if any, topic selection, peer versus professional presentation, didactic versus interactive format, and so on. Last, the field of oncology has seen a proliferation in multimedia educational and informational programs for both cancer patients and their caregivers, in such formats as videotapes, CD-ROMS and on-line programs. The lack of centralization, coupled with differences in format and content, further complicates evaluation and replication.

Goals of Counseling or Support Interventions

Several different approaches to group counseling can be identified in the literature. The most common model is called "supportive-expressive group therapy" and is characterized by mutual support, emotional expression and existential discussion (Classen et al. 2001; Kissane et al. 2004). Other approaches to group counseling include those with a cognitive behavioral approach, aimed at the acquisition of specific coping skills, and psychoeducational groups, in which the focus is on information provision. Counseling or group support intervention efforts are generally based on the assumption that caregivers will be better equipped to meet their challenges if they are given the opportunity to discuss common problems and fears with health-care professionals or others in a similar situation. Psychotherapeutic interventions are designed to reduce caregiver distress by helping caregivers adjust psychologically to the demands of caregiving (Given et al. 2001).

These interventions are typically designed to enhance morale, self-esteem, coping, and sense of control, while reducing anxiety and depression. Although providing specific information about specific aspects of patient care is frequently a component of these interventions, the focus of counseling or group support is ensuring that caregivers are equipped to meet their caregiver challenges. Caregivers with a low level of emotional support have been identified as being more depressed over time (Nijboer et al. 2001). In contrast to patient support systems, which are widely available, the sources of support for caregivers have lagged far behind those provided for patients (McCorkle and Pasacreta 2001).

Individual counseling is designed to provide caregivers with support, education and problem-solving or coping skills. However, these interventions are expensive and may prove too time-consuming for working or highly distressed caregivers (Harding and Higginson 2003).

Are Counseling or Support Interventions Effective?

Interventions designed to reduce the emotional impact of caregiving have received some attention in the literature. Interventions primarily include individual counseling and group support.

There have been few reports of the effectiveness of individual counseling in the literature. However, the data that are available suggest that individual counseling is effective in reducing caregiver burden. Emanuel et al. (1999) found that caregiver burden was significantly reduced when physicians practiced active listening. In their study, caregivers experienced less burden and distress if they felt that the treating physician listened to their needs and opinions. Toseland et al. (1990) reported that daughters and daughters-in-law who were primary caregivers of frail elderly parents had more improvement in psychological functioning and well-being with individual counseling than with group counseling. Both individual counseling and group counseling resulted in significant improvements in coping with caregiving stress. Group intervention produced greater improvements in caregivers' social supports (Toseland et al. 1990).

Goldberg and Wool (1985) reported on a support intervention for lung cancer patients and their spouses. The goals of the intervention were to provide support systems, promote emotional expression, and facilitate negotiation of the healthcare system. No difference between attendees and nonattendees was found in psychological functioning. The authors suggested that the reason for the negative findings might have been a result of the relatively positive adjustment of couples in both groups. Sabo et al. (1986) reported on a support group created for husbands of women with breast cancer. Attendance at the support group was low, only 6 of 24 husbands participated. Attendees, however, reported significantly more communication with their wives.

A more recent psychoeducational intervention for family caregivers reported mixed results. In this program, caregivers were randomized into two groups, one receiving standard care, the other receiving standard care plus the new intervention delivered through home visits, phone calls, a guidebook and an audiotape incorporating self-care strategies. Caregivers were evaluated with respect to caregiving competence, self-efficacy and anxiety. No treatment effects were reported, although caregivers in the treatment group reported a more positive caregiver experience (Hudson et al. 2005).

In summary, intervention in the support group format provides information and informal support networking for caregivers who are receptive to this type of assistance. Social support needs appear to respond best to group intervention. Some caregivers may prefer individual counseling by professionals. In addition, psychological issues may be most effectively managed with individual intervention. Therefore, the types of problems and issues specific to an individual caregiver should guide the most appropriate type of intervention.

Future research should address what factors lead caregivers to attend a support group program, and more attention should be paid to outcome measurement in caregiver support groups. Emphasis should be placed on matching the needs of caregivers to particular components of support groups. Most support groups in the United States are attended by older Caucasian women caring for spouses with cancer. Future programs should target hard-to-reach segments of the caregiver population, including men, young caregivers, and caregivers from other cultures. Lastly, individual-specific issues, such as the timing of education intervention relative to cancer diagnosis, gender, and caregiver-role, should guide future efforts in designing support interventions.

Goals of Home Hospice and Palliative Care Interventions

Hospice care involves a team-oriented approach of expert medical care, pain management, and emotional and spiritual support tailored to the patient's wishes. Emotional and spiritual support are extended to the family and generally this care is provided in the patient's home or in a home-like setting (National Hospice and Palliative Care Organization [NHPCO] 2012). Palliative care is the active total care of patients whose disease is not responsive to curative treatment. Control of pain, of other symptoms, and of psychological, social and spiritual problems is paramount. The goal of palliative care is the achievement of the best possible quality of life for patients and their families (World Health Organization [WHO] 1990). Since 1990, palliative care has arisen as a new specialty in medicine, with the goal of extending the principles of hospice care to a broader population that could benefit from this type of care earlier in the disease process. The hallmarks of both hospice and palliative care are equal attention to both the physical and psychosocial aspects of care, and involvement of the patient and caregiver as the unit of care.

As a life-threatening disease approaches the end stage, the needs of both the patient and caregiver increase. As a patient becomes more debilitated, the demands for nursing care, social support, financial resources, and spiritual care increase considerably. Extensive research has shown that caregivers providing palliative care are at risk for developing a variety of psychological and physical problems, including anxiety, depression, fatigue, reduced self-esteem, and somatic health problems (Chentsova-Dutton et al. 2000; Haley et al. 2001; Kinsella et al. 2000). Hudson et al. (2002) conducted focus groups with current lay caregivers, bereaved lay caregivers, and palliative care nurses. Participants reported that caregivers were frequently unprepared for their role and desired more guidance and support from healthcare professionals. Steele and Fitch (1996a) found that caregivers of palliative care patients required time for themselves away from the home and time for their own personal needs. In addition, caregivers reported insufficient time to rest and did not experience adequate sleep. Caregivers needed to learn ways to help patients maintain some independence. Caregivers of home hospice cancer patients have reported that effective coping strategies include learning more about the problem, keeping busy, thinking positively, and talking about the problem with family and friends (Steele and Fitch 1996b). To address caregivers' expressed needs for respite and personal time, the use of volunteers and short-term admission to inpatient facilities have been tried.

Are Home Hospice Care Interventions Effective?

Several studies suggest that participation in a hospice program is beneficial for both patients and caregivers. Jepson et al. (1999) examined changes in the psychosocial status of caregivers of cancer patients. They were particularly interested in whether the caregivers' own physical problems and the patient's participation in a home care intervention influenced caregivers' psychosocial adjustment. Patients were randomly assigned to a control group or to an intervention group in which they received a Standardized Nursing Intervention Protocol (SNIP) over a 4-week period. The intervention included a component through which caregivers were taught to problem solve, administer medications, and provide self-care behaviors. Overall, the psychosocial status of the caregivers in both groups improved. However, caregivers with physical problems of their own were found to be at risk for psychological morbidity.

In another study, terminally ill patients in a VA were randomly assigned to receive hospice care. Follow-up evaluation through the time of death showed that caregivers in the hospice program reported significantly less anxiety and greater satisfaction with care. These differences were attributed to the hospice staff better meeting caregivers' needs (Kane et al. 1986).

Other studies have demonstrated the positive influence of hospice home care on caregivers' quality of life and psychosocial status (McMillan and Mahon 1994); however, there is a surprising paucity of literature in this area. Most of the research in this area has focused on the impact of hospice care on the subsequent bereavement adjustment of caregivers. Levy et al. (1993) studied the effect of participation in a bereavement support group on adaptation in widows and widowers over 18 months. Both support group attendees and nonattendees had significant decreases in depression, anger, anxiety, subjective stress, and psychotropic medication use over the 18-month course. However, the number of support groups attended appeared to account for significant amounts of variance regarding these factors. The authors concluded that further research was required to determine the efficacy of support groups.

McCorkle et al. (1998) studied whether specialized oncology home care services provided to patients with lung cancer influenced bereavement and psychological distress among survivors. Participants were randomized to an oncology home care group, a standard home care group, or an office care control group. Spouses of patients in the oncology home care group had significantly lower psychological distress than spouses in either of the other groups. These findings have been corroborated by others.

Numerous studies have found that involvement in a hospice home care program did not influence caregiver burden or adjustment (Haley et al. 2001; Kane et al. 1986; McMillan and Mahon 1994, McMillan 1996; Meyers and Gray 2001). The lack of benefit was attributed to the strong correlation between quality of life scores for patients and their caregivers. That is, although hospice home care is thought to ameliorate some caregiver burden, the negative psychological and physical health experienced by patients at the end of life is reflected in reported caregiver burden.

Goals of Problem-Solving and Skill-Building Interventions

Throughout the caregiving process, caregivers are required to take on a variety of new and complex roles. Yet family members assuming the care of a patient with serious illness frequently lack the requisite resources or skills to undertake this role. Some caregivers may have difficulty accessing the healthcare system and utilizing support services effectively; others have difficulty making decisions and solving problems; and still others have difficulty coordinating the tasks of healthcare professionals and other family caregivers.

Schumacher et al. (2000) identified nine core caregiving processes: (1) monitoring (ensuring that changes in the patient's condition were noted), (2) interpreting (making sense of what was observed), (3) making decisions (choosing a course of action), (4) taking action (carrying out decisions and instructions), (5) providing hands-on care (carrying out nursing and medical procedures), (6) making adjustments (progressively refining caregiver actions), (7) accessing resources (obtaining what is needed), (8) working together with the patient (sharing illness-related care in a way that was sensitive to the personhood of both patient and caregiver), and (9) negotiating the healthcare system (ensuring patients needs were adequately met). Mastery of each of these caregiving processes and skills can be daunting indeed for family caregivers.

Houts et al. (1996) have developed the most widely recognized and well-studied educational model for caregiver related problem-solving and skill-building. The program, summarized by the acronym COPE (Creativity, Optimism, Planning, and Expert Information), was designed to help uninformed family caregivers assume caregiving responsibilities. The program was based on extensive research on problem-solving training and therapy. The goal of the model is to maximize the caregivers' effectiveness, sense of efficacy and satisfaction. The "Creativity" component of the program teaches caregivers to develop creative solutions to challenging situations where creativity is essential. The "Optimism" component addresses the emotional aspect of problem-solving, and combines optimism with realism, recognizing both the seriousness of the problem and the expectation that something can be done to improve the problem. The "Planning" aspect of the program addresses both problem-solving effectiveness and emotional distress, and helps caregivers develop plans to meet their individual situations. The "Expert Information" component of the program teaches caregivers what they need to do and the rationale for what they do. Houts et al. (1996) contend that their model empowers caregivers and patients for coping with illness and can help moderate caregiver stress.

Are Problem-Solving or Skill-Building Interventions Effective?

Blanchard et al. (1996) tested the effectiveness of a 6-session problem-solving intervention with spouses of cancer patients who had been diagnosed more than 3 months prior and who were not eligible for hospice care. In a randomized trial, the study compared caregivers involved in the intervention with caregivers who received usual care. A problem-solving intervention was used to help spouses solve individually identified problems. At 6 months, spouses who received the intervention were less depressed, however, there were no other effects on coping, social support, or psychological well-being. This study is significant in that the researchers studied patient-caregiver distress after a diagnosis of cancer, however, before terminal illness. In another study, 237 cancer patient/caregiver dyads were randomized into two groups, one for conventional care, and the other, a 20-week experimental group. The focus of the intervention was improvement in caregivers' symptom management ability, and reduction in their distress. However, the nursing intervention was not found to be effective in decreasing caregiver depression (Kurtz et al. 2005).

The majority of problem-solving or skill-building interventions are contained an informational or support component of the program, and are described in the next section.

Are Interventions that Incorporate Multiple Components Effective?

Several comprehensive caregiver interventions have been developed that constitute more than one type of intervention.

Heinrich and Schag (1985) developed an educational and problem-solving intervention called the Stress and Activity Management (SAM) program. This study used a randomized design where participants were assigned to a treatment group or control group. The intervention was designed to educate cancer patients and their spouses about cancer and its impact, to teach specific skills for managing stress and daily problems, and to promote problem-solving. Participants in both the control and treatment groups improved in psychological adjustment, depression, and anxiety over time; however, this was attributed to the passage of time rather than the program. The program, however, did increase participant's knowledge about cancer and coping. Caregivers in the treatment group were more satisfied with the education and support they received than caregivers in the control group.

Kaasalainen et al. (2000) designed a quasi experimental study to evaluate Caring for Aging Relatives Group (CARG), a program that provides information and support to female caregivers. Though not specifically designed to evaluate the role of an intervention in caregivers of cancer patients, results from this study are included because it provides noteworthy information in several respects. The program was a well-described, replicable intervention with a clear delineation of outcome variables. The group that received the intervention was compared with a matched comparison group regarding morale, social support, and information. The educational component of the program included providing information on the aging process, communication and problem-solving skills, stress management techniques, community resources, and issues related to relocation of the elderly. Social support was provided through leaders and other group members by encouraging caregivers to express their feelings, share experiences, and assert more control in their own situations. Results of this study were partially supportive of the usefulness of a caregiver support program. Information was gained and caregivers perceived the support program as helpful; however, morale, which was high at pretest, was maintained, but not improved, at the conclusion of the program.

Pasacreta et al. (2000) reported favorable results based on an evaluation of participant characteristics before and 4 months after attendance at a Family Caregiver Cancer Education Program (FCCEP). One component of the program focused on providing information on the medical realities of cancer such as managing symptoms, improving technical competence, and administering medication to patients in the home. The program also contained a skill-building component to address such issues as talking to the patient's physician, managing other aspects of the healthcare system, handling role and relationship changes in the family, caring for medical equipment, managing uncomfortable symptoms, talking to the children, managing other jobs and responsibilities, handling insurance and financial issues, dealing with emotional reactions, finding and asking for help, and maintaining self-care. Caregivers were invited to participate in the program during or after transition points in the patient's disease (e.g., diagnosis, initiation or cessation of treatment, recurrence, or shift from curative to palliative treatment). The number of caregivers who said they were well-informed and confident about caregiving increased after participation in the program. In addition, although the intensity of caregivers' tasks increased throughout the program, the caregivers' perceptions of burden did not increase, and perceptions of their own health improved over time.

Recommendations for the Future

To date, although an abundance of information exists regarding the needs of caregivers, there are few documented, effective strategies to guide family members caring for patients with cancer. For example, no research has compared such interventions as education, home care, counseling and problem-solving to each other. The lack of standardization, absence of scientific rigor and obstacles to the implementation of controlled research conditions under real world "messy" circumstances makes such comparisons difficult. Experimental research has only scratched the surface by testing interventions designed to meet the needs of caregivers caring for people with cancer. Clearly, examining the efficacy and effectiveness of caregiving interventions is in its infancy and much work remains to be done. Other research methods such as the use of simple, well-designed outcomes measures and single case studies can be used to further our knowledge base where randomized controlled trials are lacking.

Increasing Use of Formal Support Services A crucial area for the future would be determining why such a small number of caregivers use formal services, and how access to services can be improved. Only 15–20% of caregivers report using formal support services. Little is known about the reasons for underutilization; however, hypothesized reasons include lack of knowledge about available services or how to access them, financial constraints, fear of the stigma of accepting help, family resistance, patient refusal, and transportation problems (Shelby et al. 2002). It was noted in several studies that recruitment and retention of caregivers in intervention programs was a challenge. A number of reasons have been cited for low participation in caregiver programs, including employment, family obligations, fear of leaving the patient alone, and physical restrictions (Pasacreta et al. 2000). To increase access to existing caregiver support programs, a number of strategies can be used. First, caregiver resources can be included as a routine part of cancer treatment. Second, needed services can be established in local communities rather than major medical centers. Third, innovative technology can be used to reach caregivers where they live and where they work.

Determining an Effective Intervention "Dose" A second area for future clinical and research programs would be determining what constitutes a therapeutic "dose" of social or instrumental support for caregivers. Desired outcomes of interventions need to be clearly articulated and the "dosage" of the intervention needed for the required effect must be established. For example, the gold standard for bereavement counseling is thought to be 13 months following the death of a loved one. Managed care insurance programs may offer time-limited counseling of 6–8 weeks duration. In order to develop effective programs that will be widely implemented, programs must be feasible and cost effective. Future programs should therefore determine whether caregivers need ongoing support, or whether services are most needed at certain transition points along the illness trajectory.

Determining Whether Caregiver Burden Can Be Predicted Determining whether caregiver burden can be predicted would be enormously helpful in designing caregiver services. Factors that predict those caregivers at highest risk for distress and noncoping need to be identified. In addition, healthcare professionals must be able to easily identify caregivers who are already experiencing high levels of caregiver burden. Several risk factors for increased caregiver burden or distress have been identified in the current literature, including caregiver illness, (McCorkle and Pasacreta 2001), female gender (Yee and Schulz 2000), and lower education level (Cameron et al. 2002). Although many screening instruments exist to assess caregiver burden and distress, they are inadequate to address the entire range of dimensions affected by caregiving responsibilities among caregivers of people with cancer. Some measures are disease specific, while others examine only limited domains of caregivers' experiences. A simple way to screen caregivers for high levels of distress, stemming from depression, social isolation, physical burden, and financial strain is needed. Ideally, the tools used to screen and assess caregiver burden should be short, easy to administer, incorporate both positive and negative aspects of caregiving, and both objective and subjective burden.

Customizing Programs to Meet the Needs of Caregivers Future clinical programs must address how caregiver services can be customized to meet the needs of caregivers, rather than the needs of those for whom they care. Consideration of caregiver characteristics is a critical element in the caregiver intervention equation. Without a clear understanding of individual caregivers and their unique personal and psychological needs, interventions will be designed for the average caregiver, and will produce only average results. Interventions should be customized by gender, age, and relationship to the patient. All caregivers are not alike. For example, much of the current literature on caregiving assumes that caregivers are older than the age of 65, however, these demographics are changing. Similarly, men are notoriously reluctant to attend support groups, however, they have demonstrated the willingness to participate in programs involving the telephone, computer, or videotapes.

Developing Programs that Work Across Cultural and Ethnic Groups Ethnicity as a predictor of outcome in caregiving has been noted in the literature. Few interventions tested to date, however, have evaluated the cultural and ethnic responses to interventions. A family's social and ethnic background might influence perceptions of healthcare issues, including access to care issues and roles in caring for the patient. A comprehensive literature review of the racial, ethnic, and cultural differences in the dementia caregiving experience found that there may be differences in the stress, psychological outcomes, and variables related to service utilization among caregivers of different racial, ethnic, and cultural groups, though the reasons for the differences were unclear (Janevic and Connell 2001). Whether the same forms of education, training, and support work across cultural and ethnic groups for caregivers of cancer patients remains to be determined.

Current and Future Challenges

Public Policy Perspectives

Most family caregiving in the United States is provided in the private realm of family relationships and sense of duty. As such, public policy depends on unpaid family caregivers "doing whatever needs to be done" (Levine 2004). Only recently has federal policy recognized the service needs of family caregivers themselves (Feinberg and Newman 2004). Although this legislation is not specifically designed for caregivers of people with cancer, this subgroup of caregivers could be eligible for services in some states.

Passage of the National Family Caregiver Support Program (NFCSP) under the Older Americans Act (OAA) Amendments of 2000 marks the first federally-funded state level program to support the service needs of caregivers of older persons with illness or disability. Under these programs, local areas on aging are funded to develop support systems covering information about services; referral for services; counseling, support groups, and training for caregivers; respite care; and supplemental services, such as home care.

A recent study profiled the experience of all 50 states and the District of Columbia since the passage of the NFCSP. The report shows that only one in three states has begun providing support to caregivers of older people as a result of federal funds provided through the NFCSP. Second, less than half of the programs in this study uniformly assess caregiver needs. Rather, services are designed based on the needs of the ill or disabled person. Third, the study found wide variation in program design and interpretation among the states, leading to a lack of consistency in the services provided. Fourth, respite was the service strategy most commonly offered to caregivers. The top barriers to coordinating caregiver support programs with other programs in the states are differing eligibility requirements and service complexity and fragmentation. This leads to unevenness in services and service options for family caregivers. The major lesson learned by the states in providing family caregiver support is that "one size does not fit all"—so programs should increase the choices that families have so they can tailor available benefits to meet their specific needs (Feinberg and Newman 2004). Although this legislation was not specifically designed for families of cancer patients, some caregivers might be eligible for services if their loved ones are deemed to be eligible, i.e., older and with an illness or disability.

Another piece of legislation that affects family caregivers is the Family and Medical Leave Act of 1993 (FMLA). The FMLA allows leave for employees and their family members for serious medical conditions, while maintaining their employment status. However, the FMLA provides no services or resources for caregivers, and caregivers are not paid by their employers during the leave.

How Can Information Be Disseminated from Centers of Excellence into the Community?

Most of the published, controlled studies of caregiver interventions have taken place in university settings or centers of excellence and are likely to be considerably more intensive and expensive than caregiver support groups that are available in the community. Participation in these programs may be limited by geographical location, inconvenience, and lack of transportation. Innovative programs have designed models of collaboration, using the resources of the university settings in combination with the local expertise of community centers, senior centers, and social service agencies. This approach should be considered by funders, policy makers, and program planners.

How Can We Measure On-Line Forms of Education, Counseling and Skill-Building?

Increasingly, patients, and families are turning to the Internet to gather information on medical issues, communicate with others in similar situations, and identify resources.

Touchscreen interactive information systems, live webcasts, on-line support groups, telephone interventions, and other innovations provide convenience, confidentiality, and real-time assistance to caregivers who cannot leave their homes. Recognizing this growing trend, valid measurements to evaluate the effectiveness of these programs should be developed.

How Can We Replicate Skill-Building Programs?

In order to replicate meaningful interventions to help caregivers cope with the stress of the caregiving experience, programs must be described thoroughly. Too often, the specific content and procedural details of interventions are described in minimal detail, making it difficult to understand what was done. In addition, such programs must be made more accessible to all caregivers by increasing their cultural sensitivity, providing them free of charge, and making them available outside of work to accommodate working caregivers.

> If the major unmet needs for cancer patients and caregivers are concrete in nature (transportation = 62%, home care = 55%, financial help = 52%), why are there so few programs to address these needs?

Despite the substantial proportion of patients reporting the need for help with practical needs, few organizations currently provide this type of assistance (Shelby et al. 2002). As the use of home care for cancer patients increases, a greater demand for practical assistance will occur. Research should be conducted to demonstrate that investing the time and resources to assist families with these needs will lead to demonstrably better patient and caregiver outcomes at lower costs overall.

Conclusions

In conclusion, designing and testing caregiver interventions is a daunting task and abounds with challenges. Over the past 20 years, we have gained a solid foundation for developing effective programs as several studies have identified the needs of caregivers of patients with cancer. Less is known, however, about the effectiveness of caregiver intervention programs aimed at addressing caregivers' needs. It is time for the research focus to evolve from providing descriptions of clinical supportive efforts to providing more scientific evaluations of controlled intervention studies. To that end, it is safe to conclude that we have come a long way, and have a long way to go.

References

Agency for Health Care Policy and Research (AHCPR). (1994). *Management of cancer pain: Clinical practice guideline* (AHCPR Publication No. 94-0592). Rockville: U.S. Department of Health and Human Services.

Bass, D. M., Bowman, K., & Noelker, L. S. (1991). The influence of caregiving and bereavement support on adjusting to an older relative's death. *Gerontologist, 31*(1), 32–42.

Blanchard, C. G., Toseland, R. W., & McCallion, P. (1996). The effects of a problem-solving intervention with spouses of cancer patients. *Journal of Psychosocial Oncology, 14*(2), 1–21.

Cameron, J. I., Franche, R., Cheung, A. M., & Stewart, D. E. (2002). Lifestyle interference and emotional distress in family caregivers of advanced cancer patients. *Cancer, 94*, 521–527.

Carmody, S., Hickey, P., & Bookbinder, M. (1991). Perioperative needs of families: Results of a survey. *AORN Journal, 54*(3), 561–567.

Chentsova-Dutton, Y., Shuchter, S., Hutchin, S., Strause, L., Burns, K., & Zisook, S. (2000). The psychological and physical health of hospice caregivers. *Annals of Clinical Psychiatry, 12*(1), 19–27.

Classen, C., Butler, L. D., Koopman, C., Miller, E., DiMiceli, S., Giese-Davis, J., et al. (2001). Supportive-expressive group therapy and distress in patients with metastatic breast cancer: A randomized clinical intervention trial. *Archives of General Psychiatry, 58*(5), 494–501.

Covinsky, K. E., Eng, C., Lui, L., Sands, L. P., Sehgal, A. R., Walter, L. C., et al. (2001). Reduced employment in caregivers of frail elders: Impact of ethnicity, patient clinical characteristics, and caregiver characteristics. *Journal of Gerontology, 56*, M707–M713.

Cox, C., & Monk, A. (1996). Strain among caregivers: Comparing the experiences of African American and Hispanic caregivers of Alzheimer's relatives. *International Journal of Aging and Human Development, 43*, 93–105.

Diekmann, J. M. (1988). An evaluation of selected "I Can Cope" programs by registered participants. *Cancer Nursing, 11*(5), 274–282.

Edgar, L., Greenberg, A., & Remmer, J. (2002). Providing internet lessons to oncology patients and family members: A shared project. *Psycho-Oncology, 11*(5), 439–446.

Emanuel, E. J., Fairclough, D. L., Slutsman, J., Alpert, H., & Emanuel, L. L. (1999). Assistance from family members, friends, paid care givers, and volunteers in the care of terminally ill patients. *New England Journal of Medicine, 341*, 956–963.

Emanuel, E. J., Fairclough, D. L., Slutsman, J., & Emanuel, L. L. (2000). Understanding economic and other burdens of terminal illness: The experience of patients and their caregivers. *Annals of Internal Medicine, 132*, 451–459.

Family Caregiver Alliance. (2011). *Selected caregiver statistics.* San Francisco: Family Caregiver Alliance. Retrieved from http://www.caregiver.org/caregiver/jsp/content_node.jsp?nodeid=439.

Family Caregiver Alliance. (n.d.). *2006–2007 policy statement.* Retrieved from http://www.caregiver.org/caregiver/jsp/content_node.jsp?nodeid=882.

Feinberg, L. F., & Newman, S. L. (2004). A study of 10 states since passage of the National Family Caregiver Support Program: Policies, perceptions and program development. *Gerontologist, 44*(60), 760–769.

Ferrell, B. R., Grant, M., Chan, J., Ahn, C., & Ferrell, B. A. (1995). The impact of cancer pain education on family caregivers of elderly patients. *Oncology Nursing Forum, 22*(8), 1211–1218.

Given, B. A., Given, C. W., & Kozachik, S. (2001). Family support in advanced cancer. *CA: A Cancer Journal for Clinicians, 51*(4), 213–231.

Glajchen, M. (2003). Caregiver burden and pain control. In R. Portenoy & E. Bruera (Eds.), *Cancer pain* (pp. 467–474). New York: Cambridge University Press.

Glajchen, M. (2004). Emerging role of caregivers in cancer care. *Journal of Supportive Oncology, 2*, 145–155.

Glajchen, M., Blum, D., & Calder, K. (1995). Cancer pain management and the role of social work: Barriers and interventions. *Health and Social Work, 20*(3), 200–206.

Goldberg, R. J., & Wool, R. S. (1985). Psychotherapy for the spouses of lung cancer patients: Assessment of an intervention. *Psychotherapy Psychosomatic, 43*, 141–150.

Gordon, A. K. (1995). Deterrents to access and service for Blacks and Hispanics: The Medicare hospice benefit, healthcare utilization, and cultural barriers. In D. L. Infeld, A. K. Gordon, & B. C. Harper (Eds.), *Hospice care and cultural diversity* (pp. 65–83). Binghamton: Haworth Press.

Grahn, G., & Danielson, M. (1996). Coping with the cancer experience. II. Evaluating an education and support programme for cancer patients and their significant others. *European Journal of Cancer Care, 5*(3), 182–187.

Guarnaccia, P. J., & Parra, P. (1996). Ethnicity, social status, and families' experiences of caring for a mentally ill family member. *Community Mental Health Journal, 32*, 243–260.

Haley, W. E., LaMonde, L. A., Han, B., Narramore, S., & Schonwetter, R. (2001). Family caregiving in hospice: Effects on psychological and health functioning among spousal caregivers of hospice patients with lung cancer or dementia. *Hospice Journal, 15*(4), 1–18.

Harding, R., & Higginson, I. J. (2003). What is the best way to help caregivers in cancer and palliative care? A systematic review of interventions and their effectiveness. *Palliative Medicine, 17*, 63–74.

Heinrich, R. L., & Schag, C. C. (1985). Stress activity management: Group treatment for cancer patients and spouses. *Journal of Consulting and Clinical Psychology, 43*, 439–446.

Hickock, J. T., Morrow, G. R., Roscoe, J. A., Mustian, K., & Okunieff, P. (2005). Occurrence, severity, and longitudinal course of twelve common symptoms in 1,129 consecutive patients during radiotherapy for cancer. *Journal of Pain Symptom Management, 30*(5), 433–442.

Houts, P. S., Nezu, A. M., Nezu, C. M., & Bucher, J. A. (1996). The prepared family caregiver: A problem-solving approach to family caregiver education. *Patient Education and Counseling, 27*(1), 63–73.

Hudson, P. L., Aranda, S., & McMurray, N. (2002). Intervention development for enhanced lay palliative caregiver support: The use of focus groups. *European Journal of Cancer Care, 11*(4), 262–270.

Hudson, P. L., Aranda, S., Hayman-White, K. (2005). A psycho-educational intervention for family caregivers of patients recieving palliative care; a randomized controlled trial. *Journal of Pain and Symptom Management 30*(4), 329–341.

Hunt, G., Levine, C., & Naiditch, L. (2005). *Young caregivers in the U.S.: Report of findings*. Bethesda: National Alliance for Caregiving.

Janevic, M. R., & Connell, C. M. (2001). Racial, ethnic, and cultural differences in the dementia caregiving experience: Recent findings. *Gerontologist, 41*(3), 334–347.

Jepson, C., McCorkle, R., Adler, D., Nuamah, I., & Lusk, E. (1999). Effects of home care on caregivers' psychosocial status. *Image: Journal of Nursing Scholarship, 31*, 115–120.

Johnson, J. (1982). The effects of a patient education course on persons with a chronic illness. *Cancer Nursing, 5*(2), 117–123.

Johnson, J. L., & Norby, P. A. (1981). We can weekend: A program for cancer families. *Cancer Nursing, 4*(1), 23–28.

Juarez, G., & Ferrell, B. R. (1996). Family and caregiver involvement in pain management. *Clinics in Geriatric Medicine, 12*, 531–547.

Kaasalainen, S., Craig, D., & Wells, D. (2000). Impact of the caring for aging relatives group program: An evaluation. *Public Health Nursing, 17*(3), 169–177.

Kane, R. L., Klein, S. J., Bernstein, L., Rothenberg, R. (1986). The role of hospice in reducing the impact of bereavement. *Journal of Chronic Disease, 39*(9), 735–742.

Kinsella, G., Cooper, B., Picton, C., & Murtagh, D. (2000). Factors influencing outcomes for family caregivers of persons receiving palliative care: Toward an integrated model. *Journal of Palliative Care, 16*(3), 46–54.

Kissane, D. W., Grabsch, B., Clarke, D. M., Christie, G., Clifton, D., Gold, S., et al. (2004). Supportive-expressive group therapy: The transformation of existential ambivalence into creative living while enhancing adherence to anti-cancer therapies. *Psycho-Oncology, 13*(11), 755–768.

Kozachik, S. L., Given, C. W., Given, B. A., Pierce, S. J., Azzouz, F., Rawl, S. M., et al. (2001). Improving depressive symptoms among caregivers of patients with cancer: Results of a randomized clinical trial. *Oncology Nursing Forum, 28*(7), 1149–1157.

Kurtz, M. E., Kurtz, J. C., Given, C. W., & Given, B. (2005). A randomized controlled trial of a patient/caregiver symptom control intervention: Effects on depressive symptomatology of caregivers of cancer patients. *Journal of Pain and Symptom Management, 20*(2), 112–122.

Levine, C. (2004). *Family caregivers on the job: Moving beyond ADLs and IADLs*. New York: United Hospital Fund.

Levy, L. H., Derby, J. F., & Martinkowski, K. S. (1993). Effects of membership in bereavement support groups on adaptation to conjugal bereavement. *American Journal of Community Psychology, 21*, 361–381.

Lewis, F. M., Casey, S. M., Brandt, P. A., Shands, M. E., & Zahlis, E. H. (2005, October 10). The enhancing connections program: Pilot study of a cognitive-behavioral intervention for mothers and children affected by breast cancer. *Psycho-oncology, 14*, 1–12.

McCorkle, R., & Pasacreta, J. V. (2001). Enhancing caregiver outcomes in palliative care. *Cancer Control, 8*(1), 36–45.

McCorkle, R., Robinson, L., Nuamah, I., Lev, E., & Benoliel, J. Q. (1998). The effects of home nursing care for patients during terminal illness on the bereaved's psychological distress. *Nursing Research, 47*, 2–10.

McMillan, S. C. (1996). Quality of life of primary caregivers of hospice patients with cancer. *Cancer Practice, 4*(4), 191–198.

McMillan, S. C., & Mahon, M. (1994). The impact of hospice services on the quality of life of primary caregivers. *Oncology Nursing Forum, 21*(7), 1189–1195.

Meyers, J. L., & Gray, L. N. (2001). The relationships between family primary caregiver characteristics and satisfaction with hospice care, quality of life, and burden. *Oncology Nursing Forum, 28*(1), 73–82.

Miaskowski, C., Kragness, L., Dibble, S., & Wallhagen, M. (1997). Differences in mood states, health status and caregiver strain between family caregivers of oncology patients with and without cancer-related pain. *Journal of Pain and Symptom Management, 13*, 138–147.

Montbriand, M. J. (1994). An overview of alternative therapies chosen by patients with cancer. *Oncology Nursing Forum, 21*, 1547–1554.

National Cancer Institute. (2010). *Cancer trends progress report: 2009–2010 update*. Bethesda: National Cancer Institute, National Institutes of Health, Department of Health and Human Services. Retrieved from http://progressreport.cancer.gov.

National Hospice and Palliative Care Organization (NHPCO). (2012). *Caring connections: Caregiving*. Washington: National Hospice and Palliative Care Organization. Retrieved from http://www.caringinfo.org/i4a/pages/index.cfm?pageid=3279.

Nijboer, C., Tempelaar, R., Triemstra, M., van den Bos, G. A. M., & Sanderman, R. (2001). The role of social and psychologic resources in caregiving of cancer patients. *Cancer, 91*, 1029–1039.

Northouse, L. L., Walker, J., Schafenacker, A., Mood, D., Mellon, S., Galvin, E., et al. (2002). A family-based program of care for women with recurrent breast cancer and their family members. *Oncology Nursing Forum, 29*(10), 1411–1419.

Pasacreta, J. V., & McCorkle, R. (2000). Cancer care: Impact of interventions on caregiver outcomes. *Annual Review of Nursing Research, 18*, 127–148.

Pasacreta, J. V., Barg, F., Nuamah, I., & McCorkle, R. (2000). Participant characteristics before and 4 months after attendance at a family caregiver cancer education program. *Cancer Nursing, 23*(4), 295–303.

Reele, B. L. (1994). Effect of counseling on quality of life for individuals with cancer and their families. *Cancer Nursing, 17*(2), 101–112.

Robinson, K. D., Angeletti, K. A., Barg, F. K., Pasacreta, J. V., McCorkle, R., & Yasko, J. M. (1998). The development of a family caregiver cancer education program. *Journal of Cancer Education, 13*(2), 116–121.

Sabo, D., Brown, J., & Smith, C. (1986). The male role and mastectomy: Support groups and men's adjustment. *Journal of Psychosocial Oncology, 4*, 19–31.

Sands, R. G., Goldberg-Glen, R., & Thornton, P. L. (2005). Factors associated with the positive well-being of grandparents caring for their grandchildren. *Gerontology Social Work, 45*(4), 65–82.

Schulz, R., & Beach, S. R. (1999). Caregiving as a risk factor for mortality: The caregiver health effects study. *Journal of the American Medical Association, 282*, 2215–2219.

Schumacher, K. L., Stewart, B. J., Archbold, P. G., Dodd, M. J., & Dibble, S. L. (2000). Family caregiving skill: Development of the concept. *Research in Nursing & Health, 23*, 191–203.

Shelby, R. A., Taylor, K. L., Kerner, J. F., Coleman, E., & Blum, D. (2002). The role of community-based and philanthropic organizations in meeting cancer patient and caregiver needs. *CA: A Cancer Journal for Clinicians, 52*, 229–246.

Steele, R. G., & Fitch, M. I. (1996a). Needs of family caregivers of patients receiving home hospice care for cancer. *Oncology Nursing Forum, 23*(5), 823–828.

Steele, R. G., & Fitch, M. I. (1996b). Coping strategies of family caregivers of home hospice patients with cancer. *Oncology Nursing Forum, 23*(6), 955–960.

Toseland, R. W., Rossiter C. M., Peak, T., & Smith, G. C. (1990). Comparative effectiveness of individual and group interventions to support family caregivers. *Social Work, 35*(3), 209–217.

United Hospital Fund. (2000). A survey of family caregivers in New York City: Findings and implications for the health care system. New York: United Hospital Fund.

Vachon, M. L. S. (1998). Psychosocial needs of patients and families. *Journal of Palliative Care, 14*(3), 49–56.

Valdimarsdóttir, U., Helgason, Á. R., Fürst, C. J., Adolfsoon, J., & Steineck, G. (2002). The unrecognised cost of cancer patients' unrelieved symptoms: A nationwide follow-up of their surviving partners. *British Journal of Cancer, 86,* 1540–1545.

Warner, J. E. (1992). Involvement of families in pain control of terminally ill patients. *Hospice Journal, 8*(1–2), 155–170.

Weitzner, M. A., McMillan, S., & Jacobsen, P. B. (1999). Family caregiver quality of life: Differences between curative and palliative cancer treatment settings. *Journal of Pain and Symptom Management, 17,* 418–428.

Wong, R. K. S., Franssen, E., Szumacher, E., Connolly, R., Evans, M., Page, B., et al. (2002). What do patients living with advanced cancer and their carers want to know? A needs assessment. *Supportive Care in Cancer, 10,* 408–415.

World Health Organization (WHO). (1990). *Cancer pain and palliative care* (Technical Report Series 804). Geneva: World Health Organization.

Yee, J. L., & Schulz, R. (2000). Gender differences in psychiatric morbidity among family caregivers: A review and analysis. *Gerontologist, 40*(2), 147–164.

Chapter 6
What Professionals in Healthcare Can Do: Family Caregivers as Members of the Treatment Team

Walter F. Baile, Phyddy Tacchi and Joann Aaron

Changes in healthcare delivery in the United States have left their mark on oncology services, the most significant being the shift in patient care from inpatient to outpatient and ambulatory settings. As a result, the family and other caregivers must now assume an expanded role in providing assistance for cancer patients especially at home (Given et al. 2001; Glajhen 2004; Northouse and Northouse 1987).

Evidence suggests that altered family roles and the burden placed on family caregivers could negatively affect the quality of life of the patients with cancer and their caregivers, particularly during advanced stages of the disease (Grunfeld et al. 2004; Pasacreta et al. 2000). Professional care providers of patients with cancer are increasingly challenged to respond by evaluating the patient's support system, and assuming the role of consultant, manager, or even counselor for families, while guiding the patient and caregiver through treatment (Northouse 2005).

Promoting Family Involvement and Functioning: Essential Concepts

The Family as a Resource

Cancer is not only a physical illness, its effect on the dynamics of family functioning is considerable (Isaksen et al. 2003). The family must not only process the sudden

W. F. Baile (✉)
Department of Behavioral Science, M.D. Anderson Cancer Center,
The University of Texas, 1515 Holocombe Blvd, Houston, TX 77030-1402, USA
e-mail: wbaile@mdanderson.org

P. Tacchi
Department of Psychiatry, M.D. Anderson Cancer Center,
The University of Texas, 1515 Holocombe Blvd, Houston, TX 77030, USA

J. Aaron
Department of Community Oncology, M.D. Anderson Cancer Center,
The University of Texas, 1515 Holocombe Blvd, Houston, TX 77030, USA

R. C. Talley et al. (eds.), *Cancer Caregiving in the United States,*
Caregiving: Research, Practice, Policy,
DOI 10.1007/978-1-4614-3154-1_6, © Springer Science+Business Media, LLC 2012

impact of the cancer diagnosis but make an ongoing adjustment to the slow-motion movement of the treatment process (Gray-Price and Szczesny 1985) which for some cancers now are likely to last for years (Tummala and Maguire 2005). Also, the declining death rates for cancer suggest that it will be useful in the future to view cancer as a chronic illness rather than as an acute one (Edwards et al. 2005; Jacobs (Chap. 8)). Speice et al. (2000) delineated how the family can be an invaluable resource for the cancer patient and treatment team. Family members can function as an extra set of ears for patients who often find it difficult to recall information and store details when they are trying to deal with the impact of the cancer diagnosis and treatment. Family members through their presence, concrete assistance and listening and empathic connection can serve as sources of emotional support for the patient so that cancer becomes a "we" experience. Family members are also resources for patients when critical decisions about treatment have to be made and some cultures rely in a model of family "shared decision-making" to make choices about treatments (Blackhall et al. 1995).

Since the late 1970s, the family along with the patient has been considered as "a unit of treatment." This means that promoting optimal care of patients requires that the needs of family members also be identified and addressed (Speice et al. 2000; Quinn and Herndon 1986). However, as Pasacreta et al. (2000) conclude from their study of perceived needs of 83 family caregivers, family members may feel inadequately prepared to provide care for their sick relatives in the home because of a number of informational and skill deficits (Pasacreta et al. 2000).

Improved cancer care that embraces family members as caregivers rests upon the treatment team understanding the resources that the family brings, empowering the family to be part of the treatment team and conveying information. Fitch (2000) notes that addressing the concerns of the caregiver and supporting the family through the crisis of cancer necessitates the use of good communication and interpersonal skills (Baile and Aaron 2005). Training in this area has generally not been included as part of the curriculum in medical school or postgraduate medical programs. On the other hand, poor communication between the treatment team, patient, and family has been shown to cause significant distress in cancer patients and their families (Thomas and Morris 2002).

It is important to recognize the stresses on the family. First the financial impact of cancer is far reaching and includes costs beyond what many medical insurance plans cover (Brown et al. 2001). This is especially true today when many employers are restricting health insurance coverage or are mandating employees to pay for the increased costs of health care. Unemployed people under the age of 65, including children, often have no access to health insurance and this is becoming an increasing national crisis[1]. Studies report that financial concerns are often the greatest burdens faced by cancer caregivers (Brown et al. 2001; Siegel et al. 1991; Yun et al. 2005).

As new, expensive cancer treatments allow patients with complex medical problems to live longer, financial concerns expand exponentially to meet health needs

---

[1] Even programs that do exist are undersubscribed. For example, in many states of the United States, the Children's Health Insurance Program (CHIP) provides health insurance for children at an affordable cost and yet there is limited enrollment these health plans.

for medication, medical equipment, and extraneous necessities such as transportation, child care, home care services, extra or specific foods, and lost income and wages (Hampton 2005; Shelby et al. 2002). Other stresses include demands such as maintaining employment outside the home and competing family roles. Together, accumulated stressors complicate and compromise the emotional and physical health status of family caregivers. Family members are frequently concerned about their abilities to balance the demands of care with other ongoing responsibilities and worry what the immediate and long-term effects of dealing with cancer will be on their future (Given et al. 2001). The increased responsibilities of the family in providing short and long-term cancer care with limited support and insufficient medical training and the impact on the patient and family are critical challenges for clinicians (Pasacreta et al. 2000; Lewis et al. 1989) and for social policy makers.

The Cancer Crisis and Family Structure

Despite treatment advances in the field of oncology, a diagnosis of cancer continues to be perceived by many as an announcement of impending death, and one that unconsciously signifies the mortality of the family unit. This perception can lead to a state of acute crisis. Reviewing the literature, Mishel et al. (1984) found that a cancer diagnosis produces a more alarming response than the diagnosis of other diseases. Cancer creates anxiety, disequilibrium, and uncertainty leading to crisis. It can disorganize social processes, daily functioning, and mental stability, producing an adverse effect on the quality of life (Mills and Sullivan 1999). Few words can evoke such an immediate, life-threatening reaction as the word "cancer." A serious illness can also lead to a crisis by heightening anxiety and the couple's use of misinterpreted interchanges, or by weakening restraints such as established routines, role identities, or physical reserve. In the face of such a crisis, social and psychological interventions can positively affect the quality of life of the patients with cancer and their families (McMillan et al. 2006), and have even been thought to influence immune function (Adler 2002).

Addressing Crises

An important goal of intervention can be to help the family maintain an equilibrium, which takes into account the reality of the illness. When facing a stressful event such as cancer that disrupts its homeostatic steady state restoring balance to a family can minimize the emotional impact. As early as 1888, Henri-Lewis Le Chatelier, a French industrial chemist, made observations on the nature of systems in equilibrium, which may be applied to the relational balance in a family. He wrote, "any change in one of the variables that determines the state of a system in equilibrium causes a shift in the position of equilibrium in a direction that tends to counteract the change in the variable under consideration" (Le Chatelier 1888, p. 786) so that the entire system

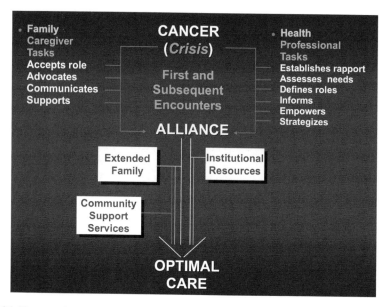

Fig. 6.1 Therapeutic alliance

needs to shift until a new equilibrium is reached. For the family disequilibrium is caused by the new energies required by the demands of cancer care. This threat can lead to anxiety and disorganization that can occur in the family until a plan is adopted to address the problem. Appropriate utilization of crisis intervention techniques by the treatment team can return the individual or family in crisis to at least the precrisis level of functioning (Gray-Price and Szczesny 1985). Four critical moments in the cancer process have been defined. These are diagnosis, end of first treatment, first recurrence, and transition to palliative care (Morris and Thomas 2001). It is at these stages that the family is likely to experience crisis and reach out for help.

The Therapeutic Alliance

Following on the discussion of crisis intervention, the healthcare team could best support the patient's caregivers if it shifts from a perspective of the traditional patient–doctor relationship, which views the role of the physician as diagnosing disease and prescribing treatment, to embrace the concept of "therapeutic alliance" , which encompasses the patient, the treatment team, and the patient's family (see Fig. 6.1). The participants in a therapeutic alliance work together as a group with a shared purpose of combining resources toward a common goal: curing the cancer and minimizing its medical and psychosocial side effects (Engel 1983; Masera et al. 1998). This therapeutic alliance functions by applying positive energies to counteract the negative forces elicited by the cancer experience. Morris and Thomas (2001) consider

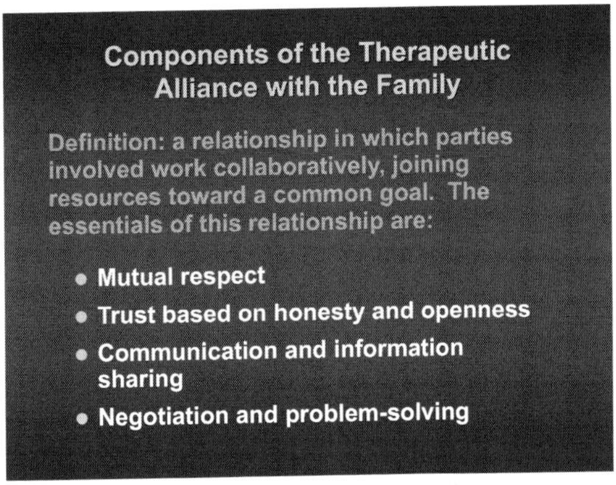

Fig. 6.2 Components of the
therapeutic alliance with the
family

**Components of the Therapeutic
Alliance with the Family**

Definition: a relationship in which parties
involved work collaboratively, joining
resources toward a common goal. The
essentials of this relationship are:

- **Mutual respect**
- **Trust based on honesty and openness**
- **Communication and information
  sharing**
- **Negotiation and problem-solving**

"carerhood" as a process, rather than a fixed state, and one in which competing needs vie for recognition. The findings of their study also suggest that carers must negotiate and make legitimate their own position as the part of this complicated process.

The International Society of Pediatric Oncology (SIOP) Psychosocial Committee has described the essential character of a therapeutic alliance between family and staff as a two-way cooperative partnership in which each party in the alliance—patient, family, healthcare staff—has particular obligations and responsibilities in the therapeutic alliance (Masera et al. 1998; see Fig. 6.2). They include:

1. *Mutual respect of the specific and different skills, experiences, and interests of the patient, family, and staff.* Mutual respect between physicians and healthcare team members and patients and caregivers and their particular value systems and skills is implicit in a therapeutic alliance. While the medical staff has expertise in the disease and its treatment, parents and family members are experts on their needs and concerns. They should describe their own role in medical care, identify important contact persons within the medical team, and elicit patient and family members concerns. Communicating the collaborative nature of the cancer treatment and encouraging family members to verbalize their concerns will signal the importance of the communication channel with the family.

2. *Communication and information sharing.* Providing information to patients and their caregivers can enhance coping (Jefford and Tattersall 2002). Information is in itself an organizing tool in that the amorphousness, the unknown, and common fears associated with a cancer diagnosis are given a voice and thus a form with known boundaries. The magnitude of free-floating emotions is compressed into words, which can limit terror and contain fantasies which may lead to helplessness and despair, impart a degree of control to the patient and family, and lessen the impact of the cancer crisis. Information about cancer treatment can provide a cognitive "road map" (Back et al. 2005), which like any map, points the way, provides signposts, and structures time and distance to travel allowing the family to anticipate resources that will be needed along the treatment trajectory.

Fig. 6.3 Five steps in establishing the therapeutic alliance

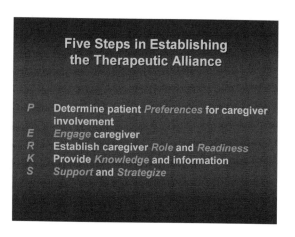

The role of family members in an alliance is also to ensure that free communication exists between family members; to seek information from the staff; to treat the staff with respect for their expertise and skills; to provide relevant information for medical and psychosocial intervention. Families as a group and the healthcare team as a group assume the mutual obligation in a therapeutic alliance to dedicate time, energy, and creativity to collaborate.

3. *Negotiation and problem solving.* Negotiation is a central skill in establishing and maintaining a therapeutic alliance. Through negotiation, collaborations are developed, conflicts are resolved, and the needs and perspectives of all the parties involved in decision-making are incorporated, although integrating the complex needs of the patient and family members with the skills and practice styles of the oncology team can be difficult at times (Speice et al. 2000). Negotiation when successful leads to increased confidence, trust, and a sense of partnership.

Establishing the Therapeutic Alliance with Caregivers—*P E R K S*

The process of establishing a therapeutic alliance is facilitated by three principles of crisis theory, which stems from observations of the behavior of individuals in crisis (Caplan 1970). It states that they are likely to: (a) reach out to others for help; (b) to accept suggestions from others to help overcome the crisis; and (c) form strong bonds with those providing assistance (see Fig. 6.3). Professional caregivers, by promoting trust, collaboration, and confidence, by providing expert advice and by reinforcing the inherent coping strengths of the patient and family are able to positively influence their coping and enhance cooperation with treatment. We propose the following strategies for establishing a therapeutic alliance in the context of cancer care. The steps are signaled by the acronym PERKS—Preferences, Engagement, Readiness for role, Knowledge and Information, and Strategy and Summary. They are outlined below.

P Determine Patient Preferences for Caregiver Involvement Many patients want the company of a close friend or family member when their diagnosis is presented. However, some patients prefer to be alone with their physician at that time. The safest path to addressing these preferences is to ask the patient beforehand who should be in attendance when the diagnosis (Sardell and Trierweiler 1993) and ensuing treatment approaches are discussed. This approach also resolves the issue of confidentiality of information. This may require a brief visit with the patient alone at the time of the office visit. An office nurse can early determine this during the time of triage by asking. . . ., "I see you came with several family members today. Whom would you like to be present when we talk about your illness and the treatment plan?"

E Engage the Caregiver Many consultations take place in environments that are not conducive to the development of a "connexial" relationship with the patient and family (Matthews et al. 1993) and are marred by disruptions from telephone calls, other healthcare professionals entering the room, and insufficient privacy (Fallowfield and Jenkins 1999; Parker et al. 2001). In a study conducted by Sardell and Trierweiler (1993), cancer patients surveyed indicated that a cancer diagnosis should be disclosed in a manner suggesting personal individuality, intimacy, and privacy. Patients want to receive a diagnosis in a face-to-face encounter. Moreover, patients want to have some prior connection with the physician who presents the diagnosis. In most cases, this refers to the primary or family physician (Parker et al. 2001; Sardell and Trierweiler 1993). Creating an hospitable environment is essential (Parker et al. 2001) and can be accomplished by choosing a suitable place with quiet and privacy for discussions and encouraging patients who wish to include family members at appointments. It is also helpful for the treatment team to inquire about family members' names and to note details about their relationship with the patient. Attentive listening to the family's concerns is a corollary that is key to providing useful assistance and engaging the caregiver(s). In addition, it is important to identify the most pressing needs, family's priorities, obstacles needing navigation, and potentially available resources. A useful approach is to offer information, providing an environment that invites questions as caregivers face new issues and are ready to absorb new information (Lunney 2000).

R Establish Caregiver Role and Readiness The caregiving role is based on the demands of the caregiving situation. These include:

Direct Care—Care carried out directly with the patient: Administration of medications; Titrating doses of medication; Observing for side effects; Observing for complications; Keeping records of symptoms and medications; Reporting untoward effects and treatment effectiveness; Determining need for Medication adjustments; Providing wound care and dressings; Bathing; Dressing; Assistance with mobility, transportation, child care; Emotional support.

Indirect Care—Care carried out on behalf of the patient: Obtaining medications; Scheduling appointments and coordinating care; Assistance with medical bills and general finances; Observing for side effects; Supervising care; Standing by (Vigilance).

Important information to establish for the caregiver role and readiness for that role is—knowledge about the disease and treatment as well as symptom management;

expected treatment trajectory; financial management; challenges such as dealing with patient mobility (Given et al. 2001). Indirect care: Providing support to the patient through listening, validating emotions, providing suggestions, and relating to the patient with positive regard.

It is impractical to expect that caregivers will have a total picture of what may be required of them and unrealistic to expect that families can meet all caregiver obligations. Hopefully, however, many will have been in a caregiver role previously so some of the aspects of the role will be familiar. Those who have not will need more extensive support.

Barriers to caregiving should be openly identified and discussed so that a proactive approach can be adopted. Lack of appropriate caregivers multiply other demands, as caregivers, etc., will identify problems and obstacles in an area where solutions need to be worked on.

K Provide Knowledge and Information A cancer diagnosis and ensuing treatment phases are highly traumatic. The person is catapulted into an unfamiliar learning environment, where there is little or no time to emotionally or psychologically accept the diagnosis of a life-threatening illness before being asked to consider treatment options and deal with the physical impact of the chosen treatment. This rapid succession of events can diminish the individual's sense of mastery and induce feelings of powerlessness and helplessness. The negative spiral of events threatens the person's whole psychosocial well-being. These points emphasize the crisis state that many patients and their families are in at such a time and demonstrate the need for support, including supplying appropriate information to the patient and family (Mills and Sullivan 1999). As previously mentioned, there is a growing awareness regarding the importance of receiving information for family/caregivers and patients alike. Mills and Sullivan point out the various functions of information to patients and family caregivers, such as helping them gain control, reducing anxiety, improving compliance, creating realistic expectations, promoting self-care and participation, generating feelings of safety and security. The literature consistently highlights the need to receive information about the dimensions of care, such as information and assistance regarding the actual disease; physical care; comfort measures; what symptoms to expect, their causes, and how to manage them; treatment regimens; expectations for future care; patients' emotional responses; household management procedures; finances; and community resources (Fitch 2000; Given et al. 2001; Mossman et al. 1999). Symptom control is a particular area of concern and can become a major struggle for patients, particularly those with advanced disease, and their family caregivers. Pain management often becomes a pervasive and intractable problem for family caregivers, contributing to care demands as well as to their own distress. Thus, healthcare professionals need to provide caregivers with information about how to manage patients' physical and emotional symptoms within the context of the caregiver's level of knowledge and ability to identify symptoms (Given et al. 2001).

Various forms of information have been assessed and many have been found to be useful. However, while verbal information is often seen as the cornerstone of information giving, an inherent problem is that most of the information available involves novel concepts and often frightening language for patients. Supplemental written information has the benefit that if patients are too anxious at diagnosis or consultation to retain the information they are given, the written data serve as a reference that can be used to refresh their memories. Furthermore, written information may be particularly beneficial to patients in the current milieu of clinical practice, when shorter hospital stays reduce the amount of time doctors and nurses have to spend discussing concerns and providing salient facts (Mills and Sullivan 1999). Recent studies show that allowing caregivers to audiotape clinical encounters or providing them with follow-up letters summarizing the essentials for the encounters, be a unique source of information as patients and caregivers can refer to it as necessary and share it with all potential caregivers (Hack et al. 2003). Video representations of caregiver experiences in cancer care can be another helpful intervention (Kettler and Baile 2005).

S Support and Strategize The therapeutic alliance is an important factor in providing support for family caregivers. In this discussion, the term "support" describes meeting family caregivers' needs for assistance in providing optimal care to the patient with cancer. As such, the focus is not only on the disease and treatment, but also on the interplay between how the disease affects the patient and the demands it imposes on the caregiver. Support from healthcare professionals, family, and friends can help family caregivers enhance their resiliency and expand their capacities to respond to care demands. The goals of support should be to enable family caregivers to maintain the patient's comfort and enhance the patient's quality of life, and to prevent or minimize unnecessary caregiver fatigue and distress. Generally, support should balance the psychosocial needs of the caregiver and promote the caregiver's physical and emotional well-being so that he or she can more effectively attend to the physical and emotional needs of the patient with cancer (Given et al. 2001). Psychoeducational interventions are an important source of support and may be easily carried out by the oncology team. Maintaining an attitude of hopefulness, encouraging spouses or family members to accompany patients to visits, stressing the importance of communication among family members, and underlining the important role that family support has in patient recovery can be effective strategies (Dorval et al. 2005).

Caregivers of terminally ill cancer patients have diverse needs. Some need help and reassurance making difficult decisions; others have problems communicating with the patient or with other family members. All caregivers must learn to cope with complex and sometimes conflicting emotional responses, including fear, guilt, and anger. Many require assistance securing appropriate healthcare services or eliciting needed personal and social support (Lev 1985; Nijboer et al. 2001). In addition to these functions, caregivers must navigate unfamiliar legal and business matters, and, ultimately, may have to make funeral arrangements (Lunney 2000).

Caregivers generally undergo adjustment difficulties and great stress from the caregiving demands placed on them. The results of elevated stress are depression, anxiety, a feeling of being burdened, role conflict, uncertainty, fatigue, insomnia, decline in physical health, lack of exercise, poor nutrition, use of medications, and morbidity (Given et al. 2001; Thomas and Morris 2002). Changes in the degree of distress and adjustment problems tend to become more intense for the caregiver as the patient's condition deteriorates. At such times, a serious assessment of the family caregiver's support needs should be documented and the capacity to care for the patient evaluated. Appropriate support from healthcare providers and others may help families to prioritize and manage patients' problems, while at the same time lowering the burdens associated with the uncertainty of caring. If families can acknowledge the value of their care, their sense of burden is likely to be lessened (Engel 1983; Given et al. 2001).

Attention should be paid to the quality of life of caregivers. Caregivers commonly perceive that they do not have time to breathe, let alone do anything else for themselves. It is essential to help them understand that they must make time to care for themselves, even in small ways. Helping caregivers establish a plan of care for themselves is as important as organizing care plans for patients (Lunney 2000) and without such a plan, it will be difficult to act in the role of caregiver in a state of readiness.

The oncology healthcare team can improve patient outcomes and reduce caregivers' anxiety, depression, and sense of frustration by dealing with practical exigencies. These can include identifying patients' home care needs, plans of care specific to each patient and family, and instructing family members about how to implement the parameters of the plan. Also, the team must assume that family members' capacities to provide care vary; these variations must be considered and interventions tailored for each situation. The interventions designed by oncologists and delivered to family caregivers should emphasize improving patient comfort and satisfaction, reducing unnecessary hospitalizations, and managing patient care across the advanced disease trajectory (Given et al. 2001).

When trying to reestablish equilibrium to families in cancer crisis, a useful approach is to make mountains manageable for today, tonight, or this week (Rickel 1987). Once the crisis has eased and the patient has returned to a precrisis level of functioning, referrals may allow the patient to work through present or other major problems in a more directed manner. In planning with a patient in crisis, it is helpful for the treatment team to: (1) list the problems as they see them; (2) have the patient/family list their problems as they see them; and (3) have each group place them into three categories. The patient/family will place them into: (1) Things I can change soon; (2) Things I may be able to change in time; and (3) Things I cannot change. The treatment team will do the same, however, the categories will be: (1) Life-threatening; (2) I can assist; and (3) I can get assistance (Rickel 1987).

Outcomes of a Therapeutic Alliance

The therapeutic benefit of the relationship with the family becomes more obvious when the clinical team is alone to conceptualize and embrace it as a journey in which they provide "safe passage." Physicians can nurture and encourage a fighting spirit in patients and encourage patients and caregivers to take control of their situation and to accept some degree of personal responsibility for the healing process. For example, physicians can suggest to patients that each day they survive allows them to take advantage of new developments in treatment. Other patients may want to actively participate in their healing through supportive activities such as exercise programs, special diets, visualization, or psychotherapy (Sardell and Trierweiler 1993).

The benefits of the supportive nature and hopeful spirit of the therapeutic alliance are:

- Reduction of the distress in handling uncertainty.
- Providing accurate information.
- Increased compliance with treatment.
- Improved satisfaction with care.
- Enhanced psychological adjustment.
- Receipt of clearly understood informed consent.
- Improved decision-making.

Involvement of Caregivers in the Treatment Team: Current Status and Future Lines of Investigation

Practice Now

Caregivers are variably involved in patient care and face limitations imposed by time and resources. Areas of concern are in training professionals and in the treatment team in allying with and empowering patients and families.

- Limitations most often reported by cancer patients and caregivers include those related to personal adjustment to illness, psychosocial support, transportation issues, financial assistance, home care, medical information (Shelby et al. 2002).
- As a first step in developing a care plan with family members, the treatment team might benefit from completing a self-assessment of their own personal and professional boundaries, as well as areas of strength and limitations in working with families (Speice et al. 2000).

Practice Needs for the Future

As cancer becomes a more chronic disease and the caregiver burden may extend well beyond the acute phase of the illness. Thus, the future practice of oncology will likely prioritize engaging/partnering with caregivers. An especially interesting aspect of family involvement revolves around managing difficult family dynamics. These can be discussed in professional team meetings, however, will require psychosocial specialists trained in this area. A particular challenge facing oncology clinicians is to understand how much a presenting problem is due to a troubled individual or to a troubled relationship (Peteet and Greenberg 1995). Various behaviors can provide clues to the existence of a high-risk family, including denial, anger, guilt, detachment, emotional and/or geographical distance, and demanding to know why certain services have not been provided, why certain procedures have been used, or staff overly bonding with the family (Welch-McCaffrey 1988).

For a therapeutic alliance to be established, families should be evaluated for functional versus dysfunctional characteristics. The emotional system of a functional family encourages independence, promotes self-esteem, exhibits positive resolution of conflicts, and promotes the ability to adapt to change. Functional families have relationships that foster emotional maturity where the individuals are able to separate thought from feelings and demonstrate a sense of separateness among family members. In functional families, differences of opinions are encouraged and there are mutual problem-solving behaviors that generate solutions to problems. Family members are flexible in relation to each other.

In contrast, dysfunctional families encourage dependence, identify one person as the problem or patient, experience negative conflict resolution, and display a rigid use of repetitive and ineffective coping. Dysfunctional families are characterized by a lack of differentiation among family members. Emotional immaturity is fostered, feelings and thoughts are enmeshed, a sense of constricting fusion among family members where differences of opinion are not acceptable exists, and family members demonstrate an inability to resolve problems through alternative solutions (Heiney 1988). In the dysfunctional family, three patterns signal that individuals are having difficulty with conflict resolution and problem solving, further complicating and intensifying the crisis of cancer. These are excessive marital conflict, overadequate compensation and inadequate reciprocity of behaviors, and the process of projection of emotions whereby one party displaces his/her emotional interpretation of events onto another party. When there is excessive marital conflict and their child is ill, parents cannot resolve issues or problems. Arguments are repeated over and over and, despite their historic ineffectiveness, the same solutions are used time after time in an attempt to resolve recurring problems. This pattern can escalate into abuse. In relationships marked by an over-adequate/inadequate reciprocal pattern, one spouse functions at the expense of the other or depletes energy from the other (Heiney 1988). For optimal and efficacious treatment, the members of the therapeutic alliance should be aware of these debilitating mechanisms and devise a plan to cope with their effects.

Studies of family functioning and illness have used theoretically-based instruments such as the Moos Family Environmental Scale (FES), the Circomplex Model of Family Functioning (FACES), the Family Paradigm, the MacMaster Family Assessment Device (FAD), and other family measures. However, the degree of correlation among measures remains uncertain (Ell 1996). This is an excellent area for future investigation.

Problem-solving therapy (PST) has been documented as an effective way to assist patients and families in coping with cancer. It has been shown to reduce distress and to increase a sense of control among persons with cancer and their family members (Scott et al. 2004). Unfortunately, PST is not widely available because counselors are not routinely prepared to offer this specialized education and are not routinely employed in medical settings. In addition, many patients with cancer and their families are reluctant to seek out the services of counselors or therapists as a way to cope with their problems. Therefore, while PST is highly effective, its widespread adoption as an education source is limited by pragmatic considerations. Fortunately, key elements of its approach are educational in nature and can be learned, adapted, and added to the array of useful psychoeducational programs for patients with cancer and their families (Bucher et al. 2001).

The process of transforming PST into an educational model began in 1992. The content for the skills-building program was derived from what counselors teach in one-on-one PST counseling sessions. Their six-step problem-solving approach was condensed into four topical areas and relabeled as the COPE model of problem solving. COPE stands for the application of: creativity (brainstorming of ideas to create a plan to solve a problem or to gather more information about the problem), optimism (feeling hopeful that one can succeed in solving the selected problem), planning (creating a systematic plan to attack the problem and also prevent its reoccurrence), and expert information (gathering information from written sources and expert professionals). Initial field-testing of the COPE educational adaptation of PST for families affected by cancer was funded by the Pennsylvania Department of Health and was conducted primarily in community settings such as churches. Program evaluation revealed that patients, families, and interested community members were receptive to the intervention.

Problem-solving education is a new form of psychoeducational education. The evaluation of its use with families affected by advanced cancer suggests that the education is well received by patients and their families and can be delivered in busy clinic settings. Experimental and control group comparisons are needed to test its effects rigorously; however, there is a growing body of literature that suggests that problem-solving education is an effective psychosocial intervention. Patients with advanced cancer and particularly their caregivers may benefit from such an educational approach (Bucher et al. 2001).

Education/Training Now

Progress in this area is variable with some disciplines having formal training, e.g., social work family assessment, nurse biopsychosocial model of care, and physicians learning informally through experience. Limitations that need to be addressed are:

- *Communication*—Communication is essential for efficacious therapeutic alliances and all aspects of interaction in the cancer setting (Baile and Aaron 2005; Parker et al. 2001). Communication should be viewed as a core clinical skill that merits a considerable investment of time and resources in training. Unfortunately, few oncologists, nurses, or medical students receive adequate formal education in communication skills using methods likely to promote change, confidence, and competence (Baile et al. 2000; Fallowfield and Jenkins 1999; Maguire et al. 1986). Effective communication during a consultation influences the range and number of symptoms elicited, permits a more precise assessment of the efficacy of therapy, affects adherence to treatment recommendations, impacts the patient's and family's emotional and physical well-being, and contributes to both patient and healthcare satisfaction (Fallowfield and Jenkins 1999; Garg et al. 1997; Maguire et al. 1986). Good communication is also associated with many important and meaningful health outcomes, including adherence to drug regimens and diets, pain control, resolution of physical and functional symptoms, improvements to physiological measures such as control of blood sugar and hypertension, and good psychological functioning of patients. Trust in the doctor is a primary motivating factor in the acceptance of clinical trial participation (Albrecht et al. 2003; Fallowfield and Jenkins 1999).

- *Burn-out*—Clinicians specializing in cancer acknowledge that insufficient training in communication and management skills is a major factor contributing to their stress, lack of job satisfaction, and emotional burnout (Fallowfield and Jenkins 1999). Enhanced communication among members of the treatment team may provide some buffer against burnout (Fallowfield 2005).

Education/Training in the Future

Paradoxically, institutional changes are occurring at a time when the needs of caregivers are becoming more complex. This may become increasingly burdensome to the family, treatment team, and society. Education and training are needed in the aspects specific to the illness of cancer and caregiver/family concerns in these areas. Wong et al. (2002) found the management of common symptoms, including pain, nausea, weakness, and fatigue, and the types of services that were available to facilitate the care of the patients at home were the major concerns of patients with advanced cancer and their families. There is a need for education and support in this realm for caregivers. In light of dramatic changes occurring in healthcare delivery throughout the country, innovative strategies for disseminating information and support to caregivers and the professionals that assist them are critically needed so that caregiver education and support will ultimately become a routine standard of care (Pasacreta et al. 2000).

Guidelines for Recognition and Treatment of Burnout As Spinetta et al. (2000) note, health care professionals are increasingly aware of the problem of burnout and are concerned with its impact on the healthcare team. Burnout can ultimately affect the care provided to the patient and family by creating indifference, emotional exhaustion, and a sense of professional and personal failure. They provide useful suggestions for identifying and addressing factors in the work environment and personal issues which are frequently echoed by experts in dealing with stress-related symptoms and personal renewal (Shanafelt 2005; Shanafelt et al. 2006).

- Training in basic and advanced communication skills. It has been pointed out how vital communication is for treatment to be biopsychosocially valid (Parker et al. 2001). Good communication skills are not only essential for forging a helpful alliance between the patient, the family caregiver, and the treatment team, they are equally as necessary for the treatment team to be effective, with the patient and with each other (Frankel and Steven 2001). A problem within oncology that impacts care in part concerns the quality of the communication within the multidisciplinary team. Poor communication between different specialists and departments can add to the confusion about the diagnosis, test results, and management (Fallowfield and Jenkins 1999; Garg et al. 1997; Maguire et al. 1986). In addition, communication is a vital conduit for providing support and enhancing family communication. There is convincing evidence that family members repeatedly express a need for information from health professionals, however, experience difficulty in obtaining the information (Keller 2001). Lack of information not only deprives the family of an important coping resource, but also contributes to family stress, and may lead to family conflict and misguided patient support (Ell 1996). Clearly research in this area is needed as is research in how to improve the communication skills of patients, particularly in interviews with the treatment team (Cegala et al. 2000).

- Training in conducting family interviews. In general, patients want physicians to adopt an attitude of confident openness and to act as supportive and encouraging coaches rather than as detached clinicians or consoling caretakers (Sardell and Trierweiler 1993). For patients, the physician's ability to maintain an attitude of hope and confidence in the face of the grim facts of cancer is a critical aspect of diagnostic disclosure and one warranting further study (Sardell and Trierweiler 1993).
- Lipkin (1996) delineates useful suggestions for the order and structural elements of an interview, which would likely be useful if widely adopted. These are (1) preparing oneself to listen and attend, (2) preparing the environment, (3) greeting the patient, (4) opening with introduction of self and purpose, (5) generation of hypotheses, (6) surveying problems, (7) picking a priority problem, (8) developing the narrative thread, (9) training the patient, (10) detailing the story of the illness, (11) use of safety net question lists, (12) the physical examination, (13) summarizing, (14) planning the next steps, and (15) closing. It would be interesting to design a study to assess the effects of this method.
- A physician's appropriate physical contact with the patient (e.g., holding a hand, a pat on the shoulder, a hug) goes a long way toward reducing the feeling of being emotionally and physically devalued as a consequence of the cancer. Touch is a powerful communicator and empathic gesture. Moreover, a physician's careful use of light humor demonstrates that solemnity is not the only way to get through life's catastrophes and that one can take a cognitive leap in the face of disaster and engage humor as an ally in the cancer war. Studies have shown that laughter has a healing benefit. Finally, patients reported greater hope when they were able to talk with their physicians as partners in the fight and as confidants to whom they could relate their feelings (Sardell and Trierweiler 1993).

Research Now

Devising efficacious strategies for promoting caregiver involvement requires ongoing research into the areas of social support; provision of information; study design; relationship between age, place in the family, and gender on the caregiving role; and other pertinent areas.

- Thus far, research in promoting family involvement has focused mostly on increasing professional caregivers' ability to detect family caregiver distress. Some promising intervention studies to promote caregiver involvement in patient care include a randomized controlled trial of a prompt list, which helped advanced cancer patients and their caregivers ask questions about prognosis and end of life care (Clayton et al. 2007) and one of the several studies using audiotapes of clinical encounters to help families and patients discuss information about their visit (Ong et al. 2000). Some intervention studies have been conducted. While there is a substantial body of literature dealing with family caregiver issues, serious limitations exist, both in the negative as well as positive aspects of caring for a loved one.

Research in the Future

- There is limited empirical evidence documenting the efficacy of standardized intervention strategies specifically for cancer caregivers (Pasacreta et al. 2000). This would be a useful line of investigation, including defining windows of opportunity for specific interventions to be used during each phase of the cancer care trajectory.
- Most research reflects family caregivers' abilities to help patients through the early phases of diagnosis and initial treatment and on the demands faced by family caregivers at the end of the patients' lives, few descriptions of the actual care requirements for patients with chronic advanced and recurrent disease exist (Given et al. 2001).
- The lack of methodological rigor of many of the previous caregiver intervention studies and the equivocal results suggest that additional studies are warranted (Toseland et al. 1995) with cogent study designs and statistical validation.
- The majority of the relatively few studies of family caregiver stress have particularly underlined the considerable impact that cancer has on the dynamics of the marital relationship (Ferrario et al. 2003). Studies to further examine this issue and the effects on other family members such as the "well sibling" are warranted.
- Future research is necessary into how to prepare family caregivers for their roles and in devising ongoing support programs for caregiver distress, especially in view of evidence that healthcare practitioners often misunderstand the emotional needs of the family. Findings that spouses experience social isolation, especially when occupied with long-term caregiving activities underscores their potential

reduced access to social network support. Family caregivers, however, have been shown to be reluctant to request assistance until their need becomes severe, such as when the caregiver's health declines (Ell 1996).

- Measures that capture the processes by which families give and take support await further development. The most difficult assessments will involve attempts to examine support and family processes over time, as during the chronic exacerbations and remissions associated with chronic conditions (Ell 1996).
- An important area for future research is an increased understanding of how to enhance family dynamics, how to refer distressed families, and how to handle ethical issues such as confidentiality.

Policy Now

While the family is often recognized as being an essential component in patient care, most guidelines for involving family members are informal and specific to individual institutions. An exception to this oversight is the SIOP guidelines (Masera et al. 1998) for creating a therapeutic alliance which serves as an excellent model for incorporating the family into the treatment team. Resources such as "Elder Care Online" (http://www.ec-online.net), which is an online community for helping caregivers of the elderly, are often resourced by members of the healthcare team, such as social workers, however, may not be as well known by nurses or other members of the medical team. In addition, the Joint Commission on Hospital Accreditation (2004) encourages the assessment of the impact of the illness on the family, and this could be expanded to specifically promote expansion of the patient care model to include the family.

Policy in the Future

- Expand standards of care to emphasize caregiver involvement. Caregivers are increasingly informally recognized as essential components of patient care, however, their needs are regarded as secondary to those of patients, who remain the primary users of health and social care. However, some ambiguity about whether caregivers are providers or users of services has been noted in the policy literature (Morris and Thomas 2001). Prior to the 1980s, caregivers in cancer were little-remarked providers of assistance to the patient, generally subsumed under the heading of "family," however, in their incipient role as users of services, they have become potential "clients" and need to be evaluated for levels of psychological distress (Morris and Thomas 2001).
- One of the important reasons for the lack of progress in policy development and service implementation has been the paucity of relevant data about the patterns

of supportive caregiver needs over time and the resultant utilization of services (Fitch 2000).

- Establish guidelines and pathways for health professionals providing cancer care in how to provide caregivers with assistance.
- Involve public/professional organizations, e.g., National Cancer Institute, American Society of Clinical Oncology, Oncology Nursing Association, National Association of Oncology Social Workers, National and International Societies of Psychooncology, to participate in training, policy, and advocacy.
- Liaison with patient advocacy groups to lobby for caregiver issues such as empowering the employed caregiver by identifying changes that can be made in employment law in addition to the federal Family and Medical Leave Act of 1993 (FMLA).
- Establish statement of cancer caregiver rights and responsibilities, e.g., institutional mission statements.
- The argument that future social support research should be conducted from a family systems perspective is particularly compelling because it expands a narrow focus on the patient to include examination of the primary caregivers as well as the social interactions that characterize day-to-day coping within families dealing with illness. There is a need for longitudinal studies of support over time (Ell 1996). If support groups or other forms of grafted support such as use of lay volunteers to meet with patients serve as an adequate substitute for or enhance family support is unknown. If, and in what ways, traditional counseling approaches is effective for helping families, particularly the spouse, is worthy of future studies (Ell 1996).
- Caregiving has traditionally been viewed as a woman's responsibility, and the investigators hypothesized that men would have more difficulty in the caregiving role than women. The relation between gender and the caregiving role needs to be addressed in future research (Pasacreta et al. 2000).
- The focus on shared medical decision-making and the greater demands placed on caregivers providing home care has increased the need for treatment-related cancer information (Shelby et al. 2002). A preponderance of the literature related to caregiving and cancer focuses on the incredible importance that being appropriately informed along the way is to cancer patients and their families and continued research is necessary to monitor and answer this need.

Conclusions

The family is increasingly recognized as an important source of support for the patient and an extension of the medical team in assessing patient well-being, promoting compliance, and advocating for the patient. The time is long past due for a proactive approach that incorporates family caregivers in patient care. Activities for a care team that embraces professional and family caregivers working together are multiple. They encompass responding to the patient's wishes and desires as the care recipient, supporting the family's strengths and responding to the needs of the family caregivers, and assessing, and if necessary, realigning care team interventions. Development of a therapeutic alliance that promotes the goals of care can best be accomplished by addressing the multiple levels of needed action: research on evidence-based interventions, research-based policy development, and implementation of caregiver education programs and supports of known empirical value. Accomplishing these steps requires parallel collaboration among clinicians as professional caregivers, care facilities as care settings, family advocates as both family caregivers and public advocates, and policy makers as the guardians of public policy on caregiving issues to bring about needed changes.

References

Adler, H. M. (2002). The sociophysiology of caring in the doctor-patient relationship. *Journal of General Internal Medicine, 17*(11), 874–881.

Albrecht, T. L., Penner, L. A., & Ruckdeschel, J. C. (2003). Understanding patient decisions about clinical trials. *Journal of Cancer Education, 18*(4), 210–214.

Back, A. L., Arnold, R. M., Baile, W. F., Fryer-Edwards, K., & Tulsky, J. (2005). Approaching difficult communication tasks in oncology. *CA: A Cancer Journal for Clinicians, 55*(3), 164–177.

Baile, W. F., & Aaron, J. (2005). Patient-physician communication in oncology: Past, present, and future. *Current Opinion in Oncology, 17*(14), 331–335.

Baile, W. F., Buckman, R., Lenzi, R., Glober, G, Beale, E. A., & Kudelka, A. (2000). SPIKES: A six-step protocol for delivering bad news: Application to the patient with cancer. *Oncologist, 5*(4), 302–311.

Blackhall, L. G., Murphy, S. T., Gelya, F., Michel, V., & Azen, S. (1995). Ethnicity and attitudes toward patient autonomy. *Journal of the American Medical Association, 274*(10), 820–825.

Brown, M. L., Lipscomb, J., & Snyder, C. (2001). The burden of illness of cancer: Economic cost and quality of life. *Annual Review of Public Health, 22,* 91–113.

Bucher, J. A., Loscalzo, M., Zabora, J., Houts, P. S., Hooker, C., & Brintzenhofeszoc, K. (2001). Problem-solving cancer care education for patients and caregivers. *Cancer Practice, 9*(2), 66–70.

Caplan, G. (1970). The theory and practice of mental health consultation. New York: Basic Books.

Cegala, D. J., McClure, L., Marinelli, T. M., & Post, D. M. (2000). The effects of communication skills training on patients' participation during medical interviews. *Patient Education and Counseling, 41*(2), 209–222.

Clayton, J. M., Butow, P. N., Tattersall, M. H., Devine, R. J., Simpson, J. M., Aggarwal, G., et al. (2007). Randomized controlled trial of a prompt list to help advanced cancer patients and their caregivers to ask questions about prognosis and end-of-life care. *Journal of Clinical Oncology, 25*(6), 715–723.

Dorval, M., Guay, S., Mondor, M., Masse, B., Falardeau, M., Robidoux, A., et al. (2005). Couples who get closer after breast cancer: Frequency and predictors in a prospective investigation. *Journal of Clinical Oncology, 23*(15), 588–596.

Edwards, B. K., Brown, M. L., Wingo, P. A., Howe, H. L., Ward, E., Ries, L. A., et al. (2005). Annual report to the nation on the status of cancer, 1975–2002, featuring population-based trends in cancer treatment. *Journal of the National Cancer Institute, 97*(19), 1407–1427.

Ell, K. (1996). Social networks, social support and coping with serious illness: The family connection. *Social Science Medicine, 42*(2), 173–183.

Engel, G. L. (1983). The biopsychosocial model and family medicine. *Journal of Family Practice, 16*(2), 409, 412–413.

Fallowfield, L., & Jenkins, V. (1999). Effective communication skills are the key to good cancer care. *European Journal of Cancer, 35*(110), 1592–1597.

Ferrario, S. R., Zotti, A. M., Massara, G., & Nuvolone, G. (2003). A comparative assessment of psychological and psychosocial characteristics of cancer patients and their caregivers. *Psycho-Oncology, 12,* 1–7.

Fitch, M. (2000). Supportive care for cancer patients. *Hospital Quarterly, 3*(4), 39–46.

Frankel, R. M., & Steven, T. (2001). Getting the most out of the clinical encounters: The four habits model. *Journal of Medical Practice Management, 16*(4), 184–191.

Garg, A., Buckman, R., & Kason, Y. (1997). Teaching medical students how to break bad news. *Canadian Medical Association Journal, 156*(8), 1159–1164.

Given, B. A., Given, C. W., & Kozachik, S. (2001). Family support in advanced cancer. *CA: A Cancer Journal for Clinicians, 51*(4), 213–231.

Glajhen, M. (2004). The emerging role and needs of family caregivers in cancer care. *Journal of Supportive Oncology, 2*(2), 145–155.

Gray-Price, H., & Szczesny, S. (1985). Crisis intervention with families of cancer patients: A developmental approach. *Topics in Clinical Nursing, 7*(1), 58–70.

Grunfeld, E., Coyle, D., Whelan, T., Clinch, J., Reyno, L., Earle, C. C., et al. (2004). Family caregiver burden: Results of a longitudinal study of breast cancer patients and their principal caregivers. *Canadian Medical Association Journal, 170*(12), 1811–1812.

Hack, T. F., Pickles, T., Bultz, B. D., Reuther, J. D., Weir, L. M., Degner, L. F., et al. (2003). Impact of providing audiotapes of primary adjuvant treatment consultations to women with breast cancer: A multi-site, randomized, controlled trial. *Journal of Clinical Oncology, 21*(22), 4138–4144.

Hampton, T. H. (2005). Cancer treatment's trade-off: Years of added life can have long term costs. *Journal of the American Medical Association, 94*(2), 167–168.

Heiney, S. (1988). Assessing and intervening with dysfunctional families. *Oncology Nursing Forum, 15*(5), 585–590.

Isaksen, A. S., Thuen, F., & Hanestad, B. (2003). Patients with cancer and their close relatives: Experiences with treatment, care, and support. *Cancer Nursing, 26*(1), 68–74.

Jefford, M., & Tattersall, M. H. N. (2002). Informing and involving cancer patients in their own care. *The Lancet Oncology, 3*(10), 629–637.

Joint Commission on Accreditation of Hospitals. (2004). *Spiritual assessment.* Retrieved from http://www.jointcommission.org/AccreditationPrograms/Hospitals/Standards/FAQs/Provision+of+Care/Assessment/Spiritual_Assessment.htm. Accessed Feb 2009.

Keller, M. (2001). Information supplied to cancer patients and their caregivers: No more unmet needs? *Supportive Care in Cancer, 9*(8), 563–564.

Kettler, P. J., & Baile, W. F. (2005). Caring for the cancer patient: The caregiver's perspective. *Psycho-Oncology, 14,* S55.

Le Chatelier, H. L. (1888). A general statement of the laws of equilibrium. *Comptee Rendus, 99,* 786–789.

Lev, E. L. (1985). Community support for oncology patient and family. *Topics in Clinical Nursing, 7*(1), 71–78.

Lewis F. M., Woods N. F., Hough E. E., & Bensley L. S. (1989). The family's functioning with chronic illness in the mother: The spouse's perspective. *Social Science Medicine, 29,* 1261–1269.

Lipkin, M. (1996). Patient education and counseling in the context of modern patient-physician-family communication. *Patient Education and Counseling, 27*(1), 5–11.

Lunney, J. R. (2000). Resources for caregivers of terminally ill cancer patients. *Cancer Practice, 8*(2), 99–100.

Maguire, P., Fairbairn, S., & Fletcher, C. (1986). Consultation skills of young doctors: I—Benefits of feedback training in interviewing as students persist. *British Medical Journal, 292*(6535), 1573–1576.

Masera, G., Spinetta, J. J., Jankovic, M., Ablin, A. R., Buchwall, I., Van Dongen-Melman, J., et al. (1998). Guidelines for a therapeutic alliance between families and staff: A report of the

SIOP working committee on psychosocial issues in pediatric oncology. *Medical and Pediatric Oncology, 30*(3), 183–186.

Matthews, D. A., Suchman, A., & Branch, W. T. (1993). Making "connexions": Enhancing the therapeutic potential of patient-clinician relationships. *Annals of Internal Medicine, 118*(12), 973–977.

McMillan, S. C., Small, B. J., Weitzner, M., Schonwetter, R., Tittle, M., Moody, L., et al. (2006). Impact of coping skills intervention with family caregivers of hospice patients with cancer. *Cancer, 106*(1), 214–222.

Mills, M. E., & Sullivan, K. (1999). The importance of information giving for patients newly diagnosed with cancer: A review of the literature. *Journal of Clinical Nursing, 8*(6), 631–642.

Mishel, M., Hostetter, T., King, B., & Graham, V. (1984). Predictors of psychosocial adjustment in patients newly diagnosed with gynecological cancer. *Cancer Nursing, 7*(4), 291–299.

Morris, S. M., & Thomas, C. (2001). The carer's place in the cancer situation: Where does the carer stand in the medical setting? *European Journal of Cancer Care, 10*(2), 87–95.

Mossman, J., Boudioni, M., & Slevin, M. L. (1999). Cancer information: A cost-effective intervention. *European Journal of Cancer, 35*(11), 1587–1591.

Nijboer, C., Tempelaar, R., Triemestra, M., van den Bos, G. A. M., & Sanderman R. (2001). The role of social and psychologic resources in caregiving of cancer patients. *Cancer, 91*(5), 1029–1039.

Northouse, L. L. (2005). Helping families of patients with cancer. *Oncology Nursing Forum, 32*(4), 743–750.

Northouse, P. G., & Northouse, L. L. (1987). Communication and cancer: Issues confronting patients, health professionals, and family members. *Journal of Psychosocial Oncology, 5*(3), 17–46.

Ong, L. M., Visser, M. R., Lammes, F. B., van Der Velden, J., Kuenen, B. C., de Haes, J. C. (2000). Effect of providing cancer patients with the audiotaped initial consultation on satisfaction, recall and quality of life: A randomized, double-blind study. *Journal of Clinical Oncology, 18*(16), 3052–3060.

Parker, P. A., Baile, W. F., de Moor, C., Lenzi, R., Kudelka, A. P., & Cohen, L. (2001). Breaking bad news about cancer: Patients' preferences for communication. *Journal of Clinical Oncology, 19*(7), 2049–2056.

Pasacreta, J. V., Barg, F., Nuamah, I., & McCorkle, R. (2000). Participant characteristics before and 4 months after attendance at a family caregiver cancer education program. *Cancer Nursing, 23*(4), 295–303.

Peteet, J., & Greenberg, B. (1995). Marital crisis in oncology patients: An approach to initial intervention by primary clinicians. *General Hospital Psychiatry, 17*(3), 201–207.

Quinn, W. H., & Herndon, A. (1986). The family ecology of cancer. *Journal of Psychosocial Oncology, 4*(1/2), 45–59.

Rickel, L. M. (1987). Making mountains manageable: Maximizing quality of life through crisis intervention. *Oncology Nursing Forum, 14*(4), 29–34.

Sardell, A. N., & Trierweiler, S. J. (1993). Disclosing the cancer diagnosis: Procedures that influence patient hopefulness. *Cancer, 72*(11), 3355–3365.

Scott, J. L., Halford, W. K., & Ward, B. G. (2004). United we stand? The effects of a couple coping intervention and adjustment to early stage breast gynecological cancer. *Journal of Consulting Clinical Psychology, 72*(6), 1122–1135.

Shanafelt, T. (2005). Finding meaning, balance and personal satisfaction in the practice of oncology. *Journal of Supportive Oncology, 3*(2), 157–162.

Shanafelt, T., Chung, H., White, H., & Lyckholm, L. J. (2006). Shaping your career to maximize personal satisfaction in the practice of oncology. *Journal of Clinical Oncology, 24*(24), 4020–4026.

Shelby, R. A., Taylor, K. L., Kerner, J. F., Coleman, E., & Blum, D. (2002). The role of community-based and philanthropic organizations in meeting cancer patient and caregiver needs. *CA: A Cancer Journal for Clinicians, 52*(4), 229–246.

Siegel, K., Raveis, V. H., Mor, V., & Houts, P. (1991). The relationship of spousal caregiver burden to patient disease and treatment-related conditions. *Annals of Oncology, 2*(7), 511–516.

Speice, J., Harkness, J., Laneri, H., Frankel, R., Roiter, D., Kornblith, A. B., et al. (2000). Involving family members in cancer care: Focus group considerations of patients and oncological providers. *Psycho-Oncology, 9*(2), 101–112.

Spinetta, J. J., Jankovic, M., Ben Arush, M. W., Eden, T., Epelman, C., Greenberg, M. L., et al. (2000). Guidelines for the recognition, prevention and remediation of burnout in health care professionals participating in the care of children with cancer: Report of the SIOP working committee on psychosocial issues in pediatric oncology. *Medical and Pediatric Oncology, 35*(2), 122–125.

Thomas, C., & Morris, S. M. (2002). Informal carers in cancer contexts. *European Journal of Cancer Care, 11*, 178–182.

Toseland, R. W., Blanchard, C. G., & McCallion, P. (1995). A problem solving intervention for caregivers of cancer patients. *Social Science Medicine, 40*(4), 517–528.

Tummala, M. K., & Maguire, W. P. (2005). Recurrent ovarian cancer. *Clinical Advances in Hematology & Oncology, 3*(9), 723–736.

Welch-McCaffrey, D. (1988). Family issues in cancer care: Current dilemmas and future directions. *Journal of Psychosocial Oncology, 6*(1/2), 199–211.

Wong, R. K. S., Franssen, E., Szumacher, E., Connolly, R., Evans, M., Page, B., et al. (2002). What do patients living with advanced cancer and their carers want to know? A needs assessment. *Supportive Care in Cancer, 10*(5), 408–415.

Yun, Y. H., Rhee, Y. S., Kang, I. O., Lee, J. S., Bang, S. M., Lee, W. S., et al. (2005). Economic burdens and quality of life of family caregivers of cancer patients. *Oncology, 68*(2–3), 107–114.

Part II
Issues in Providing Direct Care

Chapter 7
Issues Faced by Family Caregivers in Providing Appropriate Care for Cancer Patients with Short-Term/Intermittent Care Needs

Robert Bergamini and Karrie Cummings Hendrickson

The diagnosis of cancer is a devastating event, both for individuals with cancer and for their families. Providing necessary care for a loved one or friend can have a substantial impact on both the physical and mental health of the caregiver. The migration of cancer treatment from an inpatient to an outpatient setting has had many benefits for the patient and family; however, at the same time, that change also has resulted in a significant increase in the care responsibilities of the person with cancer and for the caregiver (Given et al. 2001; Hayman et al. 2001; Weitzner et al. 2000). While much attention has been paid to the needs of the patient, there has been less attention given to the needs of the caregiver. Lack of attention to the caregiver's needs may lead to complications that compromise the physical and mental health of the caregiver, and can interfere with the healthcare of the person with cancer (Jensen and Given 1991; Nijboer et al. 2000; Schumacher et al. 2000).

Following the diagnosis—and over the ensuing months and/or years—the responsibilities thrust upon the caregiver include:

- Emotional support to the patient and participation in medical decision-making,
- Education and training in medical treatments,
- Insurance issues (many would say battles),
- Financial issues, including operation and maintenance of the household,
- Transportation,
- Coordination of care from multiple healthcare providers,

R. Bergamini (✉)
Unity Physician Hospital Organization, 607 S New Ballas Road,
St. Louis, MO 63141, USA
e-mail: drbobstl@yahoo.com

K. C. Hendrickson
Decision Support, Yale-New Haven Health System,
Yale University, 20 York St., New Haven, CT 06510, USA
e-mail: karrie.hendrickson@yale.edu

R. C. Talley et al. (eds.), *Cancer Caregiving in the United States,*
Caregiving: Research, Practice, Policy,
DOI 10.1007/978-1-4614-3154-1_7, © Springer Science+Business Media, LLC 2012

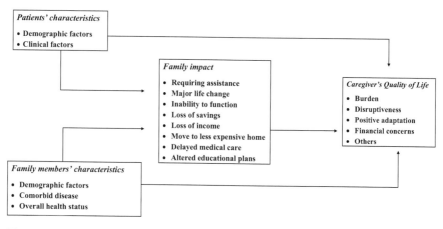

Fig. 7.1 Conceptual research model for studying burdens and quality of life of family caregivers of cancer patients (Yun et al. 2005)

- Assistance with activities of daily living (e.g., bathing), and
- Maintenance of the caregiver's own life and needs (job, school, etc.), despite significantly increased demands on the caregiver's time.

Even for short-term or intermittent care needs, the caregiver will be challenged by fatigue; conflicts with work or school; a sense of being overwhelmed by the volume of tasks to be performed; doubts of personal skill, stamina, and knowledge; and issues related to the caregiver's own individual life (Chan and Chang 1999; Hardwick and Lawson 1995; Laizner et al. 1993; Pasacreta et al. 2000). The magnitude of the impact on a patient and family cannot be minimized.

Yun et al. (2005) present a useful and informative model that will guide the discussion of caregiver experiences in this chapter (Fig. 7.1). They suggest that the burdens associated with caregiving are inversely related to the quality of life of the caregiver.

As the needs of the patient vary over time, the resultant demands and burdens on the caregiver also change and their quality of life is affected. In this chapter, we discuss the challenges caregivers encounter when managing the care of a person with cancer in the home. We examine obstacles encountered by caregivers during the phases of cancer (diagnosis, treatment and recovery, and disease progression and terminal care), along with special concerns for caregivers of children with cancer and young caregivers of adults with cancer. Finally, we review the current state and future directions of healthcare education, research, and public policy with regard to caregivers of people with cancer.

Diagnosis

At the time of diagnosis—and for about 100 days afterward—the patient, primary caregiver, and extended family are faced with a multifaceted crisis, which has been called the "existential plight of cancer" (Raveis and Pretter 2005; Weisman and Worden 1977). During this time, regardless of educational or professional background, the caregiver is thrust into an important supporting role, while at the same time, struggling with individual emotions, and dealing with the disruption, uncertainty, and turmoil caused by the diagnosis of cancer (Harden et al. 2002; Sherman and Simonton 2001; Veach and Nicholas 1998). Healthcare professionals focus on the patient's needs and direct resources to ensure that those needs are met. The caregiver is assumed willing to accept the supporting role demanded, without any significant assessment of caregiver skills or needs. The nature of cancer and its treatment is such that the demands placed on the caregiver are ambiguous and unpredictable. There are, however, several issues that uniformly emerge immediately.

Emotional Support and Acceptance Approximately 70% of caregivers for adults with cancer are spouses and many others are their adult children (Bakas et al. 2001; Hayman et al. 2001; Weitzner et al. 2000); and virtually all initial primary caregivers of children with cancer are parents. Laizner et al. (1993) found that many of these caregivers believe that they must focus on the physical and emotional needs of the patient, and not voice their personal doubts and insecurities, which they fear could upset or adversely affect their loved one.

The complexity and depth of support required varies widely among caregivers, however, many report that at the time of diagnosis, the amount of support required usually exceeds anything ever previously experienced by the primary caregiver and/or the extended family. The medical situation is often unstable and evolving rapidly (especially when children are the patients), leaving no option for a leisurely learning curve (Hardwick and Lawson 1995; Laizner et al. 1993; Rivera 1997; Stetz and Brown 1997).

This illustrates the Yun et al. (2005) model well. Caregivers sacrifice their own needs (to express feelings and receive emotional support) for the good of the loved one with cancer (needs positive attitude), and in so doing caregivers sacrifice some of their quality of life.

Medical Training The rapid movement of patients from inpatient treatment settings to outpatient treatment mandates caregiver training and involvement in many medically related aspects of care (Hayman et al. 2001; Weitzner et al. 2000). This has been shown to cause considerable apprehension in caregivers (Hardwick and Lawson 1995; Nijboer et al. 1999). With ever shortening lengths of (inpatient) stay, this education and training must now begin almost immediately after diagnosis (Pasacreta et al. 2000). Necessary education will almost certainly include central line care, administration of intravenous fluids and medication, and administration of pain medication (by a variety of routes). It can also include wound care, stoma care, inhalation treatments, and other aspects of physical care to the person's body. The assumption of these medically related tasks can be overwhelming at best, and terror provoking at worst.

One specific area of grave concern for many caregivers is providing or assisting their family member with personal hygiene activities, such as bathing and catheter care (Bakas et al. 2001; Oberst et al. 1989). As Yun's model (2005) suggests, the caregiver's concern and distress increase as the level of the body care required increases. Caregivers may find themselves routinely performing care tasks that were once considered repulsive or embarrassing.

Caregiver Education Caregivers work to identify information about the person with cancer's specific diagnosis and proposed treatment after diagnosis (Harden et al. 2002; Nijboer et al. 1999; Schumacher 1996; Stetz and Brown 1997). Often this task takes the form of asking questions of the oncologist, but because each individual needs and desires different types of information, persons with cancer and their caregivers often do not get the information they need. The shocking nature of the diagnosis along with limited appointment times in busy oncology offices result in many questions going unasked and unanswered, leaving the family unprepared to provide care at home (Harden et al. 2002). This point was clearly illustrated by Harden et al. (2002), who interviewed 20 couples living with prostate cancer and found that the dyads believed it would have been helpful for a trained clinician to spend some time with them answering questions and tailoring information to the specific needs of their family situation.

Because many caregivers do not receive the education they need at the time of diagnosis, many also conduct private research on the Internet (Lewis et al. 2005). The easy availability and volume of information obtainable on the Internet and other electronic sources can overload both the person with cancer and caregiver. The caregiver then needs to filter through legitimate medical information and other information which is from nonstandard, nonreviewed, and unconfirmed sources (Dahl and Portenoy 2004). The medical team must be willing and available to interpret and explain electronic and other literature to help prevent their patients and families from falling victim to so-called "miracle cures," such as St. John's Wort, which may interfere with certain types of chemotherapy, and ice caps or scalp tourniquets (marketed to prevent hair loss), which simply do not work.

Pain Control Much has been written about the inadequate pain control of cancer patients. Over 80% of patients with advanced cancer will experience significant pain during the course of their illness (Walsh 2000; Wolfe et al. 2000). Adequate pain control is vitally important to both mental and physical health, and is necessary for optimal patient care. In the period immediately following diagnosis, the person with cancer may experience pain associated with diagnostic or therapeutic surgery, the cancer itself, or treatment via radiation or chemotherapy (such as the jaw pain experienced with Vincristine).

In most cases, the caregiver will be asked to assume a significant role in the management of the cancer pain symptoms, but they face many potential barriers to effective pain management, and many caregivers will never gain confidence in pain management (Kimberlin et al. 2004). Barriers to effective pain management include fear of drug addiction and side effects, lack of understanding of the implications of drug tolerance, fear of respiratory depression, and a lack of understanding of the mechanisms involved in persistent pain (Aranda et al. 2004). Caregivers describe pain management as emotionally draining and requiring significant psychological adjustment, however, studies have shown that the family caregivers' attitudes about the management of cancer pain greatly influence the person with cancer's experience of the disease (Aranda et al. 2004; Given et al. 2001).

From the caregiver perspective, the emotional aspects of seeing a loved one suffer in pain cannot be underestimated. However, traditional societal norms admonish against the use of narcotics and warn of the dangers of addiction, and some even suggest that there is an implied physical and mental weakness associated with the continued use of narcotics (Aranda et al. 2004). These norms may contribute both to the person with cancer's willingness to report pain accurately and the caregivers willingness to administer pain medication (Kimberlin et al. 2004). Focused instruction of the caregiver in the management of cancer pain, however, has resulted in improved management of pain, so clinicians must be willing to provide caregivers with adequate information and support to facilitate appropriate cancer pain management of their loved one.

Kimberlin et al. (2004) interviewed 22 cancer patients and 15 caregivers. Their findings suggest that improved support of caregivers in pain management will involve clinicians answering questions thoroughly, providing complete information about what to expect from the medication and the disease, providing written information, avoiding jargon, and verifying patient (and family) understanding (Kimberlin et al. 2004).

Insurance Issues Compliance with insurance company contract requirements can be difficult and confusing. In one extreme case, a specific company required that the insured (father) leave the bedside of his intubated, critically ill child to initiate the certification process. The company steadfastly refused to speak with any healthcare personnel until the father made the initiating call. Other companies may be less demanding, but interactions with an insurance company can be overwhelming, and if not managed effectively, can, as Yun's model suggests, contribute to a decline in the caregiver's quality of life.

The caregiver is often thrust into a situation that rapidly becomes confrontational in nature. While the patient and caregiver usually do not have to deal with issues related to the hospital stay, outpatient therapies and prescriptions rapidly become an increasing source of frustration and difficulty. Responsibility for the coordination of home care services, durable medical equipment deliveries, and picking up prescriptions often falls solely on the caregiver, and if not managed successfully, a delay in care may be the only option, as most services are far too expensive for the cost to be born out of pocket.

In an effort to prevent problems with insurance and service management, the insurance company may assign a case manager (in-house or through an oncology management company) to the patient. While the initial contact will be with the patient, the caregiver often assumes responsibility for communication with the case manager. Many people are not familiar with the concept of case management and are fearful of the intrusion of this stranger in their lives.

For the elderly patient, Medicare presents a unique set of issues. The caregiver often finds that complex rules that govern the provision of care and the coverage are significantly different than that provided by commercial insurance. Some patients and caregivers will also be concerned with Medigap Insurance and its associated rules. Outpatient and ancillary service coverage under Medicare is not necessarily intuitive or predictable, and the complex payment rules may be a source of frustration and confusion to both patients and caregivers.

Financial Issues Informal caregiving costs account for a significant portion of the direct nonmedical costs associated with a cancer diagnosis (Hayman et al. 2001). The caregiver must assume responsibility for financial matters, including payment of scheduled debts (mortgage, rent, etc.) and allocation of financial resources to other responsibilities (food, utilities, and now, medically related expenses). Outpatient medications, if not covered by insurance, can represent a substantial and overwhelming burden. Zofran (or any of its competitors) can cost $200 for ten doses (3 days' worth of medication). The stories of families being forced to choose between medication and other needs can become a tragic reality in an instant.

Family Issues Depending on the age of the patient and family members, the stage of the family's development (newly forming family, young family, aging family), and the dynamics of the family, the effects of a cancer diagnosis on the family unit will vary (Harden 2005; Nijboer et al. 2000; Sherman and Simonton 2001; Veach and Nicholas 1998). These family characteristics affect who will assume the role of the primary caregiver (parent, spouse, sibling, or child), the tasks associated with caregiving, and the family's ability to cope effectively with the diagnosis. One study by Nijboer et al. (2000) found that women, younger caregivers, and caregivers with high socioeconomic status tend to experience caregiving negatively, while others may experience it in a more positive light. Veach and Nicholas (1998) suggest that oncology clinicians can improve the caregiving experience by doing what Yun's model suggests, thus decreasing caregiver burden. They further propose that caregiver burden can be reduced if healthcare providers more effectively tailor treatments to meet the needs of their patients and caregivers by performing a psychosocial assessment on the family unit.

Treatment and Recovery

While medical personnel may be upbeat, delighted, and encouraged by the fact that the duration of newer chemotherapy regimens is measured in months instead of years, a patient and/or caregiver can easily be overwhelmed by a proposed treatment protocol of several months' duration. One father, when told that his son would be receiving treatment for 9 months and close follow-up thereafter dryly noted that a highly publicized repeat felon had just received a shorter "sentence." He openly expressed concern about the quality of his son's life, and his (the father's) own ability to cope with seeing his child repeatedly receiving chemotherapy treatments. His comments underscore the apprehension and emotions that accompany the realization that a loved one has an illness that will not be cured with a short course of antibiotics.

Once past the initial diagnostic period, the demands placed on the caregiver will change (Nijboer et al. 2000). Most caregivers report that the most time-consuming tasks during treatment and recovery are emotional support, transportation to various medical appointments, and monitoring symptoms (Bakas et al. 2001; Sarna and McCorkle 1996; Sherman and Simonton 2001). Other issues include ongoing insurance problems, operation and maintenance of the household, assistance with activities of daily living, maintenance of the caregiver's own life and needs, and fatigue (Jepson et al. 1999; Toseland et al. 1995).

Emotional Support Spouses identify emotional support as the most time-consuming aspect of care (Bakas et al. 2001). While the psychosocial status of caregivers tends to improve and distress seems to diminish over the first 3 to 6 months following diagnosis (Sherman and Simonton 2001), the provision of emotional support to the person with cancer remains a significant task during therapy and recovery. Caregivers, in assessing their ability to provide emotional support for patients, have identified that they, themselves, have educational needs in the area of interpersonal relations, communication, and provision of emotional support (Jepson et al. 1999; Kimberlin et al. 2004). No matter how strong the existing relationship between the caregiver and the person with cancer is, the demands for emotional support (due to fears about the effectiveness of therapy, side effects, and the possibility of relapse) in the setting of cancer therapy and recovery are significant and, as Yun's model implies, will likely exceed the experience of the caregiver.

Transportation Nonspousal caregivers (usually adult children or siblings of adults with cancer and parents of children with cancer) have identified transportation as the most time-consuming aspect of care provision (Bakas et al. 2001). These caregivers often have multiple responsibilities, including families and children, who place other demands on time, vehicles, and availability. Therefore, the caregivers are often placed in the difficult situation of choosing between two or more competing priorities.

Transportation of the cancer patient often involves much more than physical movement of the patient from place to place. Many outpatient chemotherapy regimens incorporate home infusion therapy, which requires a backpack (which may be pulled on wheels as opposed to worn on the back), weighing more than 30 lbs, to which the patient is continuously attached. Many patients and caregivers report that there is no easy way to secure these items on a wheelchair, walker, or in an automobile. Similarly, IV tubing is easily twisted, kinked, or even broken, during transport.

Other issues that may affect transportation must be addressed, including the physical stability, gait, and size of the person with cancer. Many cancer medications, such as lorazepam (used to control nausea and vomiting), can adversely affect stability. In addition, chemotherapy agents, such as vincristine and cisplatin, can cause peripheral neuropathy, which makes walking difficult and produces an unsteady gait. Finally, the size of the patient plays a large part in whether or not a caregiver can safely transport him (or her) to therapy. A petite spouse may be injured when a much larger patient loses balance and the caregiver tries to prevent a fall.

Monitoring Symptoms Monitoring symptoms, with the implications for medical care involved, is time consuming and emotionally burdensome for the caregiver (Bakas et al. 2001; Toseland et al. 1995). The caregiver must first learn a certain amount of medical information and accept the responsibility (emotionally, if not legally) for errors in judgment, and must accept the impact those errors might have on the patient's health, well-being, and chances of survival.

Caregivers often express concern during treatment and recovery that certain symptoms are indicative of disease progression. This concern is not always communicated to the patient and may not be communicated to the treating physician. Worsening pain is the most common symptom that causes this concern, however, any symptom, from a change in neurologic status to new lymphadenopathy, will provoke concern (Aranda et al. 2004).

Pain Control Pain, if present past the initial diagnosis period, requires different interventions and places different responsibilities on the caregiver (Cleeland et al. 1994; Walsh 2000). The caregiver must be taught management techniques to deal with pain associated with treatment (Ferrell et al. 1995). Drug tolerance becomes a more important issue and chronic pain may require ongoing narcotic administration, via an intravenous patient-controlled analgesia (PCA) pump, epidural catheter, sustained release oral preparations, or transdermal administration (Aranda et al. 2004). Management of breakthrough pain with short-acting opioids may also be necessary. While not all of these decisions belong to the caregiver alone, remembering to change transdermal patches and deciding when to give "breakthrough medications" often are the responsibilities of the caregiver and can be challenging.

In addition to the previously listed concerns surrounding the pain management, other social aspects unexpectedly emerge (Ferrell et al. 1991). For example, recent publicity surrounding the drug Oxycontin has caused substantial difficulties for patients and their caregivers (U.S. Government Accounting Office 2004). Some caregivers report experiences with pharmacists, who refused to fill legitimate Oxycontin prescriptions, and some people with cancer have reported having their medication stolen. Other people with cancer pain have stated that they fear for their own safety and hide the fact that pain medications are in their homes. Conditions such as these have caused the U.S. government to reexamine the FDA's policies on risk management in order to decrease the social dangers associated with the use of powerful opioids in people with severe pain (U.S. Government Accounting Office 2004).

Financial and Insurance Issues The caregiver, who must maintain employment outside of the home, will likely be faced with the necessity of returning to work while the patient is still receiving treatment (Hayman et al. 2001). The primary caregiver must then balance the needs of the patient, the demands of a job, and the needs involved in running a household. The Family Medical Leave Act of 1993 (FMLA; Public Law 103-3) allows 12 weeks of leave, but this is often without pay (The Family Medical Leave Act of 1993). Most caregivers utilize FMLA leave on an intermittent basis, allowing them to be present and provide care during actual treatments. They may then need to locate alternative caregivers for when the primary caregiver is at work.

Allocation of income then becomes an issue for some families, especially those with children at home (Yun et al. 2005). Up to 25% of the disposable income of a family will be consumed by medically related, nonreimbursed expenses. The patient needs may take priority over many other family needs during treatment and for months after the treatment is complete. Many families have residual financial obligations at the completion of chemotherapy.

Insurance issues may continue to pose problems for people with cancer and their caregivers during therapy and recovery. Many note the burden of a seemingly endless amount of paperwork. Rules, limitations on care, limitations on medications continue to cause confusion and fatigue in caregivers. Most caregivers do not have a concept of reinsurance and expect that it will be transparent to the patient (and, therefore, to them). This is not always the case. Reinsurance companies have their own case managers, may require that the family "start from scratch" in establishing a care plan, and may even require that some care providers be changed. This can be especially difficult on both patient and caregiver, for example, when a home care agency is changed.

Office copayments may also become a financial burden. As the provision of care is shifted to an outpatient setting, the financial burden of copayments increases significantly. Healthcare providers are contractually prohibited from waiving copayments and must make an effort to collect them. Many insurance companies include a provision in the coverage documents that stipulates that the insurance can be cancelled for failure to pay copayments. It is not unusual for a patient to require five office visits in a week that chemotherapy is administered, and $20 copayments quickly add up to a substantial financial burden.

The copayments on home care vary. While some plans cover home care at 100%, others cover only a percentage of the charges. It is important for the person with cancer and caregiver to understand the full limitations of coverage, and the patient responsibility for home care charges should be determined before agreeing to home care as part of the care management plan.

Respite care is an additional expense the family may face. The primary caregiver is often responsible for determining the availability of respite care, scheduling the care, and finding the financial resources to pay for it. Insurance companies typically do not cover the cost of respite care, therefore many families must call upon members of the extended family to assist with care on an intermittent basis. While the "respite" required in this setting may only be an evening or part of a day, meeting that need can be a daunting task for the caregiver (Jepson et al. 1999; Nijboer et al. 1998).

Stress and Fatigue Caregiver stress and fatigue is a well-documented event (Jensen and Given 1993; Nijboer et al. 1998; Nijboer et al. 1999). The basis of caregiver fatigue is multifactorial, and includes employment status, hours of caregiving required daily, health of the caregiver, emotional requirements of caregiving, and duration of the caregiving need (Gaston-Johansson et al 2004; Weitzner et al. 2000). However, none of these criteria are reliably predictable of caregiver fatigue.

Given the increasing importance of the caregiver role in the daily life of a person with cancer, medical providers must remain sensitive to the presence of caregiver stress and fatigue (Gaston-Johansson et al. 2004). Lewis (2004) reports her research on caregivers of women with breast cancer revealed that the stress of caregiving may be too much for many caregivers and they may never learn to cope or provide all types of care. In these cases, modifications of treatment regimens and home care plans may be necessary to ensure people with cancer receive the necessary home care (Lewis 2004). Due to the absence of a tool that easily measures caregiver fatigue, the healthcare providers remain responsible for an accurate assessment of caregiver status and capabilities.

Disease Progression and Terminal Care

Disease progression and terminal care may require long-term caregiving; however, they may also occur quickly or intermittently and so the caregiver needs during these phases are briefly addressed here.

When cancer recurs or progresses to advanced stages, the burdens of caregiving on the family change and can result in a decline in health of both the person with cancer and, as Yun et al. (2005) predict, the caregiver (Nijboer et al. 1998; Yun et al. 2005). Many studies report that most terminally ill cancer patients would prefer to die in their homes (Singer et al. 2005). However, achieving this goal is not as easy as it sounds. Providing terminal care at home can be physically and emotionally challenging for both the caregiver and the person with cancer. The primary concerns of recurrence and progression include symptom management, financial concerns, and emotional support for both the patient and the caregiver (Ferrario et al. 2004; Given et al. 2001).

Symptom Management As cancer progresses, treatments become less effective. During this phase, caregivers have the responsibility of identifying troublesome symptoms, deciding when to consult a clinician, and advocating for the patient's wishes (Given et al. 2001). They continue to face the stigma and fears associated with long-term use of narcotics and may be asked to master new skills and manage new routes of medication administration, such as intravenous patient-controlled analgesia (PCA).

While pain remains a tremendous concern, dyspnea, air hunger, and fatigue often become more troublesome for people as their cancer progresses (Wolfe et al. 2000). These symptoms can be difficult to manage and can contribute to fear and anxiety in the caregiver.

Financial Concerns The extended duration of the illness and the increasing intensity of care required during this period often result in caregivers quitting all work outside the home and focusing completely on the needs of the person with cancer (Pasacreta et al. 2000; Yun et al. 2005). Though the need for transportation and the copays associated with frequent medical bills may decrease, the sudden decrease in family income can create significant problems for caregivers and their families.

Emotional Support The most commonly reported emotional symptom of both care-givers and patients during disease progression is anxiety about what to expect (Singer et al. 2005). Both report the need for support and honesty from clinicians during this time. While more and more progressive disease is being managed at home with pal-liative care teams, the burden this intense care places on caregivers can put them at risk of long-term bereavement and pathologic grief (Ferrario et al. 2004). Clini-cians must assess caregivers' well-being and intervene when necessary, particularly in the area of emotional support (Bakas et al. 2001). Singer et al. (2005), however, report that though they experience great financial and emotional burdens, caregivers who provide end-of-life care at home are more likely to be satisfied with the care experience than those whose loved ones die in the hospital.

Special Concerns for Caregivers of Children with Cancer

Nearly all caregivers of children with cancer are their parents. As with adults, research on these caregivers has revealed that parent caregivers also suffer from uncertainty and physical and emotional strain (Svavarsdottir 2005). Parents report that their primary concern when providing care for a child with cancer is providing emotional support to that child. Other concerns include balancing work and caregiving activities, including transportation.

Caregivers of children with cancer are unique, however, in that many report that one of their most challenging primary concerns is providing emotional support to their partner, the child's other parent (Svavarsdottir 2005). This can place significant strain not only on the caregiver, but also on the marriage. Many couples separate or divorce during or after the serious illness or death of a child (Sirki et al. 2000). Like adult caregivers, however, caregivers of children with cancer report that their primary need is accurate information tailored specifically to the needs of their family (Lewis et al. 2005). Information would be helpful both for the caregiver role and for the family relationship.

Special Concerns for the Teenage/Young Adult Caregiver

Literature on young caregivers is sparse, and much is retrospective in nature. The incidence of children and teens caring for older adults is underestimated. There are many possible circumstances that place a child or teen in the position of a young caregiver. These include illness in a parent, grandparent, or other relative residing in the child's home. Even if the young person is not the primary caregiver, he or she may be asked to participate in care. In such instances, the young caregiver may face additional responsibilities and tasks, possible physical changes to the home environment, alterations to school schedules, and limitations on activities outside of school and the home, as well as the issues identified for adult caregivers (Gates and Lackey 1998).

The most common tasks assigned to young caregivers include running errands, household chores, assisting with meals, taking care of other children, providing companionship (not leaving an adult unattended), assistance with activities of daily living, and shopping (Gates and Lackey 1998; Hilton and Elfert 1996). A significant percentage of young caregivers are required to assist with personal care issues, including bathing, use of the bathroom, and dressing (Lackey and Gates 2001). They also administer medication. A small percentage of young caregivers have even reported that they had to deal with catheter care, colostomy care, or dressing changes (Lackey and Gates 2001).

For young caregivers, the school can be an invaluable time of respite. Many report that school is relatively protected time, and that schools in general are accommodating in meeting their specific needs. Some reported that they did have to miss a few days of school to accompany a patient for therapy or for a physician office visit, but many young caregivers also report that their school provided significant support for their situation. School is often viewed as a haven from caregiving. It is interesting to note, however, that most of the articles in the current literature pre-date the emphasis now placed on formal Individual Education Programs (IEPs) and Section 504 educational plans. The current focus in many school districts is that all accommodations of the educational process must be through these plans. The legislation establishing these plans does not address the issue of the child as a caregiver.

Fatigue is cited as the major issue for young caregivers. One study noted that the typical day for a young caregiver started at 6 A.M. and ended at 10 P.M. Most young caregivers cite the need for added rest—as opposed to tailored information—as their primary concern while serving as a caregiver.

Responsibilities of the Medical Community: Current Status and Future Direction

Education

As noted earlier in this chapter, many caregivers stress the desire to work with their physicians to create cancer treatment and home care plans that are tailored to the specific need of their families (Lewis et al. 2005). In addition, Stewart (1995) found better health outcomes in patients who had good communication with their providers than those who did not. Much of the literature suggests that new models of cancer care and new reimbursement strategies for care have placed the responsibility for identifying the needs of both patients and their family caregivers on healthcare providers (Merckaert et al. 2005). For physicians and nurses to be effective in this role, however, their educational programs must include courses on the development of excellent communication skills as well as the skills necessary to locate community resources and connect caregivers with these supports (Merckaert et al. 2005; Stewart 1995).

Currently, however, studies suggest that communication among healthcare providers and patients and/or caregivers is less than ideal (Horwitz et al. 1998;

Wissow et al. 2005). In one study, 81.1% of subjects reported that they had a psychosocial concern about a child that they thought was worthy of discussion with the child's physician, but only 41% of the subjects actually discussed the topic at the visit (Horwitz et al. 1998). Wissow et al. (2005) found that physicians may contribute to this lack of communication by dismissing or ignoring patient and/or caregiver hints of psychosocial distress. Merkert et al. (2005), however, found that communication skills training programs can be effective and highly recommended them to professionals caring for cancer patients and their families.

Research

Numerous studies have been completed or are currently under way, which examine the roles and needs of the caregivers of people with cancer. A brief OVID search yields about 600 citations (January 9, 2007). Currently, many focus on interventions which both support the caregiver in providing the needs of the ill family member and in maintaining their own health and mental/emotional well-being (Pasacreta and McCorkle 2000).

As suggested in the education section, future additional research is needed in the areas of communication between providers and caregivers as well as in identifying and providing the needs of caregivers in light of the limited resources of most healthcare practices.

Public Policy

Though much of the work of family caregivers often goes unseen, the needs of family caregivers have not gone unnoticed in the realm of public policy. Powerful lobbying groups such as the American Cancer Society have taken up the cause and addressed it with policy makers. Currently, in the 109th Congress, 75 bills mentioning caregivers, in some capacity, have been introduced into either the House or the Senate (Library of Congress 2005). Though the status of these bills is not yet resolved, updates on these and other bills can be found at http://thomas.loc.gov/.

In the realm of public law, however, one of the most significant acts affecting caregivers has been the Family Medical Leave Act of 1993 (Public Law 103–3). As mentioned earlier, this act allows 12 weeks of leave without pay ("The Family Medical Leave Act of 1993"). Most caregivers utilize FMLA leave on an intermittent basis, allowing them to be present and provide care during actual treatments without fear of losing their job.

While this has done a lot to allow families to remain financially stable while acting as caregivers, it has not provided much for the physical and emotional health of those who need to utilize it. Further public policies are needed to support the work of home caregiving and to provide much-needed respite care.

Conclusion

The discussion in this chapter has demonstrated that the medical community does not yet fully respond to the needs of caregivers or recognize the important role that they play in total patient care (Bakas et al. 2001; Given et al. 2001; Jansma et al. 2005). While virtually every article referenced on caregiving indicated the necessity for further study, it is clear that the medical community must respond to the already well-demonstrated needs of caregivers, both for the health of the primary patient as well as the health and well-being of the caregivers. As illustrated in Yun's Caregiver Burden Model, healthcare providers must work to decrease caregiver burden to improve caregiver's quality of life and thus make the caregiving experience more effective and rewarding.

The future response of the medical community to the needs of caregivers should include a concerted effort to provide:

1. Recognition that cancer is a family illness and family caregivers are a valuable part of the patient care team.
2. Quality printed educational material for patient and caregiver with appropriate, tailored emphasis for each recipient, and geared for specific stages of the disease process (diagnosis, treatment, follow-up).
3. Assessment of caregiver skills and interventions designed to improve the skills needed to provide care.
4. Advocacy support for dealing with insurance and financial issues.
5. Support groups and other interventions whose purpose is to improve the support skills of the caregiver, as well as the provision of emotional support.
6. Assessment of caregiver ability to continue to provide the level of care demanded by the patient's medical condition. Caregiver fatigue, job status, and additional family obligations must be considered and analyzed in an ongoing fashion. This will serve to protect the health of the caregiver, and the safety of the patient.

Caregivers are the often-unrecognized backbone of the healthcare team. Their participation in the care of the person with cancer is both demanded and essential. Studies have shown that with the right support, providing care for a loved one with cancer can be an overall positive experience (Singer et al. 2005; Weitzner et al. 2000). Ample research has been done to document many of the needs of these individuals, from emotional and educational support to practical assistance in the provision of transportation and running of a household. They require and deserve support for their efforts, their needs, and their own lives as they provide care and service to a family member with cancer.

References

Aranda, S., Yates, P., Edwards, H., Nash, R., Skerman, H., & McCarthy, A. (2004). Barriers to effective cancer pain management: A survey of Australian family caregivers. *European Journal of Cancer Care, 13*(4), 336–343.

Bakas, T., Lewis, R. R., & Parsons, J. E. (2001). Caregiving tasks among family caregivers of patients with lung cancer. *Oncology Nursing Forum, 28*(5), 847–854.

Chan, C. W. H., & Chang, A. M. (1999). Managing caregiver tasks among family caregivers of cancer patients in Hong Kong. *Journal of Advanced Nursing, 29*(2), 484–489.

Cleeland, C. S., Gonin, R., Hatfield, A. K., Edmonson, J. H., Blum, R. H., Stewart, J. A., et al. (1994). Pain and its treatment in outpatients with metastatic cancer. *New England Journal of Medicine, 330*(9), 592–596 (see comment).

Dahl, J. H., & Portenoy, R. K. (2004). Myths about controlling pain. Reprinted with permission of the Mayday Fund. *Journal of Pain & Palliative Care Pharmacotherapy, 18*(3), 55–58.

Ferrario, S. R., Cardillo, V., Vicario, F., Balzarini, E., & Zotti, A. M. (2004). Advanced cancer at home: Caregiving and bereavement. *Palliative Medicine, 18*(2), 129–136.

Ferrell, B. R., Cohen, M. Z., Rhiner, M., & Rozek, A. (1991). Pain as a metaphor for illness. Part ii: Family caregivers' management of pain. *Oncology Nursing Forum, 18*(8), 1315–1321.

Ferrell, B. R., Grant, M., Chan, J., Ahn, C., & Ferrell, B. A. (1995). The impact of cancer pain education on family caregivers of elderly patients. *Oncology Nursing Forum, 22*(8), 1211–1218.

Gaston-Johansson, F., Lachica, E. M., Fall-Dickson, J. M., & Kennedy, M. J. (2004). Psychological distress, fatigue, burden of care, and quality of life in primary caregivers of patients with breast cancer undergoing autologous bone marrow transplantation. *Oncology Nursing Forum, 31*(6), 1161–1169.

Gates, M. F., & Lackey, N. R. (1998). Youngsters caring for adults with cancer. *Image: The Journal of Nursing Scholarship, 30*(1), 11–15.

Given, B. A., Given, C. W., & Kozachik, S. (2001). Family support in advanced cancer. *CA: A Cancer Journal for Clinicians, 51*(4), 213–231.

Harden, J. (2005). Developmental life stage and couples' experiences with prostate cancer: A review of the literature. *Cancer Nursing, 28*(2), 85–98.

Harden, J., Schafenacker, A., Northouse, L., Mood, D., Smith, D., Pienta, K., et al. (2002). Couples' experiences with prostate cancer: Focus group research. *Oncology Nursing Forum, 29*(4), 701–709.

Hardwick, C., & Lawson, N. (1995). The information and learning needs of the caregiving family of the adult patient with cancer. *European Journal of Cancer Care, 4*(3), 118–121.

Hayman, J. A., Langa, K. M., Kabeto, M. U., Katz, S. J., DeMonner, S. M., Chernew, M. E., et al. (2001). Estimating the cost of informal caregiving for elderly patients with cancer. *Journal of Clinical Oncology, 19*(13), 3219–3225.

Hilton, B. A., & Elfert, H. (1996). Children's experiences with mothers' early breast cancer. *Cancer Practice, 4*(2), 96–104.

Horwitz, S. M., Leaf, P. J., & Leventhal, J. M. (1998). Identification of psychosocial problems in pediatric primary care: Do family attitudes make a difference? *Archives of Pediatrics & Adolescent Medicine, 152*(4), 367–371.

Jansma, F. F. I., Schure, L. M., & de Jong, B. M. (2005). Support requirements for caregivers of patients with palliative cancer. *Patient Education and Counseling, 58*(2), 182–186.

Jensen, S., & Given, B. A. (1991). Fatigue affecting family caregivers of cancer patients. *Cancer Nursing, 14*(4), 181–187.

Jensen, S., & Given, B. A. (1993). Fatigue affecting family caregivers of cancer patients. *Supportive Care in Cancer, 1*(6), 321–325 (see comment).

Jepson, C., McCorkle, R., Adler, D., Nuamah, I., & Lusk, E. (1999). Effects of home care on caregivers' psychosocial status. *Image: The Journal of Nursing Scholarship, 31*(2), 115–120.

Kimberlin, C., Brushwood, D., Allen, W., Radson, E., & Wilson, D. (2004). Cancer patient and caregiver experiences: Communication and pain management issues. *Journal of Pain and Symptom Management, 28*(6), 566–578.

Lackey, N. R., & Gates, M. F. (2001). Adults' recollections of their experiences as young caregivers of family members with chronic physical illnesses. *Journal of Advanced Nursing, 34*(3), 320–328.

Laizner, A. M., Yost, L. M. S., Barg, F. K., & McCorkle, R. (1993). Needs of family caregivers of persons with cancer: A review. *Seminars in Oncology Nursing, 9*(2), 114–120.

Lewis, F. M. (2004). Family-focused oncology nursing research. *Oncology Nursing Forum, 31*(2), 288–292.

Lewis, D., Gundwardena, S., & El Saadawi, G. (2005). Caring connection: Developing an internet resource for family caregivers of children with cancer. *CIN: Computers, Informatics, Nursing, 23*(5), 265–274.

Library of Congress. (2005). Thomas. Retrieved from http://thomas.loc.gov/. Accessed 6 Jan 2007.

Merckaert, I., Libert, Y., & Razavi, D. (2005). Communication skills training in cancer care: Where are we and where are we going? *Current Opinion in Oncology, 17*(4), 319–330.

Nijboer, C., Tempelaar, R., Sanderman, R., Triemstra, M., Spruijt, R. J., & Van Den Bos, G. A. M. (1998). Cancer and caregiving: The impact on the caregiver's health. *Psycho-Oncology, 7*(1), 3–13.

Nijboer, C., Triemstra, M., Tempelaar, R., Sanderman, R., & Van Den Bos, G. A. (1999). Determinants of caregiving experiences and mental health of partners of cancer patients. *Cancer, 86*(4), 577–588.

Nijboer, C., Triemstra, M., Tempelaar, R., Mulder, M., Sanderman, R., & Van Den Bos, G. A. (2000). Patterns of caregiver experiences among partners of cancer patients. *Gerontologist, 40*(6), 738–746.

Oberst, M. T., Thomas, S. E., Gass, K. A., & Ward, S. E. (1989). Caregiving demands and appraisal of stress among family caregivers. *Cancer Nursing, 12*(4), 209–215.

Pasacreta, J. V., & McCorkle, R. (2000). Cancer care: Impact of interventions on caregiver outcomes. *Annual Review of Nursing Research, 18,*127–148.

Pasacreta, J. V., Barg, F., Nuamah, I., & McCorkle, R. (2000). Participant characteristics before and 4 months after attendance at a family caregiver cancer education program. *Cancer Nursing, 23*(4), 295–303.

Raveis, V. H., & Pretter, S. (2005). Existential plight of adult daughters following their mother's breast cancer diagnosis. *Psycho-Oncology, 14*(1), 49–60.

Rivera, L. M. (1997). Blood cell transplantation: Its impact on one family. *Seminars in Oncology Nursing, 13*(3), 194–199.

Sarna, L., & McCorkle, R. (1996). Burden of care and lung cancer. *Cancer Practice, 4*(5), 245–251.

Schumacher, K. L. (1996). Reconceptualizing family caregiving: Family-based illness care during chemotherapy. *Research in Nursing & Health, 19*(4), 261–271.

Schumacher, K. L., Stewart, B. J., Archbold, P. G., Dodd, M. J., & Dibble, S. L. (2000). Family caregiving skill: Development of the concept. *Research in Nursing & Health, 23*(3), 191–203.

Sherman, A. C., & Simonton, S. (2001). Coping with cancer in the family. *Family Journal: Counseling and Therapy for Couples and Families, 9*(2), 193–200.

Singer, Y., Bachner, Y. G., Shvartzman, P., & Carmel, S. (2005). Home death: The caregivers' experiences. *Journal of Pain & Symptom Management, 30*(1), 70–74.

Sirki, K., Saarinen-Pihkala, U. M., & Hovi, L. (2000). Coping of parents and siblings with the death of a child with cancer: Death after terminal care compared with death during active anticancer therapy. *Acta Paediatrica, 89*(6), 717–721.

Stetz, K. M., & Brown, M. A. (1997). Taking care: Caregiving to persons with cancer and AIDS. *Cancer Nursing, 20*(1), 12–22.

Stewart, M. A. (1995). Effective physician-patient communication and health outcomes: A review. *Canadian Medical Association Journal, 152*(9), 1423–1433 (see comment).

Svavarsdottir, E. K. (2005). Caring for a child with cancer: A longitudinal perspective. *Journal of Advanced Nursing, 50*(2), 153–161.

The Family Medical Leave Act of 1993, P. L. 103-3. *United States Senate*. Retrieved from http://www.dol.gov/esa/regs/statutes/whd/fmla.htm. Accessed 6 Jan 2007.

Toseland, R. W., Blanchard, C. G., & McCallion, P. (1995). A problem solving intervention for caregivers of cancer patients. *Social Science & Medicine, 40*(4), 517–528.

U.S. Government Accounting Office. (2004). Oxycontin abuse and diversion and efforts to address the problem: Highlights of a government report. *Journal of Pain & Palliative Care Pharmacotherapy, 18*(3), 109–113.

Veach, T. A., & Nicholas, D. R. (1998). Understanding families of adults with cancer: Combining the clinical course of cancer and stages of family development. *Journal of Counseling & Development, 76*(2), 144–156.

Walsh, D. (2000). Pharmacological management of cancer pain. *Seminars in Oncology, 27*(1), 45–63.

Weisman, A. D., & Worden, J. (1977). The existential plight in cancer: Significance of the first 100 days. *International Journal of Psychiatry in Medicine, 7*(1), 1–15.

Weitzner, M. A., Haley, W. E., & Chen, H. (2000). The family caregiver of the older cancer patient. *Hematology: Oncology Clinics of North America, 14*(1), 269–281.

Wissow, L. S., Larson, S., Anderson, J., & Hadjiisky, E. (2005). Pediatric residents' responses that discourage discussion of psychosocial problems in primary care. *Pediatrics, 115*(6), 1569–1578.

Wolfe, J., Grier, H. E., Klar, N., Levin, S. B., Ellenbogen, J. M., Salem-Schatz, S., et al. (2000). Symptoms and suffering at the end of life in children with cancer. *New England Journal of Medicine, 342*(5), 326–333.

Yun, Y. H., Rhee, Y. S., Kang, I. O., Lee, J. S., Bang, S. M., Lee, W. S., et al. (2005). Economic burdens and quality of life of family caregivers of cancer patients. *Oncology, 68*(2–3), 107–114.

Chapter 8
Issues in Caregiving for Cancer Patients with Long-Term Care Needs

Barry J. Jacobs

As survival rates for even the most lethal forms of cancer have increased over the past several decades, more and more cancer survivors and their caregivers have had to live with the disease as a long-term, chronic stressor affecting the quality of their llives. This chapter will cull the research, educational and clinical literatures about long-term cancer caregiving to provide an overview of some of the key issues–including late effects of medical treatments, psychological consequences of caregiving, decreased social supports, and financial strain– with which many families have to contend. A case vignette will be used to illustrate these issues and to suggest means by which families can live as well as possible with cancer over extended periods of time.

Mrs. Lucas' husband, Bert Lucas, a retired minister, is part of an increasing cadre of Americans who are long-term survivors of cancer. Because of the progress in early detection and treatments, the number of those living with cancer and its residual effects rose sharply in the last several decades from 3 million in 1971 to over 10 million in 2002 (National Cancer Institute 2006a). According to the Annual Report to the Nation on the Status of Cancer, overall cancer death rates in the United States decreased by 1.1% per year from 1993 through 2002; for men, death rates declined for 12 of the 15 most common cancers; for women, death rates declined in 9 of the 15 most common cancers (Edwards et al. 2005). Survival rates for even the most lethal forms of cancer have increased. The patients with advanced non-small-cell lung cancer are living longer when administered newer chemotherapeutic agents and a platinum derivative (Winton et al. 2005). The use of multiple chemotherapeutic agents has also meant that patients with ovarian cancer are surviving for increasing lengths of time with periodic recurrences requiring treatments as they might with any other chronic disease (Markman 2005; Tummala and McGuire 2005).

In response to these increased survival rates, the "cancer survivorship" movement has taken shape over the past 25 years. In 1986, a group of cancer researchers and educators formed a patient-led advocacy group called the National Coalition for

B. J. Jacobs (✉)
Crozer-Keystone Family Medicine Residency Program, 1260 E. Woodland Avenue, 19094 Springfield, PA, USA
e-mail: barry.jacobs@crozer.org

R. C. Talley et al. (eds.), *Cancer Caregiving in the United States*,
Caregiving: Research, Practice, Policy,
DOI 10.1007/978-1-4614-3154-1_8, © Springer Science+Business Media, LLC 2012

Cancer Survivorship to provide support services to the growing number of patients who were living longer after being diagnosed with cancer, and to encourage the study of those cancer survivors (National Coalition for Cancer Survivorship 2006). Partly, as a result of that group's pioneering efforts, there has been an upsurge in research articles over the past 15 years on "cancer survivorship" (Aziz and Rowland 2003; Deimling et al. 2002). Many of these studies explore the "quality of life" issues faced by cancer survivors (Abendstein et al. 2005; Carver et al. 2006; Ferrell et al. 2005; Ganz et al. 2002; Northouse et al. 2002), including physical sequelae, changes in emotional well-being, spiritual meanings, and financial implications. In 1996, the National Institute of Health's National Cancer Institute formed its own Office of Cancer Survivorship "in recognition of the large number of individuals now surviving for long periods of time and their unique and poorly understood needs" (National Cancer Institute 2006b).

Just as it took time for cancer survivors to receive the attention of researchers and policymakers, the lives of those survivors' family caregivers, like Mrs. Lucas, have only begun to be studied extensively. This research is necessarily complex, attempting to understand the impact of multiple, interacting variables in order to answer the following questions: How are family caregivers affected by caring for a loved one with cancer over long periods of time? Which components of the caregiving experience have the greatest impact on family members' capacities for coping? Does the family's coping affect the patient's coping, and vice versa? Does the quality of family caregiving influence the patient's clinical outcomes and survival? Does the patient's clinical outcome affect family caregivers' long-term psychological adjustment? After arriving at their own answers to these questions, a few authors have gone on to devise specific family educational and clinical interventions to help relatives better endure cancer caregiving's arduous demands (Given et al. 2004; McMillan et al. 2006; Northouse 2005; Northouse et al. 2005).

This chapter will cull the research, educational, and clinical literatures about long-term cancer caregiving to provide an overview of some of the key issues with which family members have to contend. The conclusions that will be drawn about future directions for practice, education, research, and policy will aim to address one specific question: How can we create conditions for families like the Lucas' to live as well as possible over time with the specter of cancer in their lives?

Cancer as a Stressful Chronic Disease

There have been many aspects of her husband's ordeal with cancer over the last 4 years that have troubled Mrs. Lucas. Early on, accompanying him to the hospital for the stem cell transplant and then weeks of chemotherapy was extremely wearying. However, at least at that time, her three adult sons, along with their wives, traveled frequently from their out-of-town homes to support their parents. After the initial period of her husband's intensive treatments, however, their children became focused again on their own lives and families and visited less frequently. Mrs. Lucas began to experience a lack of family support. Unfortunately, she was reluctant to ask members of her husband's former congregation to help them for fear of imposing her burdens upon them. Instead, she took solely upon herself the many helper roles her husband needed—she became a nurse to dole him pills, a nurse's aide to help him get back and forth to the bathroom several times a night, a chauffeur to transport him from one medical office to another, a cook to make nutritious meals for him, a cheerleader to rally him, and, as often as not, a decision-maker to tell him what to do since despondency had robbed him of his self-sufficiency and confidence. She would not mind playing those roles if he were at least appreciative, but he seemed to take her efforts for granted. She consequently felt trapped in a daily grind of chores and obligations that gave her little gratification. This made her sad and resentful and caused her to question why God had chosen to punish them so.

There are many factors that appear to be affecting Mrs. Lucas' coping and her capacity for taking care of her husband, including the nature of her husband's disease and its residual effects, his mood and responses to her efforts, her degree of family and social support, her capacity for shifting to new family roles, the degree of satisfaction she derives from her relationship with her husband, her overall mood, and her appraisal of the caregiving situation. While many of them are interrelated, examining some of them separately will provide insight into the effects of long-term cancer caregiving in general.

The Disease's Severity, Course, and Late Effects

Theorists who have created conceptual models for understanding the impact of any chronic illness upon families have long posited that a disease's severity and course weigh heavily on the family's capacity for coping because sicker patients are more debilitated and need more care (Rolland 1994). In studies of the impact of cancer, numerous authors have suggested that the more advanced the stage of the disease, the greater the emotional duress suffered by the patient; this is likely due to cancer's potential threat to life and to the fact that sicker individuals need more invasive and distressing treatments (Halford et al. 2000). As the patient goes, so often go the family caregivers. Wellisch (1995) cited two studies (Cancer Care Inc. and National Cancer Foundation 1977; Koocher and O'Malley 1981) in which there was "found to be a positive correlation between length and severity of illness and measures of dysfunction in family members" (p. 389).

Recent studies of long-term cancer survivors raise other concerns for family members. In a review of the literature, Aziz and Rowland (2003) concluded that:

It is becoming an acknowledged fact that most cancer treatment options available and in use today will affect the future health and life of those diagnosed with this disease. Adverse cancer treatment-related sequelae thus carry the potential to contribute to the ongoing burden of illness, health care costs, and decrease length and quality of survival (p. 258).

This has been researched most extensively with pediatric cancer survivors. Bhatia (2005) found that, as a result of the toxicity of cancer treatments and/or an individual's genetic propensity to develop cancer, "approximately two thirds of the survivors of childhood cancer will experience at least one late effect, and about one third will experience a late effect that is severe or life-threatening." Such effects include "impairment in growth and development, neurocognitive dysfunction, cardiopulmonary compromise, endocrine dysfunction, renal impairment, gastrointestinal dysfunction, musculoskeletal sequelae, and subsequent malignancies." An overview of the Childhood Cancer Survivor Study of over 14,000 pediatric cancer survivors noted similar results, but also cited additional complications such as "pregnancy loss, giving birth to offspring with low birth weights, and decreased educational attainment" (Robison 2005). While none of these researchers directly address the implications for family caregivers, it stands to reason that the likelihood of late medical effects creates a degree of uncertainty about the future health of loved ones that negatively impact relatives' coping. The actual advent of such effects will probably increase caregivers' burden and distress.

Mrs. Lucas has had to deal with the delayed effects of her husband's cancer treatments within months of his diagnosis. While she realizes that the neuropathic pain he now suffers is not his fault, she finds his constant complaints of burning sensations and his inability to engage in physical chores both grating and burdensome. Occasionally, she becomes so frustrated that she urges him to overcome his pain and do more. That only prompts Mr. Lucas to feel misunderstood and accuse her of being uncaring. This response adds to Mrs. Lucas' frustration and sense of hopelessness.

Caregiver Factors: Personality and Appraisal

While the characteristics of the patient's disease have an impact on patient and caregiver coping, other factors may have even greater import. Compas et al. (1994) found that the severity of the cancer was only moderately related to the degree of anxiety or depression a patient suffered. Other authors have reached similar conclusions about the patient's relatives, arguing that attributes of the family members themselves, rather than the specifics of the cancer, are more predictive of difficulties of coping among caregivers (Given et al. 2004). This is consistent with the research finding that the effects of caregiving vary widely among family members even when they are dealing with similar patient medical circumstances (Braithwaite 2000).

Both personality characteristics and appraisal have been widely studied and linked with caregiver depression. In their review of the personality literature, Nijboer et al. (2001) noted that mastery, neuroticism (defined as a state of being "anxious, moody, and frequently depressed"), and extraversion are traits that have been associated with depression, especially during stressful times, and that caregivers with a greater sense of mastery and a lower degree of neuroticism were less prone to depression. In their own study of 148 colorectal cancer patients and their partners over 6 months post-hospital discharge, they found that caregivers' depression was "strongly predicted" by neuroticism and to a lesser degree by mastery and extraversion. Kim et al. (2005)

studied 120 spouses of lung cancer patients and arrived at similar results, finding that "neuroticism was directly associated with greater depressive symptoms" (Interestingly, both studies linked high neuroticism with lower levels of social support, another factor discussed below). While it would not be immediately evident that personality characteristics—stable, crystallized, long-term traits—could be amenable to change by clinical interventions, Nijboer et al. (2001) suggested that by providing caregivers with skills to give them a greater sense of mastery and ensuring that they have positive interactions with the patients, healthcare professionals can decrease rates of caregiver depression.

Other researchers have focused on a related but distinct attribute of family members: caregiver appraisal. Defined variously as the way a caregiver perceives the patient's condition and the need for caregiving or the meanings that she attributes to the medical ordeal, appraisals are seen as attitudes or beliefs that shape the ways family caregivers react emotionally and determine their quality of life (Mellon 2002; Oberst et al. 1989; Skerrett 1998). An example of a positive appraisal is viewing caregiving as an opportunity to make a crucial difference in the life of a loved one and to reinforce family bonds (Mellon 2002). Caregivers with this appraisal are more likely to feel gratified by their role and be more resilient handling its rigors over time. An example of a negative appraisal is viewing caregiving as a form of entrapment foisted upon obligated family members; caregivers who adopt this perspective are more likely to feel burdened by their duties and become depleted and depressed in the long term.

A common negative appraisal occurs when long-term cancer caregivers persistently fear that the patient's cancer is going to recur, increasing their stress and detrimentally impacting their quality of life (Mellon 2002; Mellon and Northouse 2001). Living with uncertainty of the future because of such fears can detract from the family's capacity to focus upon non-illness-related needs. The family thus loses its ability to generate hope. For example, Weihs and Reiss (2000) posted that families dealing with long-term cancer care must move between being "living centered" (i.e., focusing on all family members' developmental needs) and "cancer-centered" (i.e., devoting most of the family's resources to the patient's medical needs). Family members who appraise each of the patient's somatic complaints as a possible indication that the cancer is recurring will remain cancer-centered, thereby neglecting the developmental needs of other family members.

The concept of caregiver appraisal has clinical utility. By devising a psychometric instrument for measuring caregivers' appraisals, Cooper et al. (2006) sought a means of identifying early on those caregivers who were at greatest risk for eventually experiencing distress. They also hoped to garner content-specific information about the caregivers' beliefs in order to design interventions and promote their well-being. Mellon (2002) contended that caregivers' negative appraisals could be countered by assisting them in "finding positive meaning [to] reframe the cancer experience … and tap into spiritual beliefs and practices … to enhance family quality of life."

Mrs. Lucas' personality has always been introverted and meek with a moderate degree of neuroticism and relatively low levels of mastery. Her belief that God is unfairly punishing her and her husband is a type of negative appraisal called "negative coping" (Koenig et al. 1998). It is associated with a greater likelihood of depression and poorer health. Training in coping techniques, such as relaxation exercises and assertiveness, could decrease her propensity toward frustration and neuroticism and help her to ask her family more directly for assistance. Speaking with a pastor or healthcare professional about her cancer experience may allow her to shift her perspective to a more positive one—e.g., God is testing, not punishing, her. These interventions would have positive implications for her psychological adjustment to the chronic medical situation.

Family and Social Support

A common finding of research on adjustment to chronic illness in general is that family and social support—including assistance with activities of daily living, financial aid, and emotional support—improves the psychological status of most patients. Similar results have been found with the effects of family and social support on individuals with cancer (Grassi and Rosti 1996; Northouse 1988). It is not surprising that family caregivers of patients with a wide variety of acute and chronic illnesses also experience increased well-being as the result of receiving family and social support (Cameron et al. 2006; Raina et al. 2005). Halford et al. (2000) posited that when cancer patients and their family caregivers feel mutually supported by one another, the beneficial psychological effects appear to be greater for each of them.

Nijboer et al. (2001) found more complicated relationships between family, social support, and caregiver well-being. Their research revealed "social support ... is beneficial for caregivers and mitigates the relation between stressors (in this case, patient's depression and negative caregiver experiences) and caregiver's depression to a limited degree" (p. 1036). In specific, the authors found that "less negative interactions were predictive of a favorable caregiver outcome in the long term" and that daily emotional support acted "as a moderator of the relation between negative caregiver experiences and caregiver's depression" (p. 1036), but they hastened to add that caregivers do not perceive all support positively; it can be construed as a negative influence. Well-intended support that fails to actually provide help to the family members can actually increase caregiver psychological distress. For example, advice from others may make caregivers feel as if they are being criticized for either doing things wrong or not doing enough.

Cancer caregivers who are isolated from extended family members, friends, and neighbors and therefore lack family and social support and may have a more difficult time coping, especially over time. In the absence of helpful relatives or acquaintances, many of these caregivers come to rely upon healthcare and social service professionals to a greater degree (see "Professional Support"). Even when willing family members and friends are available though, there are several potential obstacles to the use and ongoing benefit of the support they could provide.

Shifts in Family Roles. Conflicts can arise over the shifts in family roles necessitated by the decreased functioning of the ill family member. For example, if the primary breadwinner stops working for an extended period of time to undergo intensive chemotherapy, then other family members may have to take jobs to earn money in order to make up for the loss of income due to their loved one's medical disability. Some of these relatives may have difficulty adjusting to these role changes. They may resist and resent them, particularly if the changes go on for many months and threaten to become permanent, and thereby begrudge supporting the family in that manner.

Breakdown of Communication. A second obstacle to mutual family support is the breakdown of effective communication among family members. Effective communication in cancer caregiving generally consists of openly discussing details of the disease, its treatments, and their impact upon the family in order to negotiate an equitable family caregiving plan, but as Wellisch (1995) points out, many families fighting cancer adopt a communication style that is more a "veil of silence" to protect each other and themselves from provoking unbearable feelings of fear, anger, and sadness. However, when family members do not negotiate openly in their dealings with cancer or give voice to the feelings they have, they may fail to adequately address problems, make decisions, or express the caring that is essential for weathering the prolonged medical crisis.

Quality of Relationships. A third obstacle to the provision of support may be caused by the quality of the relationships among family members and friends. This can take numerous forms. In some families and social circles, there is too little love, commitment, and cohesion prior to a patient's diagnosis with cancer to serve as a prerequisite for support once relatives and acquaintances are faced with the uncertainties and sacrifices of long-term cancer caregiving. Those who do agree to support the patient may not have enough investment in his well-being to uphold their commitment throughout the months and years in which help is needed. As a general rule, caregiving families tend to become more socially isolated over time because friends feel uncomfortable dealing with the effects of illness and consequently withdraw. Family members also tend to focus more narrowly on illness concerns over time and cease reaching out to others with whom they feel they have less in common. Rolland (1994) wrote extensively about the negative changes in family relationships, or what he called "relationship skews," that undermine intimacy and closeness when medical issues come to dominate the interactions among relatives. In an extended case study of a young couple dealing with the husband's lung cancer with brain metastases, Rolland (1997) depicted how a patient's development of cognitive impairments necessarily skewed the power, decision-making, and capacity for emotional sharing between the spouses.

Willingness to Accept Support. Caregiving family members experience varying degrees of willingness to accept or resist support (Jacobs 2006). Caregivers sometimes express reluctance to ask for help or utilize aid that is offered because they do not want "handouts"; they feel that caring for their family member is their duty and believe that accepting support would be tantamount to shirking that responsibility. It is frequently difficult to convince them that making use of family and social support would likely help them conserve their energies and render them better able to provide care to their loved one over time, especially in a long-term caregiving situation.

The fact that Mrs. Lucas' sons and their families live at a distance from her and her husband makes family support hard to come by for her caregiving efforts. This is compounded by Mr. Lucas' lack of appreciation for all that she does because he is self-absorbed by his own cancer fears. However, Mrs. Lucas' reticence about accepting the help of their former congregants and other kinds of social support is due to her own shyness and pride. By not reaching out more, she puts herself at greater risk of developing caregiver distress over the long term.

Professional Support

There is a wide array of professional services available to family caregivers to support them in their care of cancer patients, including clinical services (e.g., physicians, physical therapists, home health nurses and aides), social services (e.g., case management, Meals on Wheels, support groups, transportation programs, respite), and legal and financial services (e.g., attorneys, financial planners). The many cancer Websites, including those run by the American Cancer Society and the National Cancer Institute, provide a general overview of what these services entail, but not where to find them in local communities. Regional cancer centers are a better source of local information and referrals for patients and caregivers. To the degree that cancer caregivers are able to avail themselves of professional support, they are likely to cope better through their loved one's on-going medical predicament.

A key issue for caregivers in taking advantage of these services is how to work effectively with the available professionals. Good communication is crucial in this endeavor. Caregivers often become concerned when professionals have not communicated fully or properly to them the ramifications of different treatment options for the patient. For example, Seaburn (2001) described his anger when his father, dying from metastatic colon cancer, was transferred from an acute care to a subacute unit within the same medical center; he learned after the fact that the oncologist they had worked with for years would not continue treating his father in the new setting. It is not surprising that many guides for family caregivers include tips on how to communicate effectively with professionals in order to form partnerships or teams (National Cancer Institute 2006c; National Family Caregivers Association 2006). The professional oncology literature includes many research articles on teaching oncologists and nurses effective means of sharing medical information—such as prognoses—with patients and their family members (e.g., Baile and Aaron 2005).

While Mrs. Lucas has limited family and social support, she has garnered greater professional support. Her sons convinced her to hire a home health aide to come to her home three mornings a week to help bathe and groom her husband. (She is worried about the cost of this professional service, but is continuing it for the time being.) She has a good rapport with her husband's oncologist and feels that she can call him at any time with questions. The nurses at the cancer center have always been very friendly and supportive and have helped her maintain her morale.

Financial Strain

Many authors have noted that long-term caregiving often strains families' finances (Wagner 2004). Caregiving costs fall into three categories: out-of-pocket expenses for medical services not covered by insurance, out-of-pocket expenses for nonmedical services and items considered essential for the comfort of the ill loved one, and wages lost because the caregiver must take a leave or time off from a job in order to provide care.

For many families engaged in long-term cancer caregiving, the degree of financial strain is significant (for those families of patients who need experimental drugs not covered by any health insurance, the costs can be catastrophic). Yun et al. (2005) found that loss of family income was most strongly associated with caregiver burden and suggested that the best way of improving the quality of life of caregivers was creating means of easing their financial strain (also see Bergamini, this book). In contrast, Lauzier et al. (2005) found that the economic costs of long-term treatment for breast cancer were substantial, "but were not the most worrisome aspect of the illness during treatments." Early studies estimated that the nonmedical costs of childhood cancer patients plus family wages lost amounted to 25% of weekly family income (Lansky et al. 1979) or 38% of gross annual family income (Bloom et al. 1985). More recent research has looked at the indirect costs borne by families: receiving treatments such as chemotherapy (Moore 1998); suffering side-effects, such as toxicity (Calhoun et al. 2001) and pain (Fortner et al. 2003); falling into special populations, such as breast cancer patients (Moore 1999) and the elderly (Hayman et al. 2001); or using particular services, such as home care (Stommel et al. 1993). These researchers have found expenses that are wide-ranging but, in almost all instances, significant. When long-term cancer caregiving families use their life savings to provide for a loved one, it is likely that the resulting economic depletion will hamper their abilities to address other vital family needs.

Because Mr. Lucas had to retire early when he was diagnosed with multiple myeloma and Mrs. Lucas gave up her part-time job as caregiving duties took up her time, they are less well off financially than they had hoped to be at the time they stopped working. Now living on a fixed pension while paying for nonmedical services like a home health aide, Mrs. Lucas has to tap into her savings each month to pay the regular bills. She is plagued with the constant worry that she and her husband will run out of money before they both die.

Caregiver Distress

A major concern for family members is how the burden of long-term caregiving affects their psychological well-being. The extensive research on the topic, conducted primarily with the relatives of demented patients, has produced alarming results.

These caregivers suffer higher rates of depression and anxiety than same-age peers who are not caregivers (Schulz and Martire 2004). These effects seem to persist even after the patient has died and the caregiving has ended. In a study of surviving spouses of patients with dementia, Robinson-Whelen et al. (2001) found that, though levels of stress decreased after the patient died, levels of depression and loneliness remained high for up to 3 years. They speculated that the chronic depression is largely due to continued ruminations about the caregiving experience.

Research on the psychological effects of long-term cancer caregiving on family members has yielded mixed results. Some authors concluded that while caregivers suffer depression at the time of the patient's diagnosis and treatments, the majority of patients and family members return to premorbid levels of stress and mood (Grassi and Rosti 1996; Kupst et al. 1995). In contrast, Given et al. (2004) found caregivers' moods to reach threshold levels of clinical depression up to a year following the cancer diagnosis. They also found that caregivers' depression was most strongly associated with the patients' cancer- and treatment-related symptoms. A weaker association was discerned between caregivers' degree of depression and their relationship with the care receiver. Depression was also to some degree related to the caregiver's current employment status. Employment outside the home was found to decrease depression for spouse caregivers, but not for adult children taking care of a cancer-stricken parent. Cameron et al. (2002) concluded that cancer caregivers are most susceptible to emotional distress when their caregiving precludes their involvement in valued activities and interests.

When she noticed that she had been sleeping poorly for months and seemed sad much of the time, Mrs. Lucas made an appointment to see her family physician for an evaluation. Her family doctor thought that she was mildly depressed in response to the on-going caregiving demands and her decreased marital satisfaction. The doctor made suggestions that Mrs. Lucas accept greater social support in order to improve her mood. She also recommended that Mrs. Lucas return for a follow-up appointment in 2 months; if Mrs. Lucas is not feeling better at that time, her physician will consider recommending medication and/or counseling.

Future Needs/Directions

Practice

Even with the growing interest in cancer survivorship and quality of life issues, the bulk of healthcare resources for cancer patients and their family caregivers is still devoted to making the initial diagnosis and administering the early treatments. Families need healthcare and social service professionals to be available to them long after the early treatment stages. Living with the residual and late effects of cancer and its treatments, as well as fears of recurrence, can be a drawn-out ordeal. For example, many recent pediatric oncology articles have called for on-going "after cancer care" programs to deal with the unique health needs and risks of childhood cancer survivors

(Bhatia 2005; Hudson 2005; Robison 2005). Such after-care programs for childhood and adult survivors should use evidence-based guidelines (Hewitt et al. 2005) and include the participation of family members to identify those most vulnerable to developing difficulties over time. This is especially true for family caregivers of patients with recurrent disease (Northouse et al. 2002).

There are a number of educational and clinical programs that have been tested in recent years whose purpose is to prevent the development of coping problems in family caregivers over the long term (Halford et al. 2000; McMillan et al. 2006). Their preliminary findings suggest that they show promise, though much more study and refinement needs to be undertaken (see Haigler et al. 2011, this series.).

Education and Training

To be attuned to the needs of families dealing with long-term cancer caregiving, oncologists, nurses, social workers, and others need to be trained and made aware of the many challenges that family members face. Making them cognizant of recent research findings on the effects of long-term cancer caregiving is important. But professionals also need practical experience with getting to know families over extended periods and learning how their lives are broadly affected by cancer. To accomplish this, professionals must have the interviewing skills to engage families on the level of their appraisals/beliefs and emotions, not just to discuss biomedical concerns. These skills are being taught in American medical schools and residencies today far more extensively than a generation ago, as evidenced by the explosive growth of standardized patient training programs and research on physician-patient communication. In general, though, healthcare professionals need much more training in how to hear, understand, and respond to cancer caregivers during the acute, chronic, and palliative phases of the disease.

Research

It is heartening that empirical and qualitative studies are being conducted on cancer survivorship and long-term cancer caregiving with greater frequency and by researchers from a variety of professional disciplines. Even more research on cancer survivorship, conducted on a larger scale through National Cancer Institute-sponsored Cooperative Groups, has recently been called for by the Institute of Medicine (Hewitt et al. 2005). Specifically, the issue of quality of life is becoming a more important focus of cancer research. One weakness of the current cancer caregiving research is that much of it is being done on caregiving dyads—patient and spouse—rather than families as a whole. Future research will need to explore other family relationships to discern whether cancer caregiving has a different impact on different types of relatives, as well as those of different ages, gender, cultural backgrounds, degrees of geographic proximity, etc. The research should also further explore which preventive interventions are truly effective in helping buffer family caregivers from the potentially deleterious effects of long-term caregiving. Ultimately, a consensus of research findings should become the basis for guidelines for clinical practice to best serve patients' family members.

Policy

In the past decade, two encouraging developments have affected policy concerning cancer and caregiving. First, the National Cancer Institute's Office of Cancer Survivorship has established itself as an increasingly powerful advocate for long-term cancer patients, as well as a source of funding for research on survivorship and cancer caregiving. Second, the National Family Caregiver Support Program, administered through the U.S. Department of Aging, has disseminated over $100 million to local support programs of caregivers of elderly individuals with any illness through county-level Area Agencies on Aging. What remains to be undertaken are large-scale support programs specifically for the long-term family caregivers of cancer patients. Such programs should have educational, research, and advocacy components and provide funding to replicate successful, innovative, local support programs on a more widespread basis. They should seek to influence training standards for cancer professionals and oncological practice to include more family support. They should champion the cause of cancer caregiving in general so that no family member feels completely isolated with her burden.

Concluding Comments

As the Lucas family has demonstrated, coping with long-term cancer can negatively affect two core features of family life—the ability to generate hope for the future and maintain supportive relationships among and between members and their communities. As such, the rigors and uncertainties of cancer, experienced over months and years, can erode the basic mission of families—to foster all their members' happiness and growth. To the degree that we can counter fears and preserve relationships by providing greater understanding and support, we can buttress families to withstand cancer and deal with its aftermath.

References

Abendstein, H., Nordgren, M., Boysen, M., Jannert, M., Silander, E., Ahlner-Elmqvist, M., et al. (2005). Quality of life and head and neck cancer: A 5-year prospective study. *Laryngoscope*, *115*(12), 2183–2192.

Aziz, N. M., & Rowland, J. H. (2003). Trends and advances in cancer survivorship research: Challenges and opportunity. *Seminars in Radiation Oncology, 13*(3), 248–266.

Baile, W. F., & Aaron, J. (2005). Patient-physician communication in oncology: Past, present and future. *Current Opinions in Oncology, 17*(4), 331–335.

Bhatia, S. (2005). Cancer survivorship: Pediatric issues. *Hematology (American Society of Hematology Education Program)*, 507–515.

Bloom, B. S., Knorr, R. S., & Evans, A. E. (1985). The epidemiology of disease expenses: The costs of caring for children with cancer. *Journal of the American Medical Association, 253*(16), 2393–2397.

Braithwaite, V. (2000). Contextual or general stress outcomes: Making choices through caregiving appraisals. *Gerontologist, 40*, 707–717.

Calhoun, E. A., Chang, C. H., Welshman, E. E., Fishman, D. A., Lurain, J. R., & Bennett, C. L. (2001). Evaluating the total costs of chemotherapy-induced toxicity: Results from a pilot study with ovarian cancer patients. *Oncologist, 6*(5), 441–445.

Cameron, J. I., Franche, R. L., Cheung, A. M., & Stewart, D. E. (2002). Lifestyle interference and emotional distress in family caregivers of advanced cancer patients. *Cancer, 94*(2), 521–527.

Cameron, J. L., Herridge, M. S., Tansey, C. M., McAndrews, M. P., & Cheung, A. M. (2006). Well-being in informal caregivers of acute respiratory distress syndrome. *Critical Care Medicine, 34*(1), 81–86.

Cancer Care, Inc. & National Cancer Foundation (1977). *Listen to the children: A study of the impact on the mental health of children of a parent's catastrophic illness*. New York: Author.

Carver, C. S., Smith, R.G., Petronis, V. M., & Antoni, M. H. (2006). Quality of life among long-term survivors of breast cancer: Different types of antecedents predict different classes of outcomes. *Psychooncology, 15*(9):749-58.

Compas, B. E., Worsham, N. L., Epping-Jordan, J. E., Grant, K. E., Mireault, G., Howell, D. C., et al. (1994). When Mom or Dad has cancer: Markers of psychological distress in cancer patients, spouses, and children. *Health Psychology, 13*(6), 507–515.

Cooper, B., Kinsella, G. J., & Picton, C. (2006). Development and initial validation of a family appraisal of caregiving questionnaire for palliative care. *Psychooncology, 15*(7):613-22.

Deimling, G. T., Kahan, B., Bowman, K. F., & Schafer, M. L. (2002). Cancer survivorship and psychological distress in later life. *Psychooncology, 11*, 479–494.

Edwards, B. K., Brown, M. L., Wingo, P. A., Howe, H. L., Ward, E., Ries, L. A. G., et al. (2005). Annual report to the nation on the status of cancer, 1975–2002, featuring population-based trends in cancer treatment. *Journal of the National Cancer Institute, 97*(19), 1407–1427.

Ferrell, B., Cullinane, C. A., Ervine, K., Melancon, C., Uman, G. C., & Juarez, G. (2005). Perspectives on the impact of ovarian cancer: Women's views of quality of life. *Oncology Nursing Forum, 32*(6), 1143–1149.

Ganz, P.A., Desmond, K.A., Leedham, B., Rowland, J.H., Meyerowitz, B.E., Belin, T.R. (2002). Quality of life in long-term, disease-free survivors of breast cancer: a follow-up study. *Journal of the National Cancer Institute, 90*, 656–667.

Fortner, B. V., Demarco, G., Irving, G., Ashley, J., Keppler, G., Chavez, J., et al. (2003). Description and predictors of direct and indirect costs of pain reported by cancer patients. *Journal of Pain Symptom Management, 25*(1), 9–18.

Given, B., Wyatt, G., Given, C., Sherwood, P., Gift, A., DeVoss, D., et al. (2004). Burden and depression among caregivers of patients with cancer at the end of life. *Oncology Nursing Forum, 31*(6), 1105–1117.

Grassi, L., & Rosti, G. (1996). Psychosocial morbidity and adjustment to illness among long-term cancer survivors: A six-year follow-up study. *Psychosomatics, 37*, 523–532.

Halford, W. K., Scott, J. L., & Smythe, J. (2000). Couples and coping with cancer: Helping each other through the night. In K. B. Schmaling & T. G. Sher (Eds.), *The psychology of couples and illness: Theory, research & practice* (pp. 135–170). Washington, DC: American Psychological Association.

Hayman, J. A., Langa, K. M., Kabeto, M. U., Datz, S. J., DeMonner, S. M., Chernew, M. E., et al. (2001). Estimating the cost of informal caregiving for elderly patients with cancer. *Journal of Clinical Oncology, 19*(13), 3219–3225.

Hewitt, M., Greenfield, S., & Stovall, E. (Eds.). (2005). *From cancer patient to cancer survivor: Lost in transition.* Washington, DC: National Academies Press.

Hudson, M. M. (2005). A model for care across the cancer continuum. *Cancer, 104*(S11), 2638–2642.

Jacobs, B. J. (2006). *The emotional survival guide for caregivers: Looking after yourself and your family while helping an aging parent.* New York: Guilford.

Kim, Y., Duberstein, P. R., Sorensen, S., & Larson, M. R. (2005). Levels of depressive symptoms in spouses of people with lung cancer: Effects of personality, social support, and caregiving burden. *Psychosomatics, 46*(2), 123–130.

Koenig, H. G., Pargament, K., & Nielsen, J. (1998). Religious coping and health status in medically ill hospitalized older adults. *Journal of Nervous and Mental Disease, 186,* 513–521.

Koocher, G. P., & O'Malley, J. (1981). *The Damocles syndrome: Psychological consequences of surviving childhood cancer.* New York: McGraw-Hill.

Kupst, M. J., Natta, M. B., Richardson, C. C., Schulman, J. L., Lavigne, J. V., & Das, L. (1995). Family coping with pediatric leukemia: Ten years after treatment. *Journal of Pediatric Psychology, 20*(5), 601–617.

Lansky, S. B., Cairns, N. U., Clark, G. M., Lowman, J., Miller, L., & Trueworthy, R. (1979). Childhood cancer: Non-medical costs of the illness. *Cancer, 43*(1), 403–408.

Lauzier, S., Maunsell, E., DeKoninck, M., Drolet, M., Hebert-Croteau, N., & Robert, J. (2005). Conceptualization and source of costs form breast cancer: Findings from patient and caregiver focus groups. *Psychooncology, 14*(5), 351–360.

Markman, M. (2005). A "snapshot" of an ovarian cancer clinical practice: Evidence for viewing the malignancy as a "chronic disease." *Current Oncology Reports, 7,* 393–394.

McMillan, S. C., Small, B. J., Weitzner, M., Schonwetter, R., Tittle, M., Moody, L., et al. (2006). Impact of coping skills intervention with family caregivers of hospice patients with cancer. *Cancer, 106*(1), 214–222.

Mellon, S. (2002). Comparisons between cancer survivors and family members on meaning of the illness and family quality of life. *Oncology Nursing Forum, 29*(7), 1117–1125.

Mellon, S., & Northouse, L. L. (2001). Family survivorship and quality of life following a cancer diagnosis. *Research in Nursing & Health, 24,* 446–459.

Moore, K. A. (1998). Out-of-pocket expenditures of outpatients receiving chemotherapy. *Oncology Nursing Forum, 25*(9), 1615–1622.

Moore, K. A. (1999). Breast cancer patients' out-of-pocket expenses. *Cancer Nursing, 22*(5), 389–396.

National Cancer Institute. (2006a). *NCI health information tip sheet for writers: Cancer survivorship.* Retrieved from http://www.cancer.gov/newscenter/tip-sheet-cancer-survivorship.

National Cancer Institute. (2006b). Cancer Control and Population Sciences: Cancer Survivorship Research: About survivorship research: History. Retrieved from http://dccps.nci.nih.gov/ocs/history.html. Accessed 12 Jan 2006.

National Cancer Institute. (2006c). *When someone you love has advanced cancer—Support for caregivers.* Retrieved from http://www.cancer.gov/cancertopics/When-Someone-You-Love-Has-Advanced-Cancer/PDF. Accessed 12 Jan 2006.

National Coalition for Cancer Survivorship. (2006). *About NCCS: The organization.* Retrieved from http://www.cansearch.org/about/org. Accessed 12 Jan 2006.

National Family Caregivers Association. (2006). *Education & support: Tips & guides.* Retrieved from http://www.thefamilycaregiver.org/ed/tips.cfm. Accessed 12 Jan 2006.

Nijboer, C., Tempelaar, R., Triemstra, M., Van Den Bos, G. A. M., & Sanderman, R. (2001). The role of social and psychologic resources in caregiving of cancer patients. *Cancer, 91*(5), 1029–1039.

Northouse, L. L. (1988). Social support in patients' and husbands' adjustment to breast cancer. *Nursing Research, 37,* 91–95.

Northouse, L. L. (2005). Helping families of patients with cancer. *Oncology Nursing Forum, 32*(4), 743–750.

Northouse, L. L., Kershaw, T., Mood, D., & Schafenacker, A. (2005). Effects of a family intervention on the quality of life of women with recurrent breast cancer and their family caregivers. *Psychooncology, 14*(6), 478–491.

Northouse, L. L., Mood, D., Kershaw, T., Schafenacker, A., Mellon, S., Walker, J., et al. (2002). Quality of life of women with recurrent breast cancer and their family members. *Journal of Clinical Oncology, 20*(19), 4050–4064.

Oberst, M. T., Thomas, S. E., Gass, K. A., & Ward, S. E. (1989). Caregiving demands and appraisal of stress among family caregivers. *Cancer Nursing, 12*(4), 209–215.

Raina, P., O'Donnell, M., Rosenbaum, P., Brehaut, J., Walter, S. D., Russell, D., et al. (2005). The health and well-being of caregivers of children with cerebral palsy. *Pediatrics, 115*(6), 626–636.

Robinson-Whelen, S., Tada, Y., MacCallum, R. C., McGuire, L., & Kiecolt-Glaser, J. K. (2001). Long-term caregiving: What happens when it ends? *Journal of Abnormal Psychology, 110*(4), 573–584.

Robison, L. L. (2005). The childhood cancer survivor study: A resource for research of long-term outcomes among adult survivors of childhood cancer. *Minnesota Medicine, 88*(4), 45–49.

Rolland, J. S. (1994). *Families, illness and disability: An integrative treatment model.* New York: Basic Books.

Rolland, J. S. (1997). A journey with hope, fear, and loss: Young couples and cancer. In S. H. McDaniel, J. Hepworth, & W. H. Doherty (Eds.). *The shared experience of illness: Stories of patients, families, and their therapists* (pp. 139–150). New York: Basic Books.

Schulz, R., & Martire, L. (2004). Family caregiving of persons with dementia—prevalence, health effects, and support strategies. *American Journal of Geriatric Psychiatry, 12*(3), 240–249.

Seaburn, D. (2001). In sickness and health: My father's death, part II. *Families, Systems & Health, 19*(2), 211–220.

Skerrett, K. (1998). Couple adjustment to the experience of breast cancer. *Families, Systems & Health, 16*(3), 281–298.

Stommel, M., Given, C. W., & Given, B. A. (1993). The cost of cancer home care to families. *Cancer, 71*(5), 1867–1874.

Tummala, M. K., & McGuire, W. P. (2005). Recurrent ovarian cancer. *Clinical Advances in Hematology & Oncology, 3*(9), 723–736.

Wagner, D. L. (2004). The financial impact of caregiving. In C. Levine (Ed.), *Always on call: When illness turns families into caregivers* (pp. 136–148). Nashville: Vanderbilt University Press.

Weihs, K., & Reiss, D. (2000). Family reorganization in response to cancer: A developmental perspective. In L. Baider, C. L. Cooper, & A. K. De-Nour (Eds.), *Cancer and the family* (2nd ed., pp. 17–39). New York: Wiley

Wellisch, D. K. (1995). A family systems approach to coping with cancer. In R. H. Mikesell, D. D. Lusterman, & S. H. McDaniel (Eds.), *Integrating family therapy: Handbook of family psychology and systems theory* (pp. 389–403). Washington, DC: American Psychological Association.

Winton, T., Livingston, R., Johnson, D., Rigas, J., Johnston, M., Butts, C., et al. (2005). Vinorlebine plus cisplatin vs. observation in resected non-small-cell lung cancer. *New England Journal of Medicine, 352*, 2589–2597.

Yun, Y. H., Rhee, Y. S., Kang, I. O., Lee, J. S., Bang, S. M., Lee, W. S., et al. (2005). Economic burdens and quality of life of family caregivers of cancer patients. *Oncology, 68*(2–3), 107–114.

Chapter 9
Caregiver End-of-Life Care of the Person with Cancer

Lodovico Balducci and Sheryl LaCoursiere

The road to caregiving can be very long. It is at times insidious; what one day may be assistance with an activity of daily living may over time turn into an ongoing need. Areas of needed assistance begin to accumulate; dependency begins to predominate. In some persons, the evolution of the caregiver role may be sudden and brief, in others gradual and prolonged. For the person with cancer, there may be much uncertainty over a prognosis. Although there are points in time that indicate the direction of the disease, such as blood tests and radiographic testing, in between there are only signs and symptoms. These signs and symptoms can range from a continuum of positive to negative responses. As events begin to accumulate, dependency on caregivers may accelerate.

For the person at the end-of-life, the focus of caregiving is sharper. There are questions that no longer need to be asked—the outcome is certain. Although everyone in this world, including the ill person, must die, the transition from curative to palliative care then accompanies a "death sentence" and allows caregivers a dedicated time not only to spend time with the patient, but also to accomplish certain tasks that accompany the impending loss of a loved one or significant other. This process can be enlightening, giving the caregiver new insights into his or her relationship with the cancer patient, and allow the working on "unfinished business," but can also be emotionally exhausting.

This chapter explores the caregiver of the patient at the end-of-life. First, the history of caregiving, particularly in relation to patients who are dying, is examined, followed by the current status of cancer caregivers in relation to practice, education and training, research, and policy. A summary of what is known, what is not known, and what is needed follows. Finally, future directions are explored.

L. Balducci (✉)
H. Lee Moffitt Cancer Center, College of Medicine, University of South Florida,
12902 Magnolia Drive, Tampa, FL 33612, USA
e-mail: Balducci@moffitt.usf.edu

S. LaCoursiere
University of Massachusetts Boston and Yale School of Medicine,
42 Middleway East, Waterbury, CT 06708, USA
e-mail: sheryl.lacoursiere@gmail.com

R. C. Talley et al. (eds.), *Cancer Caregiving in the United States,*
Caregiving: Research, Practice, Policy,
DOI 10.1007/978-1-4614-3154-1_9, © Springer Science+Business Media, LLC 2012

Care, Healing, and Cure

Historically, the two goals of care—healing and cure—are mediated by the same agent, the home-caregiver. It is important to remember that whether the goal is palliative care or cure of cancer, successful outcomes are rarely obtainable without the support of one or more persons willing and able to invest time and resources in the physical and emotional support of the patient with cancer (Butow et al. 2000; Cassileth et al. 1988; Ganz et al. 1993). How many successful palliative care outcomes or cancer cures would be forgone were it not for a caregiver able to foster compliance with a strenuous treatment schedule by providing transportation, home-care, timely management, encouragement, and listening?

The distinction of *healing* and *cure*, a fortunate happenstance of the English language highlights the separate, albeit interlinked domains of health care. *Healing* is the acceptance of illness, the personal experience of disease, through the recognition of a meaning to suffering and death, whereas *cure* refers to disease, a pathologic alteration in bodily functions that would lead to death or disability if left uncorrected. Unlike cure, healing is within everybody's reach (Byock 1997): The diagnosis of incurable and terminal disease represents a call to healing rather than to desperation.

The Cancer Care Recipient

Literature related to caregivers of the patients who are terminally-ill began to appear with increasing frequency in the early 1990s. Two predominant themes are represented in this early literature. These are related to the psychological status of caregivers and the environment in which the caregiving is taking place. A summary of this literature is indicated below.

Psychological Status

The concept of concern for caregivers, even those who are not taking care of patients with cancer, was documented in the early 1990s (Charlton 1992). Concern for the quality of life of caregivers encompasses care tasks as well as caregiver experiences, including burdens as well as positive aspects (Nijboer et al. 1998). In the first 4 weeks of caregiving, quality of life for caregivers is highest in social well-being. However, it is lowest in physical well-being (McMillan 1996). As time moves on, caregivers tend to adjust. Psychosocial status tends to improve in caregivers from the beginning point of caregiving to 3 months of caregiving. At this point, the effect levels off, with psychological well-being remaining the same after 6 months (Jepson et al. 1999). Quality of life can also be improved by intervention (Smeenk et al. 1998).

Environment

Palliative care, or care for a known patient who is dying, can take place in a hospital as well as home environment. The majority of caregivers were found to be family

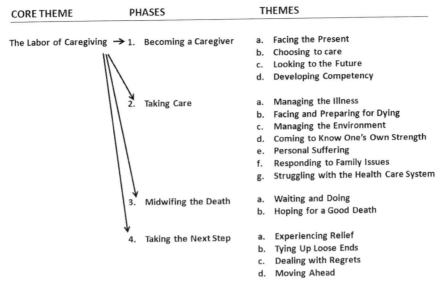

CORE THEME	PHASES	THEMES	
The Labor of Caregiving → 1.	Becoming a Caregiver	a.	Facing the Present
		b.	Choosing to care
		c.	Looking to the Future
		d.	Developing Competency
	2. Taking Care	a.	Managing the Illness
		b.	Facing and Preparing for Dying
		c.	Managing the Environment
		d.	Coming to Know One's Own Strength
		e.	Personal Suffering
		f.	Responding to Family Issues
		g.	Struggling with the Health Care System
	3. Midwifing the Death	a.	Waiting and Doing
		b.	Hoping for a Good Death
	4. Taking the Next Step	a.	Experiencing Relief
		b.	Tying Up Loose Ends
		c.	Dealing with Regrets
		d.	Moving Ahead

Fig. 9.1 The Brown and Stetz labor of caregiving model. (Brown and Stetz 1999)

members (96%) and female (72.1%; Emanuel et al. 1999). Part of the task of caregiving is negotiating with others to coordinate care for the patient, including transport, personal care, and housework. There may be a conflict with patients' wishes, leading to a call to assess caregiver needs independently (Grande et al. 1997).

At the end of the 1990s, a model of caregiving emerged. Entitled "The Labor of Caregiving Model," the framework will be used to explain the following section (Brown and Stetz 1999).

Caregivers of the Dying Cancer Patient: Current Status

Brown and Stetz: A Theoretical Framework That Can Be Used to Guide Practice, Education and Training, Research, and Policy

As the millennium occurred, the literature on caregivers rapidly expanded. There are many ways to view caregiving. The Brown and Stetz Labor of Caregiving Model (1999) is particularly helpful in that it can be used to guide not only practice, but also education and training, research, and policy related to caregivers of patients who are dying. The framework is explained next, and its applicability to the current status of caregiving is outlined in detail.

As shown in Fig. 9.1, the model outlines four phases that the caregiver of a patient who is dying goes through: *Becoming a Caregiver, Taking Care, Midwifing the Death*, and *Taking the Next Step*. These phases are explained below, and theory integrated. The majority of this chapter concentrates on the work of phase II, *Taking Care*.

Becoming a Caregiver. The first phase of caregiving has four themes: *Facing the Present, Choosing to Care, Looking to the Future,* and *Developing Competency.* In becoming a caregiver, an individual goes through a process not unlike a novice in any job. Initially, the situation is evaluated: There is a person who is dying, and the caregiver-to-be chooses that he or she is the most appropriate person to provide care, or if the person requested by the care recipient. The caregiver then attempts to look ahead and determine what tasks the patient might need assistance to manage. Then, either formally or informally, the caregiver develops expertise in needed areas (Brown and Stetz 1999).

Taking Care. The second phase of caregiving has seven themes: *Managing the Illness, Facing and Preparing for Dying, Managing the Environment, Coming to Know Ones Own Strength, Personal Suffering, Responding to Family Issues,* and *Struggling with the Health Care System.* The caregiver must supervise the patient's experience of illness, as well as make plans for the dying process. The physical environment as well as the informational environment must be managed—arranging the living space, seeking information, and coordinating with others. A realization process occurs in which the caregiver begins to know his or her own strength; however, personal suffering also occurs as the caregiver's personal resources are overwhelmed at the same time that the caregiver must face an anticipatory grieving process and deal with family and the health care system itself (Brown and Stetz 1999).

Midwifing the Death. The third phase of caregiving has two themes: *Waiting and Doing* and *Hoping for a Good Death.* In this phase, the caregiver keeps busy with the tasks of caregiving, and waits for the end to come. New skills may need to be learned, for instance, pain control. The caregiver's focus shifts from quality of life to quality of death, and encompasses wishes such as being present at the last moment. Caregivers may expect higher performance of themselves at this time, and wish to "do things right" (Brown and Stetz 1999).

Taking the Next Step. The fourth and final phase of caregiving has four themes: *Experiencing Relief, Tying Up Loose Ends, Dealing with Regrets,* and *Moving Ahead.* The caregiver may feel relief of the freedom from responsibilities, but this may be overshadowed by the grieving process. At the same time, unfinished business must be taken care of, particularly financial management of the now deceased patients' affairs. The caregiver must deal with regrets for situations they might have handled differently. Finally, postbereavement adjustment occurs, and the caregiver looks ahead to the next phase of his or her life (Brown and Stetz 1999).

Practice

In practice, the process of caregiving to the patient who is dying begins with a diagnosis, in this case terminal cancer. In the Brown and Stetz (1999) model, this would correspond to the first stage, *Becoming a Caregiver*, and proceeds into the second stage, *Taking Care.* The definition of terminal disease is elusive: for hospice purposes, terminal disease is generally considered a disease with a life expectancy of less than 6 months for which the only form of treatment is symptom management (Iwashyna et al. 2002). As a general principle, patients with terminal cancer may be expected to experience a progressive decline in their daily function as well as symptoms related to their cancer, the most distressing of which are pain and dyspnea. They will also experience a wide gamut of emotions from depression to anger to despair. They will require the support of other individuals for carrying on the instrumental activities of daily living (IADL) first and later, the activities of daily living (ADLs, Grassi and Rosti 1996; Ventafridda et al. 1991).

Under ideal circumstances, the patient becomes able to find a meaning to the approaching death by viewing it as an occasion to filter those life experiences that have had a lasting impact and crystallize life into a unique and imperishable construct. In addition, the approaching death may be an occasion to discover the affection and the devotion of friends and relatives and to unveil a new and lasting scope of intimacy. This process may take weeks to months and of necessity involves individuals close to the patient and the patient's household. The patient's "terminality" becomes the center of the family activities, interests, and reactions. In the rare condition of a well-adjusted family, the members of the household react in a unity of sorts to support each other and grow together through this painful family trajectory experience (Balducci et al. 1987). In most cases, however, a terminal disease becomes a cause of distress that may exacerbate preexisting conflicts. For instance, the highest percentage of divorces is found among parents whose children die after a prolonged admission in the pediatric intensive care unit (Miller 1996).

From this picture, the multiple roles of the family caregiver in the management of terminal cancer emerge. As shown in Table 9.1, there are five key roles of the caregiver: coordination, decision, representation, mediation, and compassion.

In addition to the roles of the individual caregiver, the demography of caregiving must also be considered. Looking at caregiving from a family perspective, within the traditional extended family, a spouse or a married daughter typically assumes the caregiving role (Balducci et al. 1987). The spouse is often an elderly person with health problems of his or her own, while the married daughter is distressed by the competing demands of her own family, her job, and the sick parent. While the family model is evolving and encompasses couples without children and unmarried individuals as well as same-sex couples, the basic model of caregiving and its inherent problems may be applied to each household. Perhaps the main change from the extended family is not so much the different family structure as it is the scarcity of helpers. Thus, the caregiver may find himself or herself in the situation of carrying on the majority of the physical work.

Caregiving may also be considered from a risk/benefit perspective. Under the best of circumstances, the caregiving experience may help the caregiver to discover a vocation endowed with unique talents that had previously remained undisclosed. A profile of the caregiver is needed. For certain personalities and personal situations, caregiving may be a source of unsurpassed *satisfaction*. Common examples may include: (a) chronically depressed individuals who may, because of their sensitivity, be able to better relate to a dying person, and who are very comfortable in dealing

Table 9.1 Key roles of the caregiver. (Weitzner et al. 2000)

Role	Key components
Coordination	The regulation and integration of various aspects of care received by the patient. This could include, for instance, who is going to take the patient for a walk, feed the patient, entertain the patient, address issues of bequeath and in general make sure that all of the patient's physical and emotional needs are addressed. Many family members and friends are willing to contribute time and resources to the patient's welfare. Without coordination, however, these efforts may be wasted and may even generate conflicts within the family. The caregiver has the task to utilize, at best, each person's talents at the more appropriate times
Decision	Terminal diseases involve painful choices, spanning from the decision to use or not use life-supporting treatment, to the need of balancing pain relief and clarity of consciousness, to the management of intercurrent infections or unexpected delirium, to funeral arrangements. While all family members should be able to express their view of these issues, the caregiver should be able to integrate different viewpoints and channel different trends toward a consensual solution. The decision not to use the treatment is just as challenging, or may be more challenging than the decision to use such treatment. The decision-maker role interdigitates very well with the next two roles, representation and mediation
Representation	The communication with health care providers may be complicated by multiple and diverging goals of different family members. In the absence of a representative of the family, the cacophony of discordant sounds may paralyze the delivery of health care. The ideal caregiver should be able to convey the messages of the family to health care providers as well as the messages of providers to the family
Mediation	It is self-evident that mediation of conflicts is the clue to consensual decisions as well as to effective representation. While the most common conflicts are those within the immediate family, the caregiver's scope may reach out of these boundaries, to the conflicts with the health care providers and to the conflicts within the private domain of each family member. It is very common, for example, that the spouse of one of the patient's children or siblings may grow irritated and resentful for the time and resources the spouse invests in the ill relative. Avoidance of an adversarial reaction by weaving together competing requests into a plan of action agreeable to all parties may make the care of the patient more effective and prevent long-term consequences of the disease, which hovers on the future of each family member
Compassion	Compassion should color each of the caregiver's activities. In the absence of compassion, even an intervention provided by the most skilled person will be mistrusted and go unheeded. In addition to the patient's discomfort and fears, compassion should embrace those members of the household that are unable to accept the patient's death or to conciliate the responsibilities toward the patient and those toward their own work and families. As compassion is the necessary background of all effective caregiving interventions, it is important to highlight the origins of the word (Patterson et al. 2002). Compassion derives from the Latin *cum pator*, meaning "to suffer together." Implicit in the word, then, is a congruence with the sufferer's situation, which means an effort to understand the origin of their discomfort and fear even when they are not our discomfort and fear. Perhaps the most effective manifestation of compassion is then the ability to listen to the patient or the distressed family members, without being judgmental, and when it is appropriate, offering solutions that are congruent with the values of the person that is listened to. Occasional eye contacts, warm touch, short comments indicating that the message is understood and accepted, may go a long way in making compassion operational

Table 9.2 Benefits of caregiving. (Haley 2003)

Satisfaction
Intimacy
Social reward
Personal growth
Self-esteem

with a person at the end-of-life who is shunned by the joyful companions of better days; (b) the nurturing individual looking for an object on whom to bestow their riches; or (c) the estranged spouse able to find in death a new occasion for intimacy. The benefits of caregiving are listed in Table 9.2.

In assessing the potential for caregiving in each situation, two principles should be followed:

• Caregiving at its best is a vocation.
• A person incapable of being a caregiver is not necessarily a callous or insensitive person. Such a person is not very different from a person who is unable to enjoy the symphony because he or she lacks music appreciation.

The best balance is obtained when the caregiving talents of a person are acknowledged and praised while those without these talents are co-opted into the management of the patients to the best of their ability under the direction of the caregiver.

Caregiving may provide new important clues to the significance of *intimacy* and in the meantime vindicate those persons who had lifelong difficulty with sexual relations. The focus on physical sexuality of our culture has privileged individuals who feel very comfortable with their own bodies. However, at the same time, it has emarginated those searching a more global, far-reaching form of intimacy. Caregiving of the dying may restitute full honor and meaning to this form of intimacy that does not hinge on sexual intercourse. In ministering to a dissolving body, the caregiver has the opportunity to respect and honor human vulnerability and in doing so, to become aware that intimacy is foremost a form of contemplation, a spiritual experience immortalized by the "Pietas" of the Renaissance artists. This contact with our spiritual nature is the quintessential form of *personal growth*. It may also provide the caregiver with lasting *self-esteem*: Spirituality is a statement that we are worthy for whom we are, not for what we do.

Last, but not least, *social reward* plays an important role in the support of the caregiver, as validation of the importance and uniqueness of a person's vocation and ministry.

The risks of caregiving have been well illustrated in the literature (see, for example, *The Multiple Dimensions of Caregiving and Disability,* this series). Another example is found in the Alzheimer disease literature, where caregivers are noted to experience earlier mortality and higher rate of depression than a population of the same age without the caregiving burden. Whereas the problems with Alzheimer disease may be extreme, it represents a useful frame of reference for the risks of caregiving in all chronic and terminal diseases. The risks of caregiving are listed in Table 9.3.

Table 9.3 Risks of
caregiving. (Haley 2003)

Depression
Mortality
Social isolation
Low self-esteem
Marital disruption
Loss of income

In addition to *depression* and potential personal *mortality*, the caregiver may suffer the same *social isolation* as the ill person. The same friends and family members that avoid the thought of death and the interaction with the person who is dying may end up skirting and dismissing the person's caregiver. This results in a vicious cycle of depression, more isolation, and more depression. A common side effect of this cycle is the disruption of personal relationships and a development of *low self-esteem*, guilt, and inadequacy. Caregivers may also risk *marital disruption* and *loss of income* because of time spent away from the spousal relationship or work.

Education and Training: Caregiver Interventions

In looking at the Brown and Stetz (1999) model, education and training encompass the first three phases of the model, beginning at *Becoming a Caregiver*, continuing into *Taking Care*, and progressing through *Midwifing the Death*. Education and training in caregiving must encompass not only health professionals, but also family caregivers.

In the preceding discussion we have established that:

- The caregiver is essential to the healing of the person who is terminally ill.
- Caregiving involves unique opportunities and rewards.
- Caregiving involves serious risks to the physical, emotional, and social welfare of the caregiver.

It behooves health care professionals to nurture caregivers as a unique health resource through education that minimizes the risk and maximizes the benefits of caregiving. Interventions that may be helpful with caregivers of the dying patient fall into four categories: *Information, Social Reward, Social Support,* and *Personal Awareness.* These areas are susceptible to modification, thus health professionals are in a unique position to assist the caregiver and, thus, ultimately benefit the patient. These areas will be explained below.

Information. Information is the backbone of effective caregiving and the initial bulwark against discouragement and burn out. The principal components that are necessary in caregiver education include information on the course of the disease, the goals of management, available resources, potential family reactions, and conflict management as well as stress management.

A major cause of concern for a caregiver who had not been previously exposed to terminal illness and death are the unknowns of the situation. "Unknowns" may take the form of many questions, particularly whether the patient is going to experience pain and other forms of discomfort, what is going to be the mechanism of death, in which situations it is appropriate to ask for medical help, and what kind of reactions the patient is going to manifest. It behooves the health care provider to assure the caregiver that the patients will not be in pain, that other forms of discomfort, especially shortness of breath, may be soothed by opioids, and to visit different possible death scenarios. In the case of diffuse liver metastases, renal failure, or hypercalcemia, it is reasonable to anticipate a peaceful outcome, through a more or less prolonged coma, generally devoid of pain. In the case of lymphangitic lung metastases or recurrent superior vena cava syndrome, it is helpful to describe the potential shortness of breath that may be ameliorated by oxygen, steroids, and opioids. When the possibility of intestinal obstruction exists, therapies that would potentially reduce the risk of obstruction should be explored, and both surgical and nonsurgical palliative options outlined. This practical description of the mechanisms of death provides the caregiver with a sense of control, and at the same time enhances confidence in the health care provider. In any case, the general attitude one wants to convey is that the patient and the family will not be abandoned, and that symptom management is taken as seriously as curative treatment by the health care provider. In addition to the description of death scenarios, it may be helpful to anticipate common and distressful reactions that may precede death. For instance, performance of apparently meaningless movements by the patient, such as "picking at things" is a common cause of concern for the family member. It may be helpful for the professional caregiver to explain to the family caregiver that these movements are common occurrences, do not seem associated with any discomfort, and are probably a form of rumination during which the patient is progressively getting ready to die. Telling caregivers and other loved ones that they may express their support by touching the patient may prevent needless anxiety and frustration.

At the same time that the process of death is illustrated, practical and realistic goals of care should be outlined. In addition to supporting the patient's welfare, these goals confirm the caregiver's role by providing meaning and expectation. Of course, the goals of care vary with the stage of the terminal disease. When the patient is still ambulatory and the cognitive function is intact, it is important to maintain the patient integrated as much as possible in the usual social context. Daily exercise, common meals, exchange of ideas, and sharing of social events, such as religious celebrations or artistic performances, are simple and effective ways to promote the socialization of the patient. However, even in the last phase of the disease, active interventions are necessary to promote the three freedoms of the patient at the end-of-life: freedom from pain, freedom from pressure ulcers, and freedom from tubes (Byock 1997). Many nonmedical and even medical people recoil to the idea of not feeding the patient. Disagreements may occur within families, and vary by culture (Phipps et al. 2003).

Awareness of the resources available to care for the patient is also important both to the delivery of effective care and to the relief of a sense of helplessness that affects many caregivers at different times. The exploration of these resources may include three parts:

- A careful description of procedures, for example, whom to call when the patient dies.
- A visit to the formal support network, including hospice, home-care, church-based and other volunteer organizations, to establish a clear outline of what they can provide.
- An examination of the patient's and caregivers' informal support network, based on family and friends. This is probably the best occasion for the caregiver to distribute the burden of caregiving among family members according to each one's special talents and availability. This distribution is essential to assure common satisfaction and a consensual approach to the management of terminal disease, while at the same time preventing or minimizing the caregiver burden. For example, a patient's child or sibling that works night shifts may stop by for breakfast in the morning before going home; the housewife with small children may dedicate one of more nights a week when her spouse is at home and able to provide childcare; the busy executive may shoulder the largest portion of the cost, and so on.

Anticipation of the reactions of different family members, with basic instructions about conflict management, is helpful to prevent painful arguments within the family. The caregiver should be aware of the occurrence and manifestations of denial, anger, bargaining, and escape (Knuti et al. 2003), to accept his or her own reactions, and to avoid passing judgment on siblings that appear callous, aloof, or discourteous. A caregiver who succeeds in not having unpleasant reactions of other family members personally will be in an advantageous position to effectively discuss the patient's needs with family members, and thus to enlist their assistance. At the same time, it is important for the caregiver to communicate personal needs to other family members to avoid being taken for granted, and mainly to make sure that these needs are being provided for in a timely manner. Among these, the need for respite, personal time, and family time are paramount. It is also important that the caregiver be able to discuss his or her own financial situation, ensure that suitable financial arrangements are made in a timely manner, and periodically review the arrangements.

Ideally, the health care provider, such as the physician or hospice nurse, should meet periodically with the family to assess the status of each member and, if necessary, act as an advocate for the caregiver. In addition to emphasizing respite as well as personal and family time, stress management should hinge on caregiver personal values. Caregivers may find important inspiration in religious beliefs (Patterson et al. 2002). Caregiving may have different representations in different religions, for instance, for the Christian assisting the patient, it may represent the comforting of Christ; for the Jew, it may suggest a good deed; for the Muslim, it may suggest a religious intervention. Even in the absence of a specific religious belief, a spiritual perspective that embraces each human life as unique colors acts of caregiving with the sense of highest human mission. The professional caregiver or health care provider should not shun the discussion of religion with the caregiver, and should be able to build the caregiver's comfort by showing congruence *with* and understanding of the caregiver's beliefs.

Social Reward. Reinforcement is the most powerful mechanism to foster compliance with any human activity, from taking medications to persist in one's profession or in one's family (Foley et al. 2002). In the case of caregiving, social reward is a critical form of reinforcement, as it provides the caregiver with status in a time of self-doubt. It behooves all family members to:

- Recognize the role of the caregiver in the healing of the loved one close to death.
- Acknowledge that the caregiver is answering to a special vocation, and is endowed with unique talents. A common but very unfortunate attitude that may undermine caregiving and plunge the caregiver into irreversible depression, is to consider caregiving a default choice for the least valuable member of a household. For example, it is common to consider a childless or unmarried child of the patient as the natural caregiver, assuming that person's time and energy are not as important as those of other family members with family responsibilities.
- Acknowledge the need for support, both emotional and financial, by the caregiver and compensate the caregiver in the most appropriate way for the investment of resources. Probably, the best way to accomplish that is for family members to meet periodically with the caregiver and to allow that person to express needs and concerns. Under the best circumstances, this experience is a powerful way to build a strong and lasting relationship between family members, and to provide meaning to being a family.

Religious ministers should be educated so that they may play an important role in rewarding caregivers, especially those who are supported in a faith that highlights caregiving as a form of ministry, by expressing the appreciation for the caregiver as well as concern for the caregiver's welfare, and by being available to the caregiver on short notice for counseling and listening. Last, health care providers may be powerful agents of caregiver rewards. In the management of terminal patients, the education of health care professionals should include reminders to never miss an opportunity to express admiration for the dedication and performance of the caregiver and concern for caregiver burden. This "less-than-a-minute-a-visit" statement of allegiance is a strong mechanism of caregiver reward.

Social Support. Social support is the concrete manifestation of allegiance to the caregiver, as already stated in different sections of this chapter. As a summary, in the context of the patient who is dying, social support may include:

- Sharing responsibilities for the management of the patient's symptoms; for this purpose both professional and family support networks are involved.
- Providing the caregiver with respite time, family time, and personal time.
- Financial reward for the loss of income.

The importance of social support cannot be underestimated as an intervention, particularly when combined with other interventions such as information and social reward.

Personal Awareness. Personal awareness is the most elusive, and at the same time most effective area of intervention education. Clearly, success of caregiving is assured only when the caregiver feels fully validated by caregiving. Promotion of personal awareness behooves everybody who interacts with the caregiver, including health care providers, family members, friends, ministerial staff, and even occasional acquaintances. While the approaches may vary, the areas of intervention should always include both the feelings and the beliefs of the caregiver.

Special emotional conditions, which can make social interactions difficult, may actually facilitate caregiving of the person at the end-of-life. This is an excellent opportunity for emphasizing the role of the "wounded healer" (Laskowski and Pellicore 2002), which explains how personal wounds may provide the experience and empathy necessary to heal other individuals. In the care of the dying, the same wounds that have handicapped the caregiver's daily life may become effective healing assets. This reverse perspective in the face of death expands and deepens the concept of normality to embrace all living experiences, including death and dying. Depressed individuals may actually be more comfortable with the thought of death than the general population: As with other illnesses, their very disease may give them an edge when dealing with patients, as they are not repulsed by the proximity of death (Gilliam and Steffen 2006). Caregivers craving a nonsexual intimacy may find their aspirations vindicated in the care of the dying. In caregiving, intimacy consists of psychological tasks such as compassionate touch and general sharing of vulnerability, as well as physical tasks such as wound care and management of incontinence. The thoughtful spectator of this challenge should congratulate the caregiver for the unique assets they bring to the situation that, for some, will validate a lifetime of isolation and sense of inadequacy.

Caregiving is also an occasion to validate one's beliefs by establishing a much needed connection between these beliefs and the practice of everyday life. Irrespective of personal religious beliefs, caregiving of the dying is a unique opportunity for manifesting human respect in action. The actions of the caring caregiver communicate the beliefs that disease and death, short of representing a waning of human life, represent a unique experience to be treasured as any other human experience.

In practice, the last step of the Brown and Stetz (1999) model, *Taking the Next Step*, may be where caregivers have the least support available to them, particularly from a health professional point of view. Because the *raison d'etre* of caregiving, the patient, is now deceased, the caregiver is in effect an ex-caregiver. In order to allow anticipation, caregiver education may include the presence of this stage, and what the caregiver might expect, such as the common emotions of relief and regret. Thus, caregiver education and training follows from the tasks at each stage of the model: *Becoming a Caregiver, Taking Care, Midwifing the Death,* and *Taking the Next Step.* Referral for additional services may be needed for those caregivers at risk for ongoing and prolonged grief.

Research

With the exception of the Brown and Stetz (1999) model, the majority of the current research related to caregiving is atheoretical. There is a schism between what is hypothesized about caregiving and what has been tested. Since the beginning of the millennium, caregiving literature has focused on the experience of the caregiver as well as their informational and support needs.

The first area of research, the *experience of the caregiver*, shows multiple lenses by which the overall trajectory of caregiving, its chronic and consuming nature, and the daily life of the caregiver can be viewed (Pasacreta et al. 2000). The experience of caregiving can produce distressing emotions that can affect a caregivers' mental and physical health (Flaskerud et al. 2000). Caregivers of persons with terminal illness are at high risk for clinical depression (Carter and Chang 2000).

The experience of the caregiver may change depending on the rapidity of patient illness. Caregivers in Sweden perceived a more meaningful involvement in caregiving when there was more time to interact with institutional staff and an opportunity for respect and connection had time to develop ("involvement in the light"), as opposed to those with a rapid illness or sudden course of death ("involvement in the dark"; Andershed and Ternestedt 2000). The experience of caregiving may be more satisfactory when a loved one dies at home, particularly when there is access to a palliative care program (Singer et al. 2005). In widows, research in Sweden indicated that a short awareness of the time of potential death may give rise to later anxiety and use of tranquilizing drugs (Valdimarsdottir et al. 2004).

Caregiving also involves the perception of burden. There may be burdens related to time and logistics as well as to physical tasks. There are emotional burdens and mental health risks as well as physical health risks (Rabow et al. 2004). In one study, the perception of burden was most alleviated by in-home nursing care, followed by family physicians, medical specialists, housekeeping, and religious support (Brazil et al. 2005). Although there is a perception of the caregiver as the primary responsibility bearer (Wennman-Larsen and Tishelman 2002), the experience of burden has also been seen as an opportunity to generate strong positive emotions, such as the expression of love (Grbich et al. 2001).

The second area of research, the *informational and support needs of the caregiver,* has been well documented. For instance, although one might suspect that the burden of caregiving might increase over time, Pasacreta et al. (2000) found that in persons that attended a family caregiving education class, the perceived burden of caregiving was not increased even when tasks increased in intensity. (For additional information on caregiver support, see *Education and Support for Caregivers*, this book.)

Caregivers need to be informed of what issues may arise in the course of caregiving. Since caregivers provide an average of 55% of needed care, communication is the primary support needed (Jansma et al. 2005). For instance, concerns may arise as to the amount of information that may be disclosed to the caregiver, particularly regarding end-of-life issues, and when negotiating family dynamics (Clayton et al. 2005). Information on the accessibility of support services is paramount (Grande et al. 2004), as well as potential role strain from both formal and informal support (Sherwood et al. 2004). The information provided must be both comprehensible and manageable (Milberg and Strang 2004). For support itself, in descending order, the most desired services are housekeeping, caregiver respite, in-home nursing care, personal support workers, and self-help/support groups (Brazil et al. 2005).

Obviously, the two main categories of research, the experience of the caregiver and the informational and support needs of the caregiver, are intertwined. The actual experience of the caregiver gives rise to informational and support needs, and the process of meeting those needs is part of the experience of caregiving. In turn, research informs policy.

Policy

Caregiving cannot be effectively promoted until society consistently acknowledges it as a meritorious societal endeavor. Current legislation is not adequate, and caregivers are disproportionately represented by traditionally vulnerable classes of people: women, the unemployed, and those without adequate insurance. When employed, caregivers miss more days of work than noncaregivers. Thus, they typically have health as well as financial vulnerability. At the federal level, there is limited policy support (Doheny 2006). However, some support is provided by the Family and Medical Leave Act of 1993 (Bell and Newman 2003; U.S. Department of Labor 2006) and the Family Caregiver Support Program under the Older Americans Act of 2001 (U.S. Department of Health and Human Services 2006).

Medicaid and Medicare are inadequate in their access to health care for caregivers and their families (Ho et al. 2005). Polices to expand Medicaid and Medicare would improve caregivers' ability to access health care for themselves and their families, as well as help eliminate the financial strain of going without health insurance. Although there is social reward for caregiving, there is little societal recognition.

Summary: What Is Known, What Is Not Known, and What Is Needed

In general, the numbers of caregivers are ever-increasing. It is known that caregivers of dying cancer patients face challenges that are both similar to and different from those experienced by other caregivers. Many times, caregivers of dying cancer patients are called on to respond to urgent needs, with a total course of illness lasting days or weeks. On the other end of the continuum, dying can be a lingering process and take place over months or years.

What is not known is the extent of the difference of these experiences, and the contextual environments in which they occur. For instance, how does the caregiver experience differ when providing care for a dying cancer patient in contrast to an individual with congestive heart failure? What are the essential "core" caregiver tasks, and which are illness-specific? More research is needed in both quantitative and qualitative domains.

Future Directions for Caregivers of Dying Cancer Patients

Applicability of Current Frameworks

The Brown and Stetz model (1999) is very applicable to the experience of caregivers of persons with cancer. It describes and acknowledges the unique stages that caregivers must pass through. Because it was developed through qualitative interview methods, it reflects the commonality of caregiver experiences. The four stages, *Becoming a Caregiver*, *Taking Care*, *Midwifing the Death*, and *Taking the Next Step*, encompass the "life-cycle" of a caregiver.

However, if one is to also examine societal forces, a caregiver model that incorporates factors external to the caregiving situation should also be examined. For instance, a more comprehensive model might include aspects of education and training, sociocultural factors, and policy. If the status of caregivers and their acknowledgement is to rise in the minds of policymakers, more formal programs should be established that present structured curricula.

Practice, Education and Training, Research, and Policy

In practice, "caregiving" is gaining momentum as a concept in the American vocabulary. Although it is not yet ubiquitous, the development of organizations such as the National Family Caregivers Association has begun to increase public awareness of the role of caregiving. However, penetration of the concept into the populations most affected, and self-identification as a caregiver, will probably take some time.

In addition, knowledge of laws and policy related to caregiving is slowly diffusing; however, more public awareness is essential to enable families to assume these added responsibilities. Although education and training opportunities are increasing for caregivers, more dissemination needs to be done about the concept of caregiving itself, and how to actually navigate the role and circumstances that might occur.

In research, more work is needed on a national as well as individual level. On a national level, aggregate data are needed to inform policy. What are the characteristics of caregivers from different regions of the United States? Are their needs different? What are the public health implications? What models can be developed that include the concept of community? On an individual level, more research is needed on the caregiver of patients at the end-of-life, and the experiences that caregivers might encounter. Together, the data should be carefully scrutinized for potential impact on policy. National trends in cancer survival should also be considered, for as the number of survivors increases, trends may become apparent in the length of dying trajectories, thus impacting the work of the caregiver.

In conclusion, the caregiver is the agent of healing for the patient who is dying. As such, the caregiver represents a unique resource that cannot be substituted or surrogated. It behooves each individual, as well as society in general, to support this precious and scarce resource. Health care professionals, patient advocates, and religious ministers all have a vested interest in preserving and nurturing the caregiver.

Maximizing the benefits and minimizing the risks of caregiving is the winning strategy. Information, social reward, social support, and promotion of self-awareness are interventions that may ease the burden of caregiving and enhance its gains. At the same time, a societal commitment to not penalize the caregiver with loss of health and income is essential. In the end, end-of-life care by caregivers of individuals with cancer is complex, and involves many layers of society, from the individual to the family and community.

Caregivers providing end-of-life care must be examined from many dimensions, in order to fully understand their evolving role in today's society. This chapter has attempted to address some of these complexities that have affected the past and present, and will undoubtedly impact the future. In order to ground the context of care, the chapter first examined the history of caregiving to individuals at the end-of-life. This was followed by the current status of cancer caregivers as both resources and participants in end-of-life care using the Brown and Stetz (1999) model. The model was used as a guide in relation to not only practice, but also education and training, research, and policy. Following this, a summary of what is known, what is not known, and what is needed in "caring for the caregiver" was examined. Finally, future directions were explored, as well as the impact of caregiving on a number of levels, from individual to societal to the policy arena.

References

Andershed, B., & Ternestedt, B. M. (2000). Being a close relative of a dying person: Development of the concepts "involvement in the light and in the dark". *Cancer Nursing, 23*(2), 151–159.

Balducci, L., Phillips, D. M., Wallace, C., & Hardy, C. (1987). Cancer chemotherapy in the elderly. *American Family Physician, 35,* 133–143.

Bell, L., & Newman. S. (2003). *Paid family & medical leave: Why we need it, how we can get it* (Policy Brief). http://www.caregiver.org/caregiver/jsp/content/pdfs/op_2003_paid_family_medical_leave.pdf. Accessed 26 March 2012.

Brazil, K., Bedard, M., Krueger, P., Abernathy, T., Lohfeld, L., & Willison, K. (2005). Service preferences among family caregivers of the terminally ill. *Journal of Palliative Medicine, 8*(1), 69–78.

Brown, M. A., & Stetz, K. (1999). The labor of caregiving: A theoretical model of caregiving during potentially fatal illness. *Qualitative Health Research, 9*(2), 182–197.

Butow, P. N., Coates, A. S., & Dunn, S. M. (2000). Psychosocial predictors of survival: Metastatic breast cancer. *Annals of Oncology, 11,* 469–474.

Byock, I. (1997). *Dying well: The prospect for growth at the end of life.* New York: Putnam.

Cassileth, B. R., Walsh, W. P., & Lusk, E. J. (1988). Psychosocial correlates of cancer survival: A subsequent report 6–8 years after cancer diagnosis. *Journal of Clinical Oncology, 6,* 1753–1759.

Carter, P. A., & Chang, B. L. (2000). Sleep and depression in cancer caregivers. *Cancer Nursing, 23*(6), 410–415.

Charlton, R. (1992). Palliative care in non-cancer patients and the neglected caregiver. *Journal of Clinical Epidemiology, 45*(12), 1447–1449.

Clayton, J. M., Butow, P. N., & Tattersall, M. H. (2005). The needs of terminally ill cancer patients versus those of caregivers for information regarding prognosis and end-of-life issues. *Cancer, 103*(9), 1957–1964.

Doheny, K. (2006). *Caregivers face major medical hurdles of their own: Survey finds many lack health care and insurance and are stressed by medical bills.* Scout News. http://news.healingwell.com/index.php?p=news1&id=527571. Accessed 26 March 2012.

Emanuel, E. J., Fairclough, D. L., Slutsman, J., Alpert, H., Baldwin, D., & Emanuel, L. L. (1999). Assistance from family members, friends, paid care givers, and volunteers in the care of terminally ill patients. *New England Journal of Medicine, 341*(13), 956–963.

Flaskerud, J. H., Carter, P. A., & Lee, P. (2000). Distressing emotions in female caregivers of people with AIDS, age-related dementias, and advanced-stage cancers. *Perspectives in Psychiatric Care, 36*(4), 121–130.

Foley, K. L., Tung, H. J., & Mutran, E. J. (2002). Self gain and self loss among African American and white caregivers. *Journals of Gerontology, Series B: Psychological Sciences and Social Sciences, 57,* s 14–22.

Ganz, P. A., Hirji, K., Sim, M. S., Schag, C. A., Fred, C., & Polinsky, M. L. (1993). Predicting psychosocial risk in patients with breast cancer. *Medical Care, 31,* 419–431.

Gilliam, C. M., & Steffen, A. M. (2006). The relationship between caregiving self-efficacy and depressive symptoms in dementia family caregivers. *Aging and Mental Health, 10*(2), 79–86.

Grbich, C., Parker, D., & Maddocks, I. (2001). The emotions and coping strategies of caregivers of family members with a terminal cancer. *Journal of Palliative Care, 17*(1), 30–36.

Grande, G. E., Farquhar, M. C., Barclay, S. I., & Todd, C. J. (2004). Valued aspects of primary palliative care: Content analysis of bereaved carers' descriptions. *British Journal of General Practice, 54*(507), 772–778.

Grande, G. E., Todd, C. J., & Barclay, S. I. (1997). Support needs in the last year of life: Patient and carer dilemmas. *Palliative Medicine, 11*(3), 202–208.

Grassi, L., & Rosti, G. (1996). Psychosocial morbidity and adjustment to illness among long-term cancer survivors. *Psychosomatics, 37,* 523–532.

Haley, W. E. (2003). The costs of family caregiving: Implications for geriatric oncology. *Critical Reviews in Oncology/Hematology, 48,* 151–158.

Ho, A., Collins, S. R., Davis, K., Doty, M. M. (2005). *A look at working-age caregivers' roles, health concerns, and need for support* (Issue Brief) (Vol. 854, pp. 1–12). New York: Commonwealth Fund.

Iwashyna, T. J., Zhang, J. X., & Christakis, N. A. (2002). Disease-specific pattern of hospice related healthcare in a cohort of seriously ill elderly patients. *Journal of Palliative Medicine, 5,* 531–538.

Jansma, F. F., Schure, L. M., & de Jong, B. M. (2005). Support requirements for caregivers of patients with palliative cancer. *Patient Education and Counseling, 58*(2), 182–186.

Jepson, C., McCorkle, R., Adler, D., Nuamah, I., & Lusk, E. (1999). Effects of home care on caregivers' psychological status. *IMAGE: Journal of Nursing Scholarship, 31(2),* 115–120.

Knuti, K. A., Wharton, R. H., Wharton, K. L., Chabner, B. A., Lynch, T. J., Jr., & Penson, R. T. (2003). Living as a cancer surpriser: A doctor tells his story. *Oncologist, 8,* 108–122.

Laskowski, C., & Pellicore, K. (2002). The wounded healer archetype: Applications to palliative are practice. *Journal of Hospice and Palliative Care, 19,* 403–407.

McMillan, S. C. (1996). Quality of life of primary caregivers of hospice patients with cancer. *Cancer Practice, 4*(4), 191–198.

Milberg, A., & Strang, P. (2004). Exploring comprehensibility and manageability in palliative home care: An interview study of dying cancer patients' informal carers. *Psycho-Oncology, 13*(9), 605–618.

Miller, R. B. (1996). Love and death in a pediatric intensive care unit. *Annual of the Society of Christian Ethics, 1996,* 21–39.

Nijboer, C., Tempelaar, R., Sanderman, R., Triemstra, M., Spruijt, R. J., & Van Den Bos, G. A. (1998). Cancer and caregiving: The impact on the caregiver's health. *Psycho-Oncology, 7*(1), 3–13.

Pasacreta, J. V., Barg, F., Nuamah, I., & McCorkle, R. (2000). Participant characteristics before and 4 months after attendance at a family caregiver cancer education program. *Cancer Nursing, 23*(4), 295–303.

Patterson, S., Balducci, L., & Meyer, R. (2002). The Book of Job: A 2,500-year-old current guide to the practice of oncology: The nexus of medicine and spirituality. *Journal of Cancer Education, 17,* 237–240.

Phipps, E., True, G., Harris, D., Chong, U., Tester, W., Chavin, S. I., & Braitman, L. E. (2003). Approaching the end of life: Attitudes, preferences, and behaviors of African-American and white patients and their family caregivers. *Journal of Clinical Oncology, 21*(3), 549–554.

Rabow, M. W., Hauser, J. M., & Adams, J. (2004). Supporting family caregivers at the end of life: "They don't know what they don't know". *Journal of the American Medical Association, 291*(4), 483–491.

Sherwood, P. R., Given, B. A., Doorenbos, A. Z., & Given, C. W. (2004). Forgotten voices: Lessons from bereaved caregivers of persons with a brain tumour. *International Journal of Palliative Nursing, 10*(2), 67–75.

Singer, Y., Bachner, Y. G., Shvartzman, P., & Carmel, S. (2005). Home death: The caregivers' experiences. *Journal of Pain & Symptom Management, 30*(1), 70–74.

Smeenk, F. W., de Witte, L. P., van Haastregt, J. C., Schipper, R. M., Biezemans, H. P., & Crebolder, H. F. (1998). Transmural care of terminal cancer patients: Effects on the quality of life of direct caregivers. *Nursing Research, 47*(3), 129–136.

U.S. Department of Health & Human Services Administration on Aging (2006). Older Americans Act. US Dept of Health and Human Services 2006. http://www.aoa.gov/AoA_programs/HCLTC/Caregiver/index.aspx. Accessed 26 March 2012.

U.S. Department of Labor Employment Standards, Administration Wage & Hour Division (2006). The Family and Medical Leave Act of 1993. http://www.dol.gov/whd/regs/statutes/fmla.htm. Accessed 26 March 2012.

Valdimarsdottir, U., Helgason, A. R., Furst, C.-J., Adolfsson, J., & Steineck, G. (2004). Awareness of husband's impending death from cancer and long-term anxiety in widowhood: A nationwide follow-up. *Palliative Medicine, 18*(5), 432–443.

Ventafridda, V., Ripamonti, C., De Conno, F., Tamburini, M., & Cassileth, B. R. (1991). Symptom prevalence and control during cancer patients' last days of life. *Journal of Palliative Care, 6,* 7–11.

Weitzner, M. A., Haley, W. E., & Chen, H. (2000). The family caregiver of the older cancer patient. *Hematology/Oncology Clinics of North America, 14,* 269–281.

Wennman-Larsen, A., & Tishelman, C. (2002). Advanced home care for cancer patients at the end of life: A qualitative study of hopes and expectations of family caregivers. *Scandinavian Journal of Caring Sciences, 16*(3), 240–247.

Chapter 10
Advances in Cancer Care Impacting Familial Caregiving

Victoria H. Raveis

More than three decades ago, the initiation of the National Cancer Act in 1971 set in motion a comprehensive national plan to reduce cancer-related morbidity and mortality (Dunn 2002). Through the years, this act has been reauthorized and updated to reflect emerging developments and priorities in cancer care and research. The activities that have been initiated through this act have contributed to the current developments in the care and management of cancer and influenced the families facing current caregiving challenges today.

Recent developments in detecting, diagnosing, treating, and managing cancer have contributed to reduced disease progression and increased survival. Overall, the cancer death rate has decreased 1.1% per year between 1992 and 2001 (Jemal et al. 2006). The current 64% 5-year relative survival rate for cancers represents a statistically significant increase in the last 20 years (American Cancer Society [ACS] 2006). This translates into over 10 million persons currently living who have been diagnosed with cancer (Hewitt et al. 2006).

As in other illness situations requiring informal support and assistance, the family is integral to the care and support provided to persons receiving treatment for cancer (Schumacher et al. 2000; see reviews by Northouse 2005; Kotkamp-Mothes et al. 2005). Families face a shared set of psychosocial challenges imposed by their relative's illness: coping with uncertainty, dealing with the losses and changes engendered by the illness, and adjusting to the caregiving situation (Raveis 2007). Caregivers are challenged in varying degrees in each of these areas at every phase of the illness.

This chapter will focus on a number of important ways that advances in understanding cancer and the developments in its treatment and management have not only impacted the structure and process of families' cancer caregiving, but also affected the positive and negative aspects of their caregiving experience and the adaptational challenges that families face. This analysis will necessarily touch upon areas that are the subject of other chapters in this volume. Following the conceptual framework on

V. H. Raveis (✉)
Psychosocial Research Unit on Health, Aging and the Community,
New York University, New York, NY 10010, USA
e-mail: victoria.raveis@nyu.edu

R. C. Talley et al. (eds.), *Cancer Caregiving in the United States,*
Caregiving: Research, Practice, Policy,
DOI 10.1007/978-1-4614-3154-1_10, © Springer Science+Business Media, LLC 2012

the cancer caregiving process developed by Nijboer et al. (1998), this review will focus primarily on two main concepts that have a central role within the caregiving situation and are posited to impact the caregiver's health: care tasks and caregiver experiences (i.e., burden and positive aspects).

Research: Current Impact

Cancer is not a single disease; it is a collection of different types, all characterized by uncontrolled growth and spread of abnormal cells. The symptoms, treatment, illness course, life expectancy, and prognosis can vary with the type of cancer and its site (i.e., body location). As a consequence, not all research and technological advances are applicable to the treatment and management of all cancers. However, a number of research developments have had a cross-cutting impact that has reshaped the caregiving situation. These are evident at each stage of the illness course—diagnosis, treatment, and survivorship.

Improved Cancer Screening Tools Enable Earlier, More Accurate Detection. A variety of technological developments in the screening and diagnosis of cancer have reduced care demands and positively impacted informal caregiving in cancer. Improvements in the precision of cancer screening tools, due to various technological advances in cancer imaging and molecular sensing, have enabled earlier cancer diagnoses. Initiating treatment at a less advanced, more curable stage enhances the likelihood that treatment will be effective (Jemal et al. 2004). In addition, treatments for early-stage cancer are usually less debilitating and extensive than for advanced disease. As a consequence, rehabilitation may be less complex and restoration of preillness functioning more feasible. This can translate into lessened caregiving demands as the extent and duration of care are reduced relative to advanced disease.

Another benefit to the increased precision in cancer screening tools is that cancers are now being detected more accurately, reducing the number of persons who unnecessarily undergo further diagnostic procedures. Providing a greater precision at the screening level reduces caregiving demands. Apart from the financial costs associated with undergoing additional diagnostic tests, the patients and families experience emotional distress and anxiety over a possible cancer diagnosis (Kash et al. 2000; Baider et al. 1999), and there are recovery-related care needs associated with invasive diagnostic procedures.

Diagnostic Procedures Are Less Invasive. Refinements in imaging technology over the last few decades have provided much clearer and more detailed images of organs and tissues. With these technological developments, the range of medical options for diagnosis has broadened. For example, advancements in computed tomography (CT) and ultrasound have made possible the insertion of long, thin needles deep within the body to biopsy organs, reducing the need for more invasive, surgical diagnostic procedures. These significant technological advances have enabled the widespread use of minimally invasive diagnostic procedures. This has reduced families' diagnostic burden as not only are inpatient stays reduced but many diagnostic procedures can now be performed on an outpatient basis. Recovery time is also shortened with a concomitant decrease in the need for practical assistance and care provision.

Criteria Have Broadened for When and Who Is a Patient. Progress in biomedical research has led to the identification of an increasing number of precancerous conditions, effectively pushing back the beginning of the disease time-line for a variety of cancers. Genetic testing is available that can identify individuals with genes associated with certain cancers, such as breast, ovarian, and pancreatic cancer. Similar diagnostics advances are expected in the future for other cancers. These various biomedical developments have broadened the number of individuals impacted by cancer and redefined cancer caregiving. Knowledge of a cancer risk precipitates a range of care tasks. Growing numbers of families are being challenged with living with the uncertainty of when or if a relative may develop cancer (Baider et al. 1999). Studies have shown that individuals are profoundly impacted and distressed by being at risk of cancer (Kelly 1983; Wellisch et al. 1991, 1992; Kash et al. 2000; Meiser et al. 2001; Raveis and Pretter 2005). Moreover, in addition to providing emotional support, family members may also be engaged in evaluating various monitoring options and preventive measures. Surveillance choices, such as "watchful waiting," may challenge families to cope with uncertainty (Wallace et al. 2004). Other options may create demands for practical support and assistance, when surgical inventions, such as prophylactic mastectomy or preventive drug therapies, are implemented.

Surgery Less Invasive or Radical. As a consequence of the refinements in imaging technology that have produced clearer and more detailed images of organs and tissues, the range of medical options for the management and treatment of cancer has expanded. Minimally invasive surgical procedures reduce inpatient stays and permit many procedures to be performed in hospitals on an outpatient basis and in physicians' offices. Use of this type of surgical procedure is also associated with reductions in the length of the recovery period and a minimization of permanent surgical changes. Progress in biomedical research has also informed the adoption of less mutilating surgical procedures. Less radical surgical approaches, such as lumpectomy, not only diminish the risk of postoperative complications such as bleeding and infection, but also cut down on the formation of scars, and reduce permanent side-effects. Clinical research has demonstrated that, compared to more radical procedures, less mutilating surgical procedures effect similar success in cancer survival (Edwards et al. 2005). These various surgical advances alleviate some of the care needs associated with surgical interventions and can translate into reduced caregiving demands. The period required for recovery is reduced and there is a greater likelihood of restoration to preillness functioning.

Treatment Side-Effects Reduced. Technological and biomedical advances have also reduced the occurrence and severity of side-effects from cancer treatments, further impacting recovery time and caregiving needs. Radiation treatments that required an inpatient stay are now routinely delivered in outpatient clinics and physicians' offices (Mor et al. 1992). These treatments are now able to be delivered with greater precision, reducing the amount of normal tissue receiving the radiation and minimizing side-effects (e.g., skin irritation, nausea, diarrhea, hair loss, loss of energy). The development of radiation implants provides for the concentrated timed delivery of radiation over a sustained interval to a limited area. This process minimizes the area affected by radiation and permits patients to remain at home during treatment, reducing the needs for multiple clinic visits.

Similar advances have been achieved with chemotherapy. Less cytotoxic chemotherapy regimes are now available that have less severe and frequent treatment side-effects, enabling more patients to be managed on an ambulatory basis (Given et al. 2001; Raveis et al. 1998). Technological developments, such as infusion pumps and vascular access devices, have also made it feasible for patients to receive complex chemotherapeutic routines while being maintained in the home (Crawley 1990). As with radiation treatment, recovery times have shortened and care needs lessened.

Biological therapies, a more recent addition to the standard cancer treatments of surgery, chemotherapy, and radiation, use the body's immune system to fight cancer and reduce or repair treatment-related side-effects. Most cancer therapies inadvertently damage or destroy some normal cells as well as cancer cells, resulting in temporary (e.g., baldness) or permanent (e.g., sterility) treatment-related side-effects. However, biological therapies selectively target the cancer cells, leaving normal cells alone. This reduces treatment-related side-effects and limits the scope and duration of patients' caregiving needs.

Medically Vulnerable Populations Receive Aggressive Treatment. The development of effective cancer treatment approaches that are less harsh and have fewer and better controlled side-effects has permitted the delivery of more aggressive cancer care to those who are medically frail or have comorbid conditions (e.g., the elderly). The burden of cancer is considerable in the elderly. In the United States, almost 60% of new cancers occur in persons over 65 (Edwards et al. 2002). Age adds a layer of complexity to cancer caregiving not present in other cancer care situations. As a consequence of the physiological changes associated with aging (e.g., decreased stamina and physical strength, frequent comorbidities, and heightened disability), the elderly are likely to have more extensive, complex, and long-term caregiving needs. Older cancer patients may require a longer period of rehabilitation from treatment, experience more severe or longer-lasting side-effects, and have a lower likelihood of restoration to preillness functioning (Balducci 2006; Carreca et al. 2005; Balducci and Yates 2000). In addition, given that the number and severity of chronic health conditions increase with age, the cancer diagnosis may not initiate the family's caregiving role, but rather expand upon or add to an already existing set of care responsibilities. With older adults, comorbid conditions are common and families may have already been providing care to their elderly relative for other health conditions when the cancer was diagnosed (Kurtz et al. 1994). Given the aging of the population, based on cancer incidence rates and U.S. Census Department population projections, it is anticipated that the number of cancer patients 65 and older will double in the next 30 years (Edwards et al. 2002). Perhaps even more significantly, the number of cancer patients aged 85 and older is expected to increase fourfold between 2000 and 2050 (Edwards et al. 2002). These projections suggest that a substantial proportion of cancer caregivers will be dealing with the added caregiving challenges associated with advanced age.

Survivorship Is Increasing. Improvements in diagnosis and advances in treating and medically managing cancer have contributed to reduced mortality and gains in cancer survival (Jemal et al. 2006). Consequently, the chronic phase or adaptation phase of the disease course, i.e., the period of survival that follows the initial medical intervention, has lengthened for an increasing number of cancer patients (Balducci and Yates 2000; Newport and Nemeroff 1998). Increased survivorship is likely to have a significant impact on caregiving demands (Lewis 2006), particularly since the number of elderly persons living with cancer is substantial. About 60% of cancer survivors are 65 or older, with 32% of the survivors 75 and older (Edwards et al. 2002).

Research: Future Impact

Biomedical Advances in Cancer Treatment May Reduce Care Needs. Emerging technological advances in biotherapy are informing the development of immuno-toxins and vaccines that utilize the immune system to attack existing cancer cells. Although the number of these drugs approved for cancer therapy is limited, a substantial number are under development. They hold a promise to significantly reduce cancer burden. Gleevec, recently approved for the treatment of chronic myeloid leukemia and gastrointestinal stomal tumors, is an example of this new class of drug therapy. Gleevec works by blocking the rapid growth of white blood cells. Its side-effects have been found to be less severe than traditional therapies and it has been shown to have a beneficial impact on patients when other treatments have failed.

A number of other ongoing areas of clinical investigation also have the potential to positively impact the scope and duration of family caregiving in the future. Developments in pharmacology show future promise for effective drug therapies that can be initiated in persons with conditions that are a precursor to cancer. Success in reducing the incidence of cancer readily translates into a reduced need for care provision. Early studies with the drug celecoxib indicated that the drug was effective in reducing the number of colon polyps in patients with a precancerous condition, familial adenomatous polyposis (FAP) (National Cancer Institute [NCI] 2006). Clinical trials are evaluating its efficacy with related conditions.

Research is also progressing on the development of a variety of cancer prevention vaccines that utilize an individual's immune system to evoke an immune response that targets cancer-causing agents. One such agent on which early clinical vaccine trials are being conducted is the sexually transmitted human papillomavirus (HPV) (Winstead 2005), which has been linked to cervical cancer. With an arsenal of effective cancer vaccines, a family's future caregiving responsibility could focus on proactive tasks, such as ensuring participation in cancer screening.

There also is continuing effort to further reduce the adverse consequences of current treatment approaches. Studies are continuing regarding a "minitransplant" option for bone marrow transplantation (NCI 2004). This experimental procedure takes advantage of the immune properties of the donor stem cells to kill the cancer cells while tolerating the patient's normal cells. A key benefit of this approach is that patients receive a much lower dose of radiation and most will be able to leave the hospital the same day as the procedure, unlike conventional bone marrow transplants in which patients are hospitalized in intensive care for 2 to 3 months. If found to be effective, it could expand the option of bone marrow therapy to include patients who are too infirm or debilitated to undergo conventional bone marrow procedures. Unlike the caregiving demands associated with traditional bone marrow transplants, the extent and intensity of caregiving demands during the briefer recovery period with minitransplants is substantially reduced.

Emerging developments in nanotechnology show promise as biodegradable carriers for therapeutic agents. Nanocarriers have been developed that directly target tumor cells, reducing damage to noncancer cells and overcoming multiple-drug resistance (NCI Alliance for Nanotechnology in Cancer 2005). The clinical application of these technological advances would further reduce cancer burden and caregiving needs.

Practice: Current Impact

Cancer and its treatment create multiple demands for caregivers as they assist patients in dealing with the physical and psychological consequences of surgery, chemotherapy, and radiation, in addition to disease-related care tasks. Informal caregiving to cancer patients can encompass emotional support, financial aid, and the provision of services ranging from instrumental aid and assistance with personal care, to health care tasks and mediation with formal care providers (Given et al. 2001; Glajchen 2004; Raveis et al. 1998; Schumacher et al. 2000). Although current practices in the treatment and management of cancer have reduced some of the caregiving demands associated with treatment delivery, recovery, rehabilitation, and adaptation, other caregiving responsibilities have increased.

Treatment Decision-Making Tasks Are Complex. The period immediately following a cancer diagnosis is a time of intense stress and crisis for patients and their families, characterized by a series of unrelenting demands, intense activity, and uncertainty (Raveis and Pretter 2005). During this time, families are confronted with needing to make numerous difficult treatment decisions that may necessitate the mastery of new information in order to make informed choices (Maliski et al. 2002). In recent years, the process of clinical decision-making has become more complex, given the ongoing advances in cancer treatment and its management, as well as the expanded access to clinical trials in community settings. The current opportunities and future promises of new therapies contribute to the uncertainties the patients and families confront when deciding among care options. Families engaged in informed decision-making are challenged with needing to search out available information and evaluate the options (Schumacher et al. 2000). Increasingly, this task may involve weighing the merits of standard practice against the uncertainty and promise of alternative or experimental treatments not routinely offered. Indeed, there is growing concern that an unintended consequence of increasing access to clinical trials is raising families' optimism and incurring unfounded hope (Sankar 2004).

Families are faced with having to weigh the risks and benefits of specific therapies (e.g., minimally invasive surgery, hormonal therapy, prophylactic therapy) in conjunction with quality-of-life considerations (e.g., the choice of potentially toxic, time-intensive interventions that might prolong life versus less aggressive measures that would improve short-term quality of life but not extend it). Implementation of a treatment choice may also require families who are intervening on behalf of the patient to ensure access to the most appropriate health care providers. These tasks represent an expansion of the health care advocacy tasks that families perform (Schumacher et al. 2000). Their performance can require a considerable investment of time and effort. The import of this responsibility is not taken casually and caregivers can find themselves challenged and stressed with the responsibility (Raveis and Pretter 2005). In addition, families may experience regret or guilt over their decision when the treatment has undesirable side-effects or the desired outcome has not been achieved; they may worry that a different choice would have been better.

Physical Environment of Care Has Changed. Several trends in health care and cancer treatment have coalesced to expand families' involvement in the care of cancer patients throughout the disease course. The national trend toward "dehospitalization" of medical care encompasses the management and treatment of cancer. The shift from the hospital to community- or home-based long-term care has transferred more care and management tasks to the family, broadening the scope of their caregiving tasks (Siegel et al. 1996). The family has become directly involved in delivery of both active treatment and rehabilitative care, a not-inconsequential expansion of their set of care responsibilities. For example, family caregivers are now directly involved in administering medications, checking proper dosage, providing pain relief, and monitoring treatment effectiveness (Given et al. 2001). They also serve as patient advocates, communicating with health professionals and other service providers for care and symptom palliation (Blanchard et al. 1997; Ferrell et al. 1991).

While the practical and emotional benefits to cancer patients of family support and assistance are readily acknowledged (Baider et al. 2003), a growing body of evidence is documenting that the costs to the caregiver of providing support and assistance are far-reaching and diverse (see Gilbar and Ben-Zur 2002; reviews by Kotkamp-Mothes et al. 2005; Given et al. 2001). The process of attending to their relative's needs for cancer-related assistance and support has been shown to be stress-inducing, imposing diverse lifestyle restrictions and engendering elevated distress levels (Cameron et al. 2002; Gilbar and Ben-Zur 2002; Given et al. 2001; Matthews et al. 2003; Northouse et al. 2000; Raveis et al. 1998).

Given the growth in the number of older adults with cancer, and the expectation that this trend will continue in the future, this shift in the physical location of the treatment and management of elderly cancer patients has direct implications for scope and duration of families' care provision. The number of families involved in caregiving for elderly cancer patients can be expected to steadily increase. Caregiving demands are likely to be more complex and time-consuming. With population aging, cancer caregivers, themselves are likely to be older as well and may simultaneously be coping with their own health conditions.

Duration of Care Has Increased. With the advent of earlier detection of cancers with effective treatments and the advances made in the medical management and treatment of the disease, survival time following the cancer diagnosis has increased (Jemal et al. 2004). The quality and quantity of survival following a cancer diagnosis is likely to have a diverse impact on the caregiving situation (Lewis 2006; Mellon and Northouse 2001). While the beneficial impact to the family of long-term survival is self-evident, awareness is growing that survivorship may present additional adaptational challenges (Houldin et al. 2006; Hewitt et al. 2006). Extended involvement in care provision increases caregivers' risk of experiencing adverse caregiving consequences. An expanding body of research investigations has documented that cancer caregiving can impact all aspects of the caregiver's life, potentially interfering with occupational, social and leisure activities; restricting privacy; imposing financial burdens; initiating conflicts with well family members; and inducing physical strain, chronic fatigue, and emotional distress (see reviews by Given et al. 2001; Kotkamp-Mothes et al. 2005; Northouse 2005). Cameron et al. (2002) observed that cancer caregivers experienced increased emotional distress, regardless of the amount of care they provided, when their care provision interfered with their lifestyle. Nijboer et al. (2001) documented similar findings in a longitudinal investigation of cancer caregivers. Caregiver depression was associated at baseline and follow-up with the perception of their schedule being disrupted due to care provision.

Coping with Treatment and Disease-Related Side-Effects. Even with advances in cancer treatment, most cancer therapies are not without some adverse health effect (i.e., nausea, pain, fatigue, weight change), that varies in controllability and duration. In addition, patients may also be experiencing disease-related symptoms. Pain and fatigue are particularly difficult for caregivers to observe, especially when efforts to manage them are ineffective. Family caregivers to cancer patients with pain have been found to experience more strain and depressive symptoms than caregivers to cancer patients without pain (Miaskowski et al. 1997). The physiological changes in organ function associated with aging place the older cancer patient at increased risk for treatment-related toxicities (Lindley et al. 1998). Comorbidities, common in older patients, also increase the risk of adverse treatment-related side-effects (Balducci et al. 2005). Elderly patients may be on other medications that can interact with cancer treatments (Edwards et al. 2002).

Substantial progress has been made in effective treatments to manage or reduce treatment or disease-related side effects, such as nausea, fatigue, and pain (Patarca-Montero 2004). Current pain management techniques include the use of patches and pumps to deliver a constant, controlled level of pain medication, enabling effective pain management in the home setting (Glajchen 2004). Despite these practice advances, barriers to effective symptom management during home care exist. Family caregivers often require information, education, and guidance in symptom management, indeed, improvement in care provision is shown following targeted intervention (Given et al. 2001; Golant et al. 2003; Pasacreta et al. 2000).

The need for symptom management does not abate when active treatment has been completed. During survivorship, the patient may experience not only the residual symptoms of the disease itself but also the sequelae of the treatment received. That is, cancer patients can be free of disease, but still experience intense symptoms posttreatment (Chang et al. 2000; Kristjanson 1993). Although some symptoms may have persisted immediately following the active treatment period, there is a growing body of evidence that symptoms associated with the cancer and its treatment can continue to emerge months to years following treatment (Hewitt et al. 2006; Houldin et al. 2006; see review by Newport and Nemeroff 1998). For example, several studies have found clinically significant cancer-related fatigue persisting several years posttreatment (Beisecker et al. 1997; Bergland et al. 1991; Broeckel et al. 1998; Cella et al. 2001). Similar findings have been reported for depression and insomnia (Breitbart 1995; Couzi et al. 1995; Meeuwesen et al. 1991; Spiegel et al. 1994).

Adaptational Challenges in Survivorship. With longer cancer survival periods, more families will have to cope with the emergence of long-term treatment-related consequences that may develop over time and necessitate further care provision. For example, as a consequence of the successes in recent decades in the treatment of childhood cancers, a growing number of adult cancer survivors are now facing a set of new health problems, including the development of new cancers related to the cancer therapies they received during childhood (Friedman and Mulhern 1991; Hewitt et al. 2006). In these instances, the total cancer-related caregiver burden may span decades and can encompass different caregiving cohorts (i.e., parental caregivers during childhood and spousal or adult child caregivers in adulthood).

In the posttreatment survivorship period, the patients and their families are living with the uncertainty centered on the treatment's efficacy and fears of disease recurrence (Li et al. 1997; Mellon and Northouse 2001). Having to live with this uncertainty and needing to adjust to disease-related changes can be highly stressful, creating heightened anxiety, depression, and demoralization among patients and their families (Jessop and Stein 1985; Li et al. 1997; see review by Kotkamp-Mothes et al. 2005). Even if the prognosis for long-term survival is good, family members may need to come to terms with disease or treatment-related changes from the patient's preillness functioning and need to adjust to losses imposed by the illness, including changes in roles and lifestyles. The shock and disbelief that family members experience during the initial diagnosis period may block out consideration of the consequences of living with cancer. Extending survival does not necessarily mean that the person is ultimately restored to a preillness level of functioning. From a care perspective, improvements in cancer survival may mean that more families are involved in a lengthier period of care provision and face the financial, insurance, and employment concerns associated with survivorship.

An emerging issue in cancer survivorship, particularly germane for elderly patients, concerns the growing awareness that survivors' noncancer health needs are not being adequately addressed. A recent analysis of Medicare claims, determined that cancer survivorship was associated with an increased likelihood of not receiving recommended care across a broad range of chronic medical conditions (Earle and Neville 2004). Given the progress in cancer survivorship, families' caregiving burden could be intensified if preventive care and treatment for comorbid conditions are not received. Comorbidities are common in older cancer survivors and this can contribute to the emergence of additional comorbidities posttreatment (Yates et al. 1980). The physiological changes in organ function associated with aging may contribute to late treatment effects on normal tissues and vital organs emerging in long-term older survivors months and years after treatment (Newport and Nemeroff 1998).

Practice: Future Impact

Aging of Population Increase Families' Cancer Burden. As the population ages, the burden of cancer, already considerable in the elderly, will continue to grow. Persons aged 50–64 have cancer rates 7 to 16 times higher than younger adults, with rates for persons aged 65–74 two to three times higher. It is anticipated, based on cancer incidence rates and U.S. Census Department population projections that the number of cancer patients 65 and older will double in the next 30 years (Edwards et al. 2002). This means that the number of persons who are likely to be involved in cancer caregiving will dramatically increase.

Financial Costs of Care. Financial costs of cancer are likely to continue to be a burden to patients and their families and may require them to face some difficult treatment choices. Cancer-related care costs are expected to increase as new, more advanced, and technologically complex therapies become routinely available (Thorpe et al. 2004). The economic costs to families of cancer care can be considerable and advances in cancer treatment may pose additional economic barriers to continued care (see review by Haley 2003). Insurance coverage may be limited for some experimental or prophylactic treatments. The high cost of drugs and medications throughout the survivorship period, or for an extensive period of time, may limit the families who could afford to provide this life-sustaining care.

Psychosocial Challenges of Cancer Survivorship. Even with advances in cancer treatments, most therapies produce some measure of adversity. With the growing number of cancer survivors, attention needs to focus on understanding and addressing the adverse effects of current and new cancer treatments, specifically with regard to the health status and quality of life of patients in their posttreatment years (Hewitt et al. 2006; Houldin et al. 2006).

Attending to the Needs of the Family Caregiver. A recent metaanalysis of distress in the cancer patient-family caregiver dyad confirmed the close relationship in distress levels (Hodges et al. 2005), supporting the value of the healthcare team viewing the patient-family caregiver dyad as the unit of care (Matthews et al. 2003; Raveis and Pretter 2005). Effort has not been routinely directed toward assisting the family in coping with the cancer experience. Rather, family caregivers have been viewed as part of the care team. Little attention has been focused on attending to families' psychosocial concerns living with a genetic risk factor for cancer. Given the emerging developments in genetic research, these issues are likely to take on added significance for families impacted by cancer.

Facilitating Informed Clinical Decision-Making. At various points in the illness continuum, patients and families are confronted with having to make decisions about treatment options. Oftentimes these decisions need to be made quickly, require assessment of complex and technical information, and weighing multiple options with varying risks and benefits against uncertain outcomes. There has been limited effort to facilitate families' involvement in the clinical decision-making process. Given the expected ongoing progress in cancer treatment and management, decision-making is likely to become even more complex in the future and procedures that can assist family in weighing options, arriving at decisions and managing their uncertainty will be critical.

Education and Training: Current Impact

An effective familial caregiver can bolster patients' well-being and alleviate demands on the health care system. However, the viability of the informal care system is not only dependent upon the willingness of the families to provide care, but also their ability to provide the needed care (i.e., task-specific skills and abilities). Deficiencies in a caregiver's performance can seriously impact the well-being of the patient and the family member, threatening the quality and sufficiency of care on a long-term basis.

Acquisition of Specialized Skills. Advances in the management and delivery of cancer treatments have not only permitted the portability of the treatment delivery (i.e., out of the hospital or clinic and into the home), but have also required the caregiver to become involved in the delivery of technical and complex care routines. These are tasks for which families may not have received prior preparation or training and initially are ill-equipped to perform. In an early study of familial caregivers to advanced cancer patients, over two-thirds of the familial caregivers reported having to learn the skills that would enable them to manage the patient's activities of daily living (i.e., assist with the patient's ambulation, handle bowel and bladder disturbances), manage the patient's pain, attend to nutritional needs and dietary requirements, and provide general comfort (Grobe et al. 1981). A recent investigation of family caregivers to end-stage cancer patients documented that this caregiver information gap still exists. Over three-quarters of the caregivers reported needing training in nursing skills and information about medical aids (Jansma et al. 2005; see review by Given et al. 2001).

Education and training programs have demonstrated efficacy in enhancing care provision. Several studies have demonstrated that patient and family education on pain management significantly decreased pain intensity ratings in cancer samples (Overcash et al. 2001; Wright et al. 2001; see review by Green et al. 2003). Cancer caregivers who participated in a course that provided education and support felt less overwhelmed, more knowledgeable, and better able to cope with caregiving (Robinson et al. 1998). Andrews (2001) noted that information was a means of increasing caregivers' feelings of efficacy and lowering perceived burden. Yates and Stetz (1999) have suggested that efforts which increase caregiver knowledge may reduce some of the ambiguity in the caregiving situation, in turn reducing caregiver distress. Coristine et al. (2003) found that caregivers caring for family members with advanced disease found it difficult to understand symptoms experienced by patients and to decide when a medical intervention was necessary. A central component of fatigue management is educating the patient and family about fatigue, i.e., the fact that management strategies exist and that it is important to report fatigue to their health care provider (Cella et al. 1998).

Technological Advances in Training Resources. While caregiver instructional materials are limited, the Internet has become an expanding resource for cancer information and education. There is a growing body of evidence that it is a viable medium for offering individualized clinical information and educational support that address families' informational and cancer caregiving needs (Lewis et al. 2005).

Informed Decision-Making. In making decisions about treatment options, families are faced with having to obtain and evaluate evidence and information that they require to make an informed choice. While efforts are being made to move toward a consolidation or synthesis of best practice approaches (Edwards et al. 2005), specialized knowledge may be necessary for family members to fully understand the clinical information about treatment options and weigh their merits and potential consequences. As cancer treatment continues to advance, families may be confronted with more complex decisions. Informed decision-making necessitates that families fully understand the level of uncertainty involved in the cancer treatment and management decisions. Interventions have been shown to be beneficial to families in managing treatment uncertainty in decision-making (Germino et al. 1998; Maliski et al. 2002; Mishel et al. 2002, 2003).

Education and Training: Future Impact

Targeted and Sustained Education Needed. Even though recent years have seen a growth in education and training opportunities for family caregivers, significantly more resources need to be provided. Caregivers' basic information needs are not sufficiently met (Chalmers et al. 2003; Iconomou et al. 2001). Training programs for family caregivers tend to be sparse and localized, usually institutionally based. Family caregivers would benefit from systematic efforts to provide education and training in basic nursing and home medical care techniques, symptom interpretation, managing treatment and illness-related side effects, as well as training in operating and maintaining in the home specialized equipment or devices. Demonstration programs which may provide specialized or targeted training and support tend to be time-limited. Instructional programs and materials for diverse caregiving groups need to be accessible throughout the disease course and updated to reflect emerging technological developments and advances in treatment and management of cancer.

Policy: Current Impact

A variety of policies implemented since the initiation of the National Cancer Act in 1971 have directly impacted how cancer care is delivered and accessed, as well as the resources available for coping and adapting to the cancer experience (Dunn 2002). As discussed below, the outcomes of these policies have shaped cancer caregiving.

Mandate to Deliver Cancer Advances to the Broader Community. During the 1980s, the National Cancer Institute (NCI) initiated a policy-driven effort to disseminate the technological developments in cancer treatment and control that are available at the major cancer centers to the broader medical community. The Community Clinical Oncology Program (CCOP) is an example of one such organizational mechanism, established by NCI, to facilitate technology transfer to community oncology programs and permit advances in cancer care to be available in community settings (Kaluzny et al. 1989). Efforts were also instituted to expand community access to NCI clinical trials. Although geographic disparities in access to quality cancer care still exist (Edwards et al. 2005), these changes have made it more feasible and less of a burden for patients to participate in clinical trials and to obtain access to the latest advances in cancer treatment while remaining in their community. Previously, clinical trial participation or access to specialized and/or state-of-the-art cancer therapies has generally only been available in major clinical and research cancer centers. Families would have to incur considerable financial expense and experience substantial time and social costs traveling to a distant treatment center for what would typically be a lengthy cancer treatment period. The National Institute of Health's policy shift to start including the elderly in most clinical trials has contributed to cancer being more aggressively treated in older adults.

Resources to Affected Groups. As part of a growing recognition on a national level of the complex challenges families face in providing adequate care or maintaining care over a lengthy time interval, a number of legislative developments have been enacted to facilitate families' management of their care burdens and demands. Examples include the Older Americans Act, which includes the National Family Caregivers

Support Program and the Family and Medical Leave Act. There has also been growing awareness over the last few decades that cancer is a family illness (Baider et al. 1999). That is, in addition to cancer affecting the patients themselves, its diagnosis, treatment, and resolution affect their family members as well, the "second-order patients" (Rait and Lederberg 1989; see review by Nijboer et al. 1998). Policy statements issued by the National Cancer Institute define cancer survivors as anyone touched by cancer (National Cancer Institute Office of Cancer Survivorship n. d.). Indeed, the National Coalition for Cancer Survivorship has stated that the patient and family should be seen as a unit of care and notes the necessity of addressing the impact and consequences of cancer care on family caregivers (Clark et al. 1996).

Policy: Future Impact

Supportive Services Needed. As advances in cancer care continue to transform cancer into a chronic disease, more individuals in the future will be living with and affected by the cancer experience. Policies that provide families with respite care, tax relief, employee caregiver assistance programs, insurance coverage for experimental procedures (including participation in clinical trials, complementary or alternative medicine), and caregiving-related "out-of-pocket" expenses, would be beneficial to family caregivers and provide relief for some caregiving burdens.

Conclusions

Family members are being increasingly relied upon as the major source of support and assistance to persons with cancer. Developments in the treatment and management of cancer are contributing to an expansion of the scope and duration of the family caregiving role. Current trends suggest that the magnitude and complexity of the caregiving situation will continue to evolve. Although advances have reduced mortality and increased cancer survival, a growing number of individuals will be living with the effect of the disease. Even though our understanding of the caregiving process is still evolving, there is a pressing need to focus more attention on addressing the challenges families face throughout the disease course.

References

American Cancer Society. (2006). *Cancer facts and figures 2006.* Atlanta: American Cancer Society.
Andrews, S. (2001). Caregiver burden and symptom distress in people with cancer receiving hospice care. *Oncology Nursing Forum, 28,* 1469–1474.
Balducci, L. (2006). Management of cancer in the elderly. *Oncology, 20*(2), 135–143.
Balducci, L., & Yates, J. (2000). General guidelines for the management of older patients with cancer. *Oncology (Huntington), 14,* 221–227.

Balducci, L., Cohen, H. J., Engstrom, P. F., Ettinger, D. S., Halter, J., Gordon, L. I., et al. (2005). Senior adult oncology clinical practice guidelines in oncology. *Journal of the National Comprehensive Cancer Network, 3*(4), 572–590.

Baider, L., Ever-Hadani, P., & Kaplan De-Nour, A. (1999). Psychological distress in healthy women with familial breast cancer: Like mother, like daughter? *International Journal of Psychiatry in Medicine, 29*(4), 411–420.

Baider, L., Ever-Hadani, P., Goldzweig, G., Wygoda, M. R., & Peretz, T. (2003). Is perceived family support a relevant variable in psychological distress? A sample of prostate and breast cancer couples. *Journal of Psychosomatic Research, 55,* 453–460.

Beisecker, A., Cook, M. R., Ashworth, J., Hayes, J., Brecheisen, M., Helmig, L., et al. (1997). Side effects of adjuvant chemotherapy: Perception of node-negative breast cancer patients. *Psycho-Oncology, 6,* 85–93.

Bergland, G., Bolund, C., Fornader, T., Rutqvist, L. E., & Sjoden, P. O. (1991). Late effects of adjuvant chemotherapy and postoperative radiotherapy on quality of life among breast cancer patients. *European Journal of Cancer, 27,* 1075–1081.

Blanchard, C. G., Albrecht, T. L., & Ruckdeschel, J. C. (1997). The crisis of cancer: Psychological impact on family caregivers. *Oncology, 11,* 189–194.

Breitbart, W. (1995). Identifying patients at risk for, and treatment of major psychiatric complications of cancer. *Supportive Care in Cancer, 3*(1), 45–60.

Broeckel, J. A., Jacobsen, P. B., Horton, J., Balducci, L., & Lyman, G. H. (1998). Characteristics and correlates of fatigue after adjuvant chemotherapy for breast cancer. *Journal of Clinical Oncology, 16,* 1689–1696.

Cameron, J. I., Franche, R. L., Cheung, A. M., & Stewart, D. E. (2002). Lifestyle interference and emotional distress in family caregivers of advanced cancer patients. *Cancer, 94,* 521–527.

Carreca, I., Balducci, L., & Extermann, M. (2005). Cancer in the older person. *Cancer Treatment Reviews, 31*(5), 380–402.

Cella, D., Peterman, A., Passik, S., Jacobsen, P., & Breitbart, W. (1998). Progress toward guidelines for the management of fatigue. *Oncology, 12*(11A), 369–377.

Cella, D., Davis, K., Breitbart, W., & Curt, G. (2001). Cancer-related fatigue: Prevalence of proposed diagnostic criteria in a United States sample of cancer survivors. *Journal of Clinical Oncology, 19*(14), 3385–3391.

Chalmers, K., Marles, S., Tataryn, D., Scott-Findlay, S., & Serkas, K. (2003). Reports of information and support needs of daughters and sisters of women with breast cancer. *European Journal of Cancer Care, 12,* 81–90.

Chang, V. T., Hwangt, S. S., Feuerman, M., & Kasimis, B. S. (2000). Symptom and quality of life survey of medical oncology patients at a Veterans Affairs Medical Center: A role for symptom management. *Cancer, 88*(5), 1175–1183.

Clark, E. J., Stovall, E. L., Leigh, S., Siu, A. L., Austin, D. K., & Rowland, J. H. (1996). *Imperatives for quality cancer care: Access, advocacy, action and accountability.* Silver Spring: National Coalition for Cancer Survivorship. http://www.canceradvocacy.org/advocacy/intro/imperatives.aspx. Accessed 14 Apr 2006.

Coristine, M., Crooks, D., Grunfeld, E., Stonebridge, C., & Christie, A. (2003). Caregiving for women with advanced breast cancer. *Psycho-Oncology, 12,* 709–719.

Couzi, R. J., Helzlsouer, K. J., & Fetting, J. H. (1995). Prevalence of menopausal symptoms among women with a history of breast cancer and attitudes towards estrogen replacement therapy. *Journal of Clinical Oncology, 13,* 2737–2744.

Crawley, M. M. (1990). Recent advances in chemotherapy: Administration and nursing implications. *Nursing Clinics of North American, 25*(2), 377–391.

Dunn, F. B. (2002). Legislators rally support for revised National Cancer Act. *Journal of National Cancer Institute, 94,* 410–411. Retrieved from http://jncicancerspectrum.oxfordjournals.org/cgi/content/full/jnci;94/6/410.

Earle, C. C., & Neville, B. A. (2004). Under use of necessary care among cancer survivors. *Cancer, 101*(8), 1712–1719.

Edwards, B. K., Howe, H. L., Ries, L. A. G., Thun, M. J., Rosenberg, H. M., Yancik, R., et al. (2002). Annual report to the nation on the status of cancer, 1973–1999: Featuring implications of age and aging on U.S. cancer burden. *Cancer, 94*(10), 2766–2792.

Edwards, B. K., Brown, M. L., Wingo, P. A., Howe, H. L., Ward, E., Ries, L. A. G., et al. (2005). Annual report to the nation on the status of cancer, 1975–2002, featuring population-based trends in cancer treatment. *Journal of the National Cancer Institute, 97,* 1407–1427.

Ferrell, B. R., Cohen, M. Z., Rhiner, M., & Rozek, A. (1991). Pain as a metaphor for illness. Part II: Family caregiver's management of pain. *Oncology Nursing Forum, 18,* 1315–1321.

Friedman, A., & Mulhern, R. (1991). Psychological adjustment among children who are long-term survivors of cancer. In J. A. Johnson & S. D. Johnson (Eds.), *Advances in child health psychology* (pp. 16–27). Gainesville: University Press of Florida Press.

Germino, B. B., Mischel, M. H., Belyea, M., Harris, L., Ware, A., & Mohler, J. (1998). Uncertainty in prostate cancer: Ethnic and family patterns. *Cancer Practice: A Multidisciplinary Journal of Cancer Care, 6*(2), 107–113.

Gilbar, O., & Ben-Zur, H. (2002). *Cancer and the family caregiver: Distress and coping.* Springfield: Charles C. Thomas, Ltd.

Given, B. A., Given, C. W., & Kozachik, S. (2001). Family support in advanced cancer. *CA: A Cancer Journal for Clinicians, 51*(4), 213–231. Retrived from http://caonline.amcancersoc.org/cgi/reprint/51/4/213.

Glajchen, M. (2004). The emerging role and needs of family caregivers in cancer care. *Journal of Supportive Oncology, 2*(2), 145–155.

Golant, M., Altman, T., & Martin, C. (2003). Managing cancer side effects to improve quality of life: A cancer psychoeducation program. *Cancer Nursing, 26*(1), 37–44.

Green, C. R., Anderson, K. O., Baker, T. A., Campbell, L. C., Decker, S., Fillingim, R. B., et al. (2003). The unequal burden of pain: Confronting racial and ethnic disparities in pain. *Pain Medicine, 4*(3), 277–294.

Grobe, M. E., Ilstrup, D. M., & Ahmann, D. L. (1981). Skills needed by family members to maintain the care of an advanced cancer patient. *Cancer Nursing, 4*(5), 371–375.

Haley, W. E. (2003). The costs of family caregiving: Implications for geriatric oncology. *Critical Reviews in Oncology/Hematology, 48,* 151–158.

Hewitt, M., Greenfield, S., & Stovall, E. (Eds.). (2006). *From cancer patient to cancer survivor: Lost in transition.* Washington: National Academies Press.

Hodges, L. J., Humphris, G. M., & Macfarlane, G. (2005). A meta-analytic investigation of the relationship between the psychological distress of cancer patients and their carers. *Social Science & Medicine, 60,* 1–12.

Houldin, A., Curtiss, C. P., & Haylock, P. J. (2006). Executive summary: The state of the science on nursing approaches to managing late and long-term sequelae of cancer and cancer treatment. *American Journal of Nursing, 106*(3 Suppl), 6–11.

Iconomou, G., Vagenakis, A. G., & Kalofonos, H. P. (2001). The informational needs, satisfaction with communication, and psychological status of primary caregivers of cancer patients receiving chemotherapy. *Support Care Cancer, 9,* 591–596.

Jansma, F. F., Schure, L. M., & de Jong, B. M. (2005). Support requirements for caregivers of patients with palliative cancer. *Patient Education and Counseling, 58,* 182–186.

Jemal, A., Clegg, L. X., Ward, E., Ries, L. A. G., Wu, X., Jamison, P. M., et al. (2004). Annual report to the nation on the status of cancer, 1975–2001, with a special feature regarding survival. *Cancer, 101*(1), 3–27.

Jemal, A., Siegel, R., Ward, E., Murray, T., Xu J., Smigal, C., & Thun, M. J. (2006). Cancer statistics, 2006. *CA: A Cancer Journal for Clinicians, 56,* 106–130. Retrieved from http://caonline.amcancersoc.org/cgi/content/full/56/2/106.

Jessop, D. J., & Stein, R. E. K. (1985). Uncertainty and its relation to the psychological and social correlates of chronic illness in children. *Social Science and Medicine, 20,* 993–999.

Kaluzny, A. D., Ricketts, III, T. Warneck, R., Ford, L., Morrissey, J., Gillings, D., et al. (1989). Evaluating organizational design to assure technology transfer: The case of the community clinical oncology Program. *Journal of the National Cancer Institute, 81*(22), 1717–1725.

Kash, K. M., Dabney, M. K., Holland, J. C., Osborne, M. P., & Miller, D. G. (2000). Familial cancer and genetics: Psychosocial and ethical aspects. In L. Baider, C. L. Cooper, & A. K. De-Nour (Eds.), *Cancer and the family* (pp. 389–401). New York: Wiley.

Kelly, P. T. (1983). "High risk" women: Breast cancer concerns and health practices. *Frontiers in Radiation Therapy Oncology, 17,* 11–15.

Kotkamp-Mothes, N., Slawinsky, D., Hindermann, S., & Strauss, B. (2005). Coping and psychological well being in families of elderly cancer patients. *Critical Reviews in Oncology/Hematology, 55*(3), 213–229.

Kristjanson, L. J. (1993). Validity and reliability testing of the FAMCARE scale: Measuring family satisfaction with advanced cancer care. *Social Science and Medicine, 36,* 693–701.

Kurtz, M. F., Given, B., Kurtz, J. C., & Given, C. W. (1994). The interaction of age, symptoms, and survival status on physical and mental health of patients with cancer and their families. *Cancer, 74,* 2071–2078.

Lewis, F. M. (2006). The effects of cancer survivorship on families and caregivers: More research is needed on long-term survivors. *American Journal of Nursing, 106*(3 suppl), 20–25.

Lewis, D., Gundwardena, S., & Saadawi, G. (2005). Caring connection: Developing an internet resource for family caregivers of children with cancer. *Computers, Informatics, Nursing, 23*(5), 265–274.

Li, L. W., Seltzer, M. M., & Greenberg, J. S. (1997). Social support and depressive symptoms: Differential patterns in wife and daughter caregivers. *Journal of Gerontology: Social Sciences, 52B*(4), S200–211.

Lindley, C., Vasa, S., Sawyer, W. T., & Winer, E. P. (1998). Quality of life and preference for treatment following systemic adjuvant therapy for early-stage breast cancer. *Journal of Clinical Oncology, 16,* 1380–1387.

Maliski, S. L., Heilemann, M. V., & McCorkle, R. (2002). From "death sentence" to "good cancer": Couples' transformation of a prostate cancer diagnosis. *Nursing Research, 51*(6), 391–397.

Matthews, B. A., Baker, F., & Spillers, R. L. (2003). Family caregivers and indicators of cancer-related stress. *Psychology, Health & Medicine, 8*(1), 45–56.

Meeuwesen, L., Schaap, C., & VanDer Staak, C. (1991). Verbal analysis of doctor-patient communication. *Social Science and Medicine, 32,* 1143–1150.

Meiser, B., Butow, P., Barratt, A., Gattas, M., Gaff, C., Haan, E., et al. (2001). Risk perceptions and knowledge of breast cancer in women at increased risk of developing hereditary breast cancer. *Psychology & Health, 16*(3), 297–311.

Mellon, S., & Northouse, L. L. (2001). Family survivorship and quality of life following a cancer diagnosis. *Research in Nursing & Health, 24,* 446–459.

Miaskowski, C., Kragness, L., Dibble, S., & Wallhagen M. (1997). Differences in mood states, health status, and caregiver strain between family caregivers of oncology outpatients with and without cancer-related pain. *Journal of Pain & Symptom Management, 13,* 138–147.

Mishel, M. H., Belyea, M., Germino, B. B., Stewart, J. L., Bailey, D. E. Jr., Robertson, C., et al. (2002). Helping patients with localized prostate carcinoma manage uncertainty and treatment side effects: Nurse-delivered psychoeducational intervention over the telephone. *Cancer, 94*(6), 1854–1866.

Mishel, M. H., Germino, B. B., Belyea, M., Stewart, J. L., Bailey, D. E. Jr., Mohler, J., et al. (2003). Moderators of an uncertainty management intervention: For men with localized prostate cancer. *Nursing Research, 52*(2), 89–97.

Mor, V., Allen, S., Siegel, K., & Houts, P. (1992). Determinants of need and unmet need among cancer patients residing at home. *Health Services Research, 27*(3), 337–360.

National Cancer Institute. (2004). Bone marrow transplantation and peripheral blood stem cell transplantation: Questions and answers. *NCI Fact Sheet: Cancer Therapy, 7*(41). Retrieved at http://www.cancer.gov/cancertopics. Accessed 12 Apr 2006.

National Cancer Institute. (2006). NCI studies using the COX-2 Inhibitor Celecoxib: Questions and answers. *NCI News Releases.* Retrieved Jan http://www.cancer.gov/newscenter/pressreleases/ Accessed 17 Dec 2004, update 4 Feb 2006.

National Cancer Institute Office of Cancer Survivorship. (n. d.). *About cancer survivorship research: Survivorship definitions.* Retrieved from http://dccps.nci.nih.gov/ocs/definitions.html. Accessed 16 Aug 2005.

NCI Alliance for Nanotechnology in Cancer. (2005, November). Nanotechnology en route from bench to bedside for cancer patients. *Monthly Feature.* http://nano.cancer.gov/news_center/monthly_feature_2005_nov.asp

Newport, D. J., & Nemeroff, C. B. (1998). Assessment and treatment of depression in cancer patients. *Journal of Psychosomatic Research, 45,* 215–237.

Nijboer, C., Tempelaar, R., Sanderman, R., Triemstra, M., Spruijt, R. J., & van den Bos, G. A. M. (1998). Cancer and caregiving: The impact on the caregiver's health. *Psycho-Oncology, 7,* 3–13.

Nijboer, C., Tempelaar, R., Triemstra, M., van den Bos, G. A., & Sanderman, R. (2001). The role of social and psychologic resources in caregiving of cancer patients. *Cancer, 91,* 1029–1039.

Northouse, L. (2005). Helping families of patients with cancer. *Oncology Nursing Forum, 32*(4), 743–750.

Northouse, L. L., Mood, D., Templin, T., Mellon, S., & George, T. (2000). Couples' patterns of adjustment to colon cancer. *Social Science and Medicine, 50*(2), 271–284.

Overcash, J., Extermann, M., Parr, J., Perry, J., & Balducci, L. (2001). Validity and reliability of the FACT-G scale for use in the older person with cancer. *American Journal of Clinical Oncology, 21*(6), 591–596.

Pasacreta, J. V., Barg, F., Nuamah, I., & McCorkle, R. (2000). Participant characteristics before and 4 months after attendance at a family caregiver cancer education program. *Cancer Nursing, 23*(4), 295–303.

Patarca-Montero, R. (2004). *Handbook of cancer-related fatigue.* New York: Haworth Medical Press.

Rait, D., & Lederberg, M. (1989). The family of the patient with cancer. In J. C. Holland & J. Rowland (Eds.), *Psychological care of the patient* (pp. 585–597). New York: Oxford University Press.

Raveis, V. H. (2007). The challenges and issues confronting family caregivers to elderly cancer patients. In S. Carmel, C. A. Morse, & F. M. Torres-Gil (Eds.), *The art of ageing well: Lessons from three nations* (pp. 85–98). New York: Baywood Press.

Raveis, V. H., & Pretter, S. (2005). Existential plight of adult daughters following their mother's breast cancer diagnosis. *Psycho-Oncology, 14,* 49–60.

Raveis, V. H., Karus, D., & Siegel, K. (1998). Correlates of depressive symptomatology among adult daughter caregivers to a parent with cancer. *Cancer, 83*(8), 1652–1663.

Robinson, K. D., Angeletti, K. A., Barg, F. K., Pasacreta, J. V., McCorkle, R., & Yasko, J. M. (1998). The development of a family caregiver cancer education program. *Journal of Cancer Education, 12*(2), 116–121.

Sankar, P. (2004). Communication and miscommunication in informed consent to research. *Medical Anthropology Quarterly, 18*(4), 429–446.

Schumacher, K. L., Stewart, B. J., Archbold, P. G., Dodd, M. J., & Dibble, S. L. (2000). Family caregiving skill: Development of the concept. *Research in Nursing and Health, 23,* 191–203.

Siegel, K., Karus, D., Raveis, V. H., Christ, G. H., & Mesagno, F. P. (1996). Depressive distress among the spouses of terminally ill cancer patients. *Cancer Practice, 4,* 25–30.

Spiegel, D., Sands, S., & Koopman, C. (1994). Pain and depression in patients with cancer. *Cancer, 74,* 2570–2578.

Thorpe, K. E., Florence, C. S., & Joski, P. (2004, August 25). Which medical conditions account for the rise in health care spending? *Health Affairs—Web Exclusive, W4,* 437–445. Accessed from http://content.healthaffairs.org/cgi/content/abstract/hlthaff.w4.437. Accessed 25 Aug 2004.

Wallace, M., Bailey, D., Jr., O'Rourke, M., & Gailbraith, M. (2004). The watchful, waiting management option for older men with prostate cancer: State of the science. *Oncology Nursing Forum, 31*(6), 1057–1066.

Wellisch, D. K, Gritz, E. R., Schain, W., Wang, H. J., & Siau, J. (1991). Psychological functioning of daughters of breast cancer patients: Part I: Daughters and comparison subjects. *Psychosomatics, 32*(3), 324–336.

Wellisch, D. K., Gritz, E. R., Schain, W., Wang, H. J., & Siau, J. (1992). Psychological functioning of daughters of breast cancer patients: Part II: Characterizing the distressed daughter of the breast cancer patient. *Psychosomatics, 33*, 171–179.

Winstead, E. R. (2005). Vaccine to prevent cervical cancer is effective. *NCI Cancer Bulletin, 39*(2), 1–2.

Wright, J. T., Jr., Cushman, W. C., Davis, B., Barzilay, J., Colon, P., Egan, D., et al. (2001). The antihypertensive and lipid lowering treatment to prevent heart attack trial (ALLHAT): Clinical center recruitment experience. *Controlled Clinical Trials, 22*(6), 659–673.

Yates, P., & Stetz, K. M. (1999). Families' awareness of and response to dying. *Oncology Nursing Forum, 26,* 113–120.

Yates, J. W., Chalmer, B., & McKegney, F. P. (1980). Evaluation of patients with advanced cancer using the Karnofsky Performance Status. *Cancer, 45*(8), 2220–2224.

Part III
Cross-Cutting Issues Impacting Caregivers and Caregiving

Chapter 11
Caregiver Stress: The Role of Spirituality in the Lives of Family/Friends and Professional Caregivers of Cancer Patients

Christina M. Puchalski

Caring for loved ones or patients who have chronic or serious illness or disability can be one of the most challenging times in a personal or professional caregiver's life. The experience is filled with so many challenging events that can result in emotional, physical, social, and spiritual changes, not only in the patient, but also in those who care for the patient. These changes can create considerable challenges for those involved in the caring process. However, the changes can also offer an opportunity for growth, fulfillment, and deepening of relationships. However, there is no simple roadmap to follow in learning how to care for others so that the positives outweigh the negatives. The changes that occur in patients and in caregivers are unpredictable; often resolutions are not easy to find.

In many ways, caring for each individual person becomes unchartered territory as each person is unique and handles his or her illness in his or her unique way. Consequently, caregivers may feel unprepared to handle the challenges as they arise. This can result in stress for the caregivers with resultant physiologic and psychological responses (Kloosterhouse 2002). This is particularly true for caregivers with a loved one with cancer. A diagnosis of cancer can cause extreme fear, helplessness, emotional and spiritual distress. The uncertainty associated with treatment choices and treatment outcome can cause tremendous anxiety and stress for patients and their loved ones.

There has been substantial anecdotal and research evidence of the physiological and emotional effects of stress on a person. Herbert Benson and others have demonstrated that stress can result in deleterious health effects, such as hypertension, cardiovascular disease, ulcers, insomnia, anxiety, depression, anger, and fatigue (Benson 1996; Selye 1978). Yet, others have identified an association between stress, the lack of psychosocial resources to deal with stressors, and immunologic disturbances. There is increasing evidence of the effect of stress on the Psychoneuroendocrine immunologic pathways—the links between the endocrine, immune, and central nervous system. Glaser et al. (1999) and Anderson et al. (1994) have shown

C. M. Puchalski (✉)
School of Medicine and Health Sciences, The George Washington University,
2300 I St NW, Suite 419, Washington, DC 20037, USA
e-mail: cpuchals@gwu.edu

R. C. Talley et al. (eds.), *Cancer Caregiving in the United States*,
Caregiving: Research, Practice, Policy,
DOI 10.1007/978-1-4614-3154-1_11, © Springer Science+Business Media, LLC 2012

that psychological stress can disrupt these pathways. The changes have been linked to adverse health effects such as cardiovascular, rheumatologic, and infectious disease. Petry et al. (1991) describe an increase in stress that is associated with higher incidences of influenza, respiratory illness, and workdays lost due to infectious disease.

Extensive research has documented the effect of caregiver burden and stress on the lives of caregivers (Brody 1981; Jivanjee 1994; Montgomery 1985; Pruchno 1989; Zarit 1986). It is well-documented that providing supportive care during the diagnosis and treatment of cancer may positively affect the mental health and stress levels of the family caregiver (Miaskowski et al. 1997; Miller et al. 1991; Schott-Baer 1993; Wyatt et al. 1999). The stress of caregiving responsibilities can result in poor health, depression, social isolation, and financial strain (Robinson 1990). Patients with serious illness often need help with their activities of daily living, personal self-care, finances, etc. This is especially true for elderly patients. Often, outside help is not readily available; only 5% of community-dwelling, long-term care recipients receive help from outside services (Ham and Slone 1992) and home care practically relieves only about 5–10 hour per week of family care. Ultimately, the responsibility of caring falls on the family, who are adult offspring, usually women or the spouse (Brakman 1994), or a combination of family and friends.

Also, having a child in the hospital usually generates a high level of stress in the family (Kloosterhouse and Ames 2002). As the family attempts to cope, transitions occur within the family system (McCubbin and Patterson 1983). As a result, family roles may get shifted; marital conflict and issues with other siblings may further add to the stress. Financial and emotional stress can further alter the family unit. Melynk and Alpert-Gillis (1998) write that parents of seriously-ill children are at high risk of experiencing a negative outcome as well as intense emotional liability. Families need resources to help them through the caregiving process, resources that are often not available. This is particularly relevant in the current climate of healthcare. As increased financial issues weaken the healthcare system, patients are cared for less in hospitals and more in the homes.

Caregivers are required to put their own lives on hold, to varying degrees, in order to care for the needs of the loved one who had cancer. Caregivers sacrifice their personal time and often their professional time with frequent absences from work (Vachon et al. 1995). Caregivers tend to feel isolated and ill-prepared to take on the task of caregiving (Beck-Friss and Stang 1993; Jones et al. 1993). Adult caregivers often neglect their own health (Lindgren 1993), which can result in increased stress for the caregiver as well as the patient (Pierce 1993). Caregivers can begin to question who they are and what gives value and meaning to their lives. However, of all these stressors, probably the greatest stress is created by the ambiguity regarding the patient's health, including the prognosis, capacity of family to provide support and care, and financial concerns (Kloosterhouse and Ames 2002; Melynk and Alpert-Gillins 1998). There is a tremendous amount of uncertainty with any illness and in life in general. While science and medicine may have some answers to many of the physical aspects of disease and illness, there are so many aspects of being ill for which there are no answers:

Table 11.1 Spiritual issues for caregivers

Loss of meaning—no time for other activities, relationships
Guilt/shame—feelings of resentment for ill persons not being able to be there 100%
Questions of faith/God
Anger at God—change in life, illness, and loved one
Sense of abandonment—caregiver feels alone, uncertain

- When will my loved one die and how?
- How long can my loved one function like this?
- Why cannot this illness be cured?
- Why is he suffering?
- Why do I feel angry with her?
- Why is he happy one day and depressed the next?
- How will I cope with her death?
- What is the meaning and purpose of my life in the midst of this caregiving experience and stress?
- Why cannot I do and be everything to another person?

These are just some of the questions that face caregivers for which there are no exact answers. Much of what caregiving involves is engaging in problem solving in situations that have clear answers for some issues and no or little answers for others. This uncertainty can lead to increased stress and suffering for both the caregivers and the patient. Caregivers are forced to change their priorities and often drastically change their life due to the lack of certainty that is inherent in any situation of a chronically-ill patient.

These questions of uncertainty, limitations, meaning, and purpose are essentially existential or spiritual questions. Burton (1998) writes, "Spirituality is the expression of self-in-relation, incorporating both material and nonmaterial realities, and reflecting the tension between the possibilities and limitations of human existence in history." Thus, caregiving will trigger spiritual questions within the caregiver as well as the patient. Some spiritual issues caregivers face are outlined in (Table 11.1). It is critical that those questions be addressed and supported.

There are many education programs for physicians and other healthcare providers that teach professionals how to address spiritual issues with cancer patients (Puchalski 2002, 2006; Puchalski and Romer 2000). It is important that those programs also extend to families and friends who are the personal caregivers as well as to professionals who are caregiving. Stress is common in the workplace, particularly for those in the healing professions (Funk 1995). Demands are frequently placed on professional caregivers that lead to an accumulation of pressure. Healthcare professionals are confronted with losing satisfaction in their work as the stresses of the changing healthcare system escalate (Remen 1977; Sulmasy 1997). There are unique stressors for professionals, including time management, boundary issues in developing relationships with patients and their families, issues of control, and battling uncertainty in the face of an educational system that teaches certainty, grief, and loss. Sulmasy writes, "Physicians are so afraid of uncertainty that they fear being generalists, fear the consequences of not doing CT scans for headaches." Montgomery

Table 11.2 Caregiver's well-being	Physical—sleep, exercise, good nutrition
	Emotional—counseling, treating depression and anxiety, grief work
	Social—support groups, talking with friends, church
	Spiritual—meditation, yoga, chaplains or spiritual directors, religious activities, deriving meaning from caregivers, forgiveness, humor, ritual

(1997) notes, "Nurses are constantly challenged to make sense of the insensible when they are confronted with inhumanity, violence, suffering, and trauma." She further goes on to postulate that the exposure to suffering and the existential questions that arise from suffering may lead to a spiritual or philosophical growth, or it may result in a "gradual wearing down of the spirit," but that the relationship with the patient facilitates spiritual growth for the professional caregiver by allowing the nurse to become part of a larger consciousness.

Since caregiving demands lead to increased stress for cancer caregivers, and stress can have deleterious health and emotional effects, self-care, therefore, becomes essential for the caregiver. However, often the needs of the cancer patient outweigh the needs of the caregivers in the process of caring for a loved one. Caregivers need to look at their own physical, social, emotional, and spiritual well-being throughout the process of caregiving (see Table 11.2). As we discuss ideal systems of care, it is critical that we give care of the cancer caregiver the same weight we assign to care of the patient with cancer. Furthermore, we need to design systems of care in which all dimensions of care—physical, emotional, social, and spiritual—are addressed.

What is Spirituality?

Spirituality is able to go beyond what is within the reach of our senses and deal with what gives meaning and substance to our lives (Puchalski and Sandoval 2003). One can ask questions such as:

- Who am I?
- What am I?
- What is my purpose?

Advanced illness is frequently characterized by suffering and distress that may manifest as these spiritual questions, and as not only physical and psychological symptoms, but also as existential or spiritual distress. Spiritual and existential distress is probably the least understood source of suffering in patients with advanced disease, for it deals with questions regarding the meaning of life, the fear of death, and the realization that one will be separated from their loved ones (Doyle 1992). Thus, illness, dying, and death are spiritual as well as physical events in the lives of patients and caregivers.

In a study of spirituality among the terminally ill, Reed (1987) defined spirituality as the relationship outside one's self: "Spirituality is defined in terms of personal views and behaviors that express a sense of relatedness to a transcendent dimension or to something greater than self." For many, these existential questions are mainly expressed in a formal religion by the belief in a deity, the theology of the religion, the concept of an afterlife, and the rituals and practices of the religion used to express those beliefs. Many religious traditions have a rich tradition and experience in giving meaning to the cause of suffering and how to restructure it into a positive experience. Sumner (1998) further defines spirituality in terms of values and "as a way of being and experiencing that comes about through the awareness of a transcendent dimension. Spirituality is characterized by certain identifiable values in regard to self, others, nature, life and whatever one considers to be the Ultimate.... It is that which gives one purpose, meaning and hope and provides a vital connection" (Sumner 1998, p. 28).

Addressing the role of religion in medicine in the first decade of the last century, William Osler wrote:

> Nothing in life is more wonderful than faith, the one great moving force, which we can neither weigh in the balance nor test in the crucible. Intangible as the ether, ineluctable as gravitation, the radium of the moral and mental spheres, mysterious, indefinable, known only by its effects, faith pours out an unfailing stream of energy while abating neither jot nor tittle of its potence (Osler 1910, p. 1471).

Osler concluded that not only did faith have important effects on health outcomes, but also that practitioners should encourage and incorporate faith as part of clinical care.

However, spirituality can be much broader than religion. People can find meaning in many different ways. One definition used in the clinical setting is:

> Spirituality is recognized as a factor that contributes to health in many persons. The concept of spirituality is found in all cultures and societies. It is expressed in an individual's search for ultimate meaning through participation in religion and/or belief in God, family, naturalism, rationalism, humanism and the arts. All of these factors can influence how patients and health care professionals perceive health and illness and how the interact with one another. (Association of American Medical Colleges 1999, p. 27)

How people find meaning and purpose in life and in the midst of suffering varies. Through one's spirituality, people develop a person roadmap that guides them through life. Whatever form spirituality takes, its active practice can help patients cope with the uncertainty of their illness, instill hope, bring comfort and support from others, and bring resolution to existential concerns, particularly the fear of death.

Humans are intrinsically spiritual beings. The 1971 White House Conference on Aging asserted that "all persons are spiritual, even if they have no use for religious institutions and practice no personal pieties. An individual's unique spirituality or spiritual style is the way he or she seeks, finds or creates, uses and expands personal meaning in the context of the entire universe" (Moberg 1971). All humans search for meaning and purpose in their lives (O'Connell 1996). Sulmasy (2002) calls this the "notion of the human person as a being in relationship." A cancer diagnosis, just as any illness, however, can disrupt any sense of meaning and purpose and affect relationships within and outside the person (Foglio and Brody 1988). Illness, including cancer, can cause people to suffer deeply. Frankl (1984) wrote, "Man is not destroyed by suffering; he is destroyed by suffering without meaning." He noted when writing about concentration camp victims that survival itself might depend on seeking and finding meaning. Spirituality, then, is one way to bring wholeness and healing to a person by a return to an integrated state where there is meaning and purpose even in the midst of suffering and loss.

In facing a serious illness such as cancer, cure may not be possible, but healing can occur. Cancer may disrupt a person's life, however, it can also offer a person the opportunity to see life in a different way. Many people with a serious and often terminal illness such as cancer talk of seeing a richness and fullness in life that they had never seen before. Some people find new priorities in their life and new appreciation for aspects of their life that they never noticed before.

Healing, then, is not synonymous with recovery, and it may occur at any time, independent of recovery from the illness of cancer. In dying, for example, restoration of wholeness may be manifested by a transcendent set of meaningful experiences while very ill, and a peaceful death. In dealing with cancer, healing may be experienced as the acceptance of limitations (Puchalski 1999). A person may look to medical care to alleviate his or her suffering and when the medical system fails to do so, begin to look toward spirituality for meaning, purpose, and understanding. It is the combination of good clinical, technical, and spiritual care that can provide the most holistic care for individuals with cancer.

The Role of Spirituality in Health

Survey Data Demonstrating Patient Need

Several national surveys have documented patients desire to have spiritual concerns addressed by their physicians. A 1990 Gallup Poll showed that religion, one expression of spirituality, plays a central role in the lives of many Americans. When asked, 95% of Americans surveyed espouse a belief in God, 57% report praying daily, and 42% report attending a worship service in the prior week (Gallup 1990). The need for attentiveness to the spiritual concerns of dying patients has been well recognized by many researchers (Conrad 1985; Moberg 1982). A survey conducted in 1997 by the George H. Gallup International Institute showed that people overwhelmingly want their spiritual needs addressed when they are close to death. In the preface to the survey report, George H. Gallup, Jr., writes: "The overarching message that emerges from this study is that the American people want to reclaim and reassert the spiritual dimensions in dying" (George H. Gallup International Institute 1997). In the 1990 Gallup survey cited previously, 75% of Americans say religion is central to their lives and a majority feels that their spiritual faith can help them recover from their illnesses. Ehman et al. (1999) found that 94% of patients with religious beliefs agreed that physicians should ask them about their beliefs if they became gravely ill; 45% of patients who denied having any religious beliefs still agreed that physicians should ask their patients about them. In this survey, 68% of patients said they would welcome a spiritual question in a medical history; only 15% said they actually recalled being asked by their physicians whether spiritual or religious beliefs would influence their decisions. In a survey of patients in a family practice outpatient clinic, 83% wanted their physicians to address their spiritual issues, citing increased trust in physician and feeling they were listened to as the benefits of such an inquiry. Patients ranked the circumstances in which they wanted to have their spiritual issues addressed as follows: 94% if seriously ill with possibility of dying, 91% if suffering from ongoing chronic illness, 83% admitted to the hospital, and 60% routine annual exam (McCord et al. 2004).

Data Documenting the Effect of Spirituality on Illness

There is a growing body of evidence documenting the relationship between patients' religious and spiritual lives and their experiences with illness including cancer (Levin and Schiller 1987). In addition to surveys demonstrating that spirituality is important to people and that a significant percentage of patients would like their physicians to discuss their spiritual beliefs with them, a number of studies show that having spiritual beliefs is beneficial to patients, particularly those with a serious illnesses such as cancer. The majority of these studies look at religion as the spiritual variable as there are more well-established measures of religiosity than spirituality. However, that is changing as newer measures of spirituality are being developed and utilized in studies (Fetzer Institute/National Institute on Aging Working Group 1999).

Reviews of the literature indicate potential associations between measures of religious commitment and health measures, including blood pressure, lower psychological distress, and morbidity and mortality, in studies of many diseases (Benson 1996; Craigie et al. 1988; Larson and Larson 1994; Larson et al. 1986; Levin et al. 1987; McKee and Chappel 1992). Religious people tend to have greater life satisfaction, marital satisfaction, well-being and altruism, coping skills, and self-esteem compared to nonreligious people (Jenkins and Pargament 1995; Saudia et al. 1991; Matthew et al. 1993; Levin and Larson 1997). Many researchers have found a strong relationship between patients' reliance on religion beliefs and practices and their coping with cancer (Brady et al. 1999; Holland 1999). Spirituality has been found as an important factor in bereavement. It has been reported that parents who have lost a child have found much support following their child's death in their spiritual beliefs (Cook and Wimberly 1983).

Spirituality is important in coping with pain and with dying. Ninety-three percent of patients with gynecologic cancers noted that their spiritual beliefs helped them cope with their cancer (Roberts 1997). In a study of patients with lung cancer and heart failure, it was found that spiritual concerns were important in both groups of patients and their caregivers. These spiritual issues included despair, feeling life is not worthwhile, feeling isolated and unsupported, feeling useless, lacking confidence, asking "why me?," and hopelessness (Murray et al. 2004). Patients with advanced cancer who found comfort in their spiritual beliefs were more satisfied with their lives, were happier, and had diminished pain (Yates et al. 1981). Hope is an important spiritual value that may mediate coping in patients and caregivers alike. Hope is particularly important for those suffering from cancer (Chang and Ji 2002). Researchers have identified hope as an influence on effective coping during time of loss, suffering, and uncertainty (Carson et al. 1990; Hockley 1993); facilitation of the coping process (Herth 1989); improved quality of life (Rustoen 1995); and positively influencing the immune system (Udelman 1991). Hopelessness is associated with an increased incidence of illness, depression, and suicidal ideation (Breitbart 2000; Gill and Gillbar 2001). In one study, hospice nurses identified hope as highly important to those they care for in their practice (Herth 1995). Many researchers believe that teaching people how to use effective coping resources, including spirituality, help them deal with stress, and have improved health. They further suggest that this may be cost-effective (Benson and Stewart 1992; Greenberg 1993).

In a questionnaire sent out by the American Pain Society, prayer was the second most common method of pain management after oral pain medications and the most common nondrug method of pain management (McNeill 1998). In a study of oncology patients by Brody et al. (1991), patients who had higher spirituality scores reported higher quality of life than patients with comparable levels of pain or fatigue who had lower spirituality scores. This spirituality may be a mediator in how patients cope with pain.

Quality of life instruments used in end-of-life care measure what is the quality of life in seriously ill and dying cancer patients. One domain in these instruments is called the existential domain, which measures purpose, meaning in life, and capacity for self-transcendence. Three items correlate with good quality of life for patients with advanced disease: if the patient's personal existence is meaningful; if the patient finds fulfillment in achieving life goals; and if life to this point is meaningful (Cohen et al. 1995). There appears to be a relationship between spirituality and religion with will to live (Tsevat et al. 2003a, b). There is a correlation between will to live in HIV patients and their intrinsic religiosity as well as spirituality in general. A study of breast cancer patients found a significant association between quality of life and spirituality (Brady et al. 1999).

Data on the Role of Spirituality in the Lives of Cancer Caregivers

Most of the studies on spirituality and religion and health focus on the patient. There is a paucity of data on the role of spirituality in personal or professional caregivers in general as well as in caregivers of patients with cancer specifically. Even in studies that describe stressors that are spiritual, little is said about spiritual support. Because of the limited studies in the area of religion and spirituality in the lives of caregivers of patients with illness, especially cancer, I will include studies broader than just cancer. However, any chronic illness, including cancer, causes stress for care access. In a study by Murray et al. (2004), spiritual needs of both patients and caregivers of lung cancer and heart failure patients were similar. So one can assume that findings could be applicable to any chronic illness, including cancer. For example, Blank et al. (1991) describe the stressors identified by caregivers included coping with added responsibilities, the fear of being alone, guilt, and limited knowledge regarding the patient's situation. Two of these, guilt and dealing with uncertainty, have to do with spiritual issues, yet the authors did not suggest any spiritual care. Wyatt et al. (1999) stress how studies have not "provided a comprehensive profile of the bereaved caregiver, including emotional, physical, spiritual, social, financial, and employment outcomes." Kloosterhouse and Ames (2002) also note that most studies have not focused on the family as the unit of analysis. However, the studies that have been done indicate the potential role for spirituality in the lives of cancer caregivers. Folkman et al. (1994) showed that increased stress motivated the engagement of religious coping in caregivers. Cupertino (1998) showed that caregivers who felt closer to God prayed frequently, believed religion to be important, and were better able to cope, also experienced less stress with their cancer caregiving demands. They felt more useful, found new meaning in life, experienced strengthened relationships and were more able to appreciate life (Cupertino et al. 1998). Jivanjee (1994) did a descriptive study of caregivers of patients with Alzheimer's disease using a naturalistic methodology. Spiritual support was consistently mentioned by all but two of the 18 participants in the study as being central to their sense of well-being and giving them the strength to cope with the demands of caregiving. Taylor (2003) did a descriptive cross-sectional, qualitative study to describe the spiritual needs of patients with cancer and family caregivers. Caregivers were observed to have similar needs to that of the patients. Seven categories of spiritual needs included:

- Needs associated with relating to an ultimate order.
- The need for positivity, hope, and gratitude.
- The need to give and receive love.
- The need to have meaning.
- The needs related to religiosity.
- The need to prepare for death.

In another study, Taylor (2006) measured the prevalence of spiritual needs and identified factors associated with spiritual needs among patients with cancer and family caregivers. She found similar prevalence and similar types of spiritual needs in patients with cancer and family caregivers. The higher the prevalence of spiritual needs, the greater the desire to receive help with those needs.

Wyatt et al. (1999) found that the caregivers of patients with cancer had more depressive symptoms than the general public. Depression was passively correlated with negative thinking and inversely correlated with positive outlook and with spirituality. Cancer caregivers endorsed the following spiritual items (See Table 11.3).

A narrative approach of cases of patients with cancer analyzed the spiritual themes that patients and families bring up in the clinical setting (Burton 1998). These narratives tend to be expressed in terms of three basic themes:

Table 11.3 Spiritual items endorsed by caregivers. (From Wyatt et al. 1999)	I believe in a power greater than myself I know what is important in life My values and beliefs help me meet daily challenges I accept the mysteries of life and death

- Power (who is in charge and loss of personal power).
- Connection (degree to which one feels related to and loved by others).
- Explanation (what the illness, loss, and life itself mean).

Ellison and Levin (1998) postulate that religion and spirituality may be a resource in coping with stressful events. Cancer caregivers who were able to find positive religious values in negative situations or found religious purpose in stress were better able to cope. Those who saw illness as a punishment from God, or saw God as an apathetic God or unfair God, did worse (Mickley et al. 1998). Religion and spirituality may help in coping with cancer because it helps alter the primary appraisal which reframes the meaning or explanation of the crisis, improves a sense of secondary control because the family feels a greater power is in control, modifies an individual's identity so the problem is less stressful and less threatening and, finally, helps people cope with the emotions arising from the crisis.

Baines (1984) demonstrated that caregiving burdens can be relieved by increasing one's spiritual perspective to reframe the experience of grief and loss. A study of families' use of religion and spirituality as a psychosocial resource found that 70% of families agreed that their religious and spiritual beliefs were important in helping them cope with having a child in the hospital. The authors hypothesize that families used their spiritual beliefs to help them appraise and give meaning to the stress of having a hospitalized child. They further found that the families own religious and spiritual beliefs had the largest positive relationship to families' use of their beliefs as a psychosocial resource.

Kaye and Robinson's (1994) study of caregivers of persons with Alzheimer's disease found that the well-being of female caregivers is affected by confronting end-of-life issues. Confronting issues of mortality and loss may enhance the importance of spirituality in the individual's life (Reed 1994). Other authors suggest that caregiving results in increased feelings of depression and need for social support (Kuhlman et al. 1991; Lindgren 1993). Spirituality was shown to improve depression and enhance social support among caregiving wives (Kaye and Robinson 1994). Robinson and Kaye further described spiritual practices that the caregivers utilized which included:

- Talking with friends and family about spiritual matters.
- Reading spiritually related material.
- Engaging in private prayer.
- Seeking spiritual guidance.

Caregivers further described spirituality as important in everyday life, forgiveness as an important part of spirituality, and feeling close to God or a higher power in prayer, worship, or important moments in life.

Table 11.4 Coping strategies. (From Pelletier-Hibbert and Sohi 2001)

Living each day as it comes
Finding positive meaning
Hoping for a good outcome
Drawing support from their faith in God

Chang et al. (1998) in a study examining the factors that influence and are influenced by religious/spiritual coping among those providing care for disabled adults, showed that religious/spiritual coping reduces symptoms of depression and role submersion. This effect is due to higher relationship quality. The authors hypothesize that religion and spirituality may play a role in sustaining human relationships that are often strained by the necessities of providing care for others. This study speaks to the relational aspects of spirituality.

Living with uncertainty, people with chronic illness including cancer, can contribute to stress in the lives of patients and caregivers. It has been shown to be a source of stress for renal patients (Ferrans and Powers 1993). The response of family members living with uncertainty associated with a chronic illness in a loved one has been negative (Pelletier-Hibbert and Sohi 2001). In one study of caregivers of patients with HIV, living in the present moment became the "anchor in the lives of many caregivers as they struggled with the uncertain future and focused on the present" (Brown and Powell-Cope 1991). The concept of living in the present moment is found in religious traditions and in spiritual programs such as the 12-step program (Alcoholics Anonymous World Services 1976). Nyamathi (1987) studied spouses of patients on hemodialysis or postmyocardial infarct and found that both groups of spouses shared two coping mechanisms: maintaining control over a situation and finding hope. Srivastava (1988) found in a study of spouses of patients on hemodialysis that accepting the situation as is, praying and finding more about the situation were the highest ranked coping strategies. A focus group analysis of family member of patients on hemo- and peritoneal-dialysis found that uncertainty related to prognosis and potential loss was the highest source of stress for the family members (Pelletier-Hibbert and Sohi 2001). Coping strategies included (Table 11.4).

Other authors have looked at the role of religion and/or spirituality as helping with coping. Segall and Wykle (1989) found religion to be the major form of coping among the Black caregivers in their study of African-American family members of patients with dementia. Richardson and Sistler's (1999) study of African-American caregivers of patients with dementia found religion to be a major coping strategy, including church attendance, prayer, belief in God, Bible study, prayer meetings, and social support. In a mixed quantitative and qualitative study, Waters et al. (2005) found that spirituality played an essential role in the spiritual and social lives of many American caregivers and in how much global caregiver role strain was experienced. Results indicate that the caregiver's level of spirituality did not affect global strain, however, the caregiver's ethnicity made a difference in the response to global strain and the level of spirituality. The caregivers noted three major themes in helping them cope with caregiving burdens:

- Biblical instruction provides guidance.
- Prayer provides inner strength.
- Morals, cultural and family values are inherent in spiritual beliefs.

The authors conclude that while the quantitative findings reveal a weak link between caregiver spirituality and global strain, the qualitative findings provide support that spiritual beliefs might moderate the cancer caregiver's overall strain.

Pierce (2001) examined caring and expressions of spirituality in African-American family caregivers of people with stroke. Caring was described as:

- A filial ethereal value.
- Self-contemplation.
- Motivation for a philosophical introspection.
- Filial piety.
- Living in the moment and hoping for the future.
- Purpose.
- Motivation that came from the approval by care recipients.
- Christian piety.

Thus, the commitment to care for a person with a chronic illness such as stroke was based on the values of commitment, love and affection, and on spiritual values of connection, religious values and meaning, and purpose. It is likely these same values are relevant in the lives of caregivers of patients with cancer. Jones et al. (2002), in a study of Asian-American women caregivers of elderly parents, found that the women approached their caregiving challenges with devout commitment to filial responsibility. They described being "grateful for the love and care their parents gave them and wanting to give back to their parents." Love and respect were a major part of the commitment. The authors show how connection with inner strength and with their life purpose might help in coping with caregiving demands. Women identified inner strength as a primary personal resource that enabled them to deal with the demands of caregiving. Moloney (1995) analyzed older women's handling of difficult situations and found that connecting with their inner selves empowered women to integrate into the caregiving experience, to derive meaning from the experience, and to grow personally. These studies reflect the importance of cultural, religious, and spiritual values in how cancer caregivers come to understand their roles and how they cope with stress.

Forbes (1994) examined the relationship between caregiver's and patient's concept of spirituality measured as spiritual well-being. She found a strong correlation between the caregiver's spiritual well-being and the caregiver's perception of the patient's spiritual well-being, suggesting the effect of the relationship of patient to caregiver as influential in the caregiver's spiritual well-being. Forbes suggests that highly significant correlations between the spiritual well-being of the caregiver and that of the patient imply that a spiritual bonding occurs. Prayer was noted as a significant coping mechanism for caregivers.

There has also been some work done in the area of compassion fatigue which is a form of burnout. It affects people who are exposed to the suffering of others, such physicians, nurses, social workers, emergency service personnel, chaplains, and those in the caring professions. Healthcare professionals with compassion fatigue find it more difficult to continue giving of themselves to their patients. They become withdrawn and find it difficult to continue being emphatic and compassionate. Some of the causes of compassion fatigue that have been cited include the increased demands of managed care, increased paperwork, longer hours, and smaller staff support (Pfifferling and Gulley 2000). Compassion fatigue can result in poor job performance, low self-esteem, increased illness, and disillusionment. Sometimes it can force people to leave their professions. Due to the intense nature of caring for an individual with cancer and the repeated or often prolonged periods of required care, this may be particularly true for professional caregivers who work with cancer patients and their families.

Some ways to deal with compassion fatigue are support groups, counseling, and talking with friends and colleagues (Joslyn 2002). Most physicians and other healthcare professionals chose medicine and healthcare because of a desire to help others and to connect to others. When system stresses force healthcare professionals to rush through patient visits, or do tasks with patients rapidly because of mounding paper work, then those professionals begin to feel they are not doing what they were called to do in the first place. Spirituality can also help healthcare professionals with compassion fatigue by giving them a way to rekindle their calling to their professional lives and by giving them a spiritual practice to help sustain them in the midst of stress. Thus, focusing on the spiritual needs of cancer patients brings healthcare professionals back to the root of their work, i.e., holistic, patient-centered care rooted in service. The attention to their own sense of meaning and purpose and the intentional integration of that meaning and purpose into their professional lives sustains them in the midst of stress. Spiritual practices, such as meditation, prayer, ritual, journaling, or experiencing beauty in the arts and music, can further nurture the healthcare professional in their lives.

Spirituality in Clinical Practice

Today, medical educators are recognizing the importance of spirituality and medicine and are beginning to ask patients and their families about their spiritual beliefs (Levin et al. 1997). There are many ethical reasons to include spirituality in the care of cancer patients and their families (Astrow et al. 2001; Post et al. 2000; Puchalski 2002). There are ethical standards in medicine, nursing, and social work that speak to the obligation of the healthcare professional to attend to all dimensions of the patient's care—the spiritual as well as the physical and psychosocial—as grounded in the biopsychosocial model of care (Sulmasy 2002). The American College of Physicians consensus panel determined that it is the physician's obligation to attend to all dimensions of a patient's suffering, including the spiritual or existential suffering (Lindgren 1993; Lo et al. 1999).

Table 11.5 The role of a chaplain. (From VandeCreek and Burton 2001)

When religious beliefs and practices are tightly interwoven with cultural contexts, chaplains constitute a powerful reminder of the healing, sustaining, guiding, and reconciling power of religious faith
Professional chaplains reach across faith group boundaries and do not proselytize
They provide supportive spiritual care through empathic listening, demonstrating an understanding of persons in distress
Professional chaplains serve as members of patient care teams
Professional chaplains design and lead religious ceremonies of worship and ritual
Professional chaplains lead or participate in healthcare ethics programs
Professional chaplains educate the healthcare team and community regarding the relationship of religious and spiritual issues to institutional services
Professional chaplains act as mediator and reconciler for those who need a voice in the healthcare system
Professional chaplains may serve as contact persons to arrange assessment for the appropriateness and coordination of complementary therapies
Professional chaplains and their certifying organizations encourage and support research activities to assess the effectiveness of providing spiritual care

It is also important to recognize that spirituality in the healthcare setting of cancer patients and their families is not in any one person's domain; physicians, nurses, social workers, psychologists, and chaplains can all deal with patient spirituality. However, most physicians are not trained to deal with complex spiritual crises and conflicts, while chaplains and other spiritual caregivers are trained in spiritual directives. Therefore, it is important that physicians and other care providers obtain a spiritual history as a way of inquiry about spiritual issues that might impact a cancer patient and also recognize when to refer to these specialists.

Nurse In the nursing code of ethics, it states that the nurse must promote an environment in which the human rights, values, customs, and spiritual beliefs of the individual, family, and community are respected (American Nurse Association 2001). It is recognized that nursing knowledge, skill, and experience are ineffectual if not accompanied by a caring attitude and one where the nurse is fully present to the patients.

Social worker Since the 1980s, social work curricula included spirituality and religion in their educational and practice guidelines because of a commitment to cultural sensitivity and because social work is grounded in a holistic view of personhood. The social work profession grew out of concerns rooted in the religious doctrine of love for one's neighbor (Loewenberg 1988). Healthcare in the United States also grew out of religious values rooted in service to others. Hence, compassionate holistic care is the foundation of healthcare in the United States.

Chaplain In recent years, the chaplain has become an increasingly important member of the cancer healthcare team. Traditionally, the role of the chaplain was sacramental, that is, to administer to the cancer patient certain prayers and rites particular to the patient's religion, such as communion or unction. Today the role of a chaplain is much broader (VandeCreek and Burton 2001; see Table 11.5). The chaplain represents an extension of the cancer patient's personal and community support system, as well as a source of spiritual support for the patient (Puchalski and Sandoval 2003). When the chaplain has a regular presence in a healthcare setting, the opportunity exists to provide support to the staff as well.

It is our spiritual side that formulates the questions dealing with ultimate meaning and purpose, questions for which medicine and science have no answers. These questions require a unique language, in which symbolism, story, and ritual are involved. It is the chaplain who has the expertise in this form of communication and, therefore, is able to address the questions. Some of these questions and concerns might be stated in the language of faith. Here, the cancer patient might invoke God and, in this instance, statements of faith would be used to deal with the questions. At other times, questions dealing with the purpose of one's life might be more appropriately answered in existential terms. The chaplain can deal with these issues in terms of how the world works, how God works, and what we consider the essence, or meaning, of life (Handzo 1990). The chaplain also ministers to the family of individuals with cancer and the professional caregivers who treat them. As mentioned above, caregiving can provoke spiritual questions in all caregivers and can give rise to stress and existential distress. By attending to the spiritual needs of personal and professional cancer caregivers, chaplains help all members of the care team cope with stress, suffering, and loss.

Finally, the inclusion of spirituality in care is central to the precepts of patient-centered care, in that spirituality and religion can impact shared decision-making, good care involves respect for cancer patients' values and beliefs, and involvement of a larger community of caregivers (such as faith-based communities) is often important in good patient care (Institute for Alternative Futures 2004).

Ethical/Clinical Considerations

There are other ethical and clinical factors that support the inclusion of spirituality into the care of patients and families. Spirituality, religion, culture, race, ethnicity, family dynamics, socioeconomic status, and education level are some of the factors that may affect one's understandings and beliefs about illness, suffering, pain, loss, dying, and coping (Talemantes and Espino 1995). People especially come to understand their health, illness, and dying as well as those of their loved ones with cancer or cancer patients through their beliefs, cultural backgrounds, past experience, and values. Lukoff et al. (1995) note, "The religious and spiritual dimensions of life are among the most important cultural factors structuring human experience, beliefs, values and behaviors as well as illness patterns." The effect of stress depends on how people, including cancer patients and their families and professional caregivers, perceive an event (McCubbin and Patterson 1983).

Religious convictions/beliefs may affect healthcare decision-making. Many medical decisions are affected by the cancer patient's religious and cultural beliefs: whether to turn a ventilator off or use of a feeding tube, blood transfusions, etc.

(University of Virginia Health Center 1997). One study found that 62% of African Americans would prefer to die at home rather than the hospital, compared to 81% of Euro Americans who would prefer to die at home (Neubauer and Hamilton 1990). In another study, ethnic/racial differences in utilization of services at St. Luke's Palliative Care Service in New York were great (Pauling-Kaplan and O'Conner 1989). Many religious organizations have published material on ethical and religious guidelines for healthcare practices (Cohen et al. 2000; United States Conference of Catholic Bishops 2001; University of Virginia Health Services 1997).

Rituals and norms surrounding the process of dying and death come from cultural, religious and family values, attitudes, and beliefs. Kagawa-Singer (1998) indicates the importance for oncology nurses to be sensitive to the diverse cultural rituals surrounding death and mourning practices. Since culture, religion, and spirituality give people beliefs, values, and ways of behaving, these can impact how death from cancer is handled and ritualized.

As discussed above, for many cancer patients, spirituality is an important dimension of their lives and a way that people cope with suffering (Puchalski 2001, 2002). So the care of the cancer patient should include spiritual care (Kavanaugh 1996; Lo et al. 2002; Puchalski 2000; Sullivan 1989). Values, wishes, and goals provide a framework for cancer treatment decisions as well as for spiritual work (O'Gorman 2002).

Clinical Implications

It is important to include a spiritual assessment or history as part of the overall clinical assessment of a cancer patient and his family. This assists in determining the cancer patient's spiritual needs and resources and the most appropriate spiritual care as well as enhancing overall caregiving (Block 2001; Bullis 1996; Lo et al. 2002). One concrete method for beginning the process of incorporating spiritual issues into one's clinical practice is to include a spiritual assessment when taking the cancer patient's social history. The acronym FICA—Faith and belief, Importance, Community, Address in care—can be helpful for structuring an interview regarding a cancer patient's or family member's spiritual views (Table 11.6; Puchalski 2000). Performing a spiritual assessment has been included in coursework on spirituality and medicine and is performed by many practicing physicians and other healthcare providers in the United States (Borneman et al. 2010). The spiritual assessment emphasizes the practice of compassion with one's patients and helps the clinician learn to integrate patient's spiritual concerns into the therapeutic plans. Clinicians are encouraged to make referrals to chaplains when appropriate. Physicians and other healthcare providers should strive to discuss cancer patient's and their familie's spiritual concerns in a respectful manner and as directed by the patient. The privacy of others regarding matters of spirituality and religion must always be respected. Care providers should not impose their beliefs on the patients and families.

Table 11.6 Spiritual assessment tool. (From Puchalski and Romer 2000, © 1996 Christina Puchalski, MD)

An acronym that can be used to remember what is asked in a spiritual history is
F: Faith or beliefs
I: Importance and influence
C: Community
A: Address
Some specific questions you can use to discuss these issues are
F: What is your faith or belief?
Do you consider yourself spiritual or religious?
What things do you believe in that give meaning to your life?
I: Is it important in your life?
What influence does it have on how you take care of yourself?
How have your beliefs influenced your behavior during this illness?
What role do your beliefs play in regaining your health?
C: Are you part of a spiritual or religious community?
Is this of support to you and how?
Is there a person or group of people you really love or who are really important to you?
A: How would you like me, your healthcare provider, to address these issues in your healthcare?
General recommendations when taking a spiritual history
Consider spirituality as a potentially important component of every patient's physical well-being and mental health
Address spirituality at each complete physical examination and continue addressing it at follow-up visits if appropriate. In patient care, spirituality is an ongoing issue
Respect a patient's privacy regarding spiritual beliefs; don't impose your beliefs on others
Make referrals to chaplains, spiritual directors, or community resources as appropriate
Be aware that your own spiritual beliefs will help you personally and will overflow in your encounters with those for whom you care to make the doctor-patient encounter a more humanistic one

Once a spiritual assessment has been made, then the appropriate spiritual intervention should be offered. While spiritual and religious interventions can be provided by any clinician, integrating a pastoral care provider in the healthcare team will ensure that the team becomes familiar with religious and spiritual issues and that patient's spiritual needs are met. Some examples of spiritual interventions are: meditation, guided imagery, art, journaling, spiritual direction, pastoral counseling, yoga, religious ritual, or prayer.

Spiritual care emphasizes the importance of the relationship between two people. The physician may be the professional expert in most of the encounters, however, the physician is still a human being. By relating from our humanness we can help to form deeper and more meaningful connections with our cancer patients. What this requires is an awareness of the healthcare provider's own values, beliefs, and attitudes, particularly toward the physician's own mortality. By confronting one's own mortality, one can be better able to understand what the cancer patient is facing. Furthermore, there needs to be recognition that a personal or professional caregiver's own cultural, religious, and spiritual beliefs and values can impact care for the patient. To be able to recognize another's spiritual-cultural values and beliefs, cancer caregivers should possess some self-awareness of their own. Thus, self-reflection on one's spiritual beliefs by family and personal caregivers as well as professional caregivers is important for understanding the cancer patient. Also, the stress of working with seriously ill and dying cancer patients can be better handled by an attentiveness to one's own spiritual and values framework. Many physicians and other healthcare providers speak of their own spiritual practices and how those practices help them in their ability to deliver good spiritual and, in fact, good medical care. They further note the importance of their own spiritual practices in self-care (Puchalski 2000).

Recommendations for Research, Education, and Clinical Practice and Policy

Research

The research to date demonstrates that spirituality, expressed in many different ways such as meaning and purpose, relationship, religion, or other spiritual beliefs, helps many cancer patients and caregivers deal with this serious illness and its caregiving demands. However, this research field is relatively new and, therefore, there is a paucity of work in the area of spirituality and caregivers. There is a lot of work on stress factors in caregiving, on what types of coping strategies cancer caregivers use, and on healthcare outcomes in cancer caregivers, but researchers have not included spirituality as one of the multiple dimensions that may enhance cancer caregiver well-being. There is little research on the role of spirituality in professional caregivers in general and of cancer patients and their families specifically. Furthermore, there are little data on the different expressions of spirituality and their effects for cancer caregivers. The more detailed mechanisms for how spirituality helps cancer caregivers and what types of spiritual interventions might work are yet to be thoroughly investigated. Some specific research questions that come from the research summarized in this document on cancer caregivers include:

- Study the various complex interrelationships among spirituality related and well-being variables.
- Investigate potential mechanisms for some of the outcomes and associations observed in studies of cancer patients and their caregivers.
- Explore cancer patient and caregiver variables, such as age, gender, ethnic or religious background, and spiritual practice patterns with their potential influences on spirituality.
- Clarify spiritually related variables, such as mediators, moderators, or main effects in cancer caregiving.
- Test specific spiritual interventions on cancer caregiver outcomes, including well-being.
- Document the effectiveness of a spiritual perspective on the lives of cancer caregivers.

- Study filial caregiving, examination of the relationships between filial values, the cancer caregiving process, and outcomes in families of diverse cultural and religious backgrounds.
- Examine the importance of finding meaning and purpose in cancer caregiving and how that affects health and stress outcomes in personal and professional cancer caregivers.
- Document the role of parish nurses in caring for and supporting cancer caregivers.
- Utilize faith or culturally based groups as helping networks for cancer caregivers.
- Document the role of volunteer lay groups as spiritual support to cancer caregivers.
- Study the roles of various professional caregivers (physicians, nurses, social workers, psychologists, chaplains, aids) in delivery of spiritual care to cancer patients and caregivers.
- Define models for living with and coping with the uncertainty of a cancer diagnosis and treatment.
- Examine the roles of spiritual, religious, and cultural rituals in cancer caregiver's lives, specifically how the strategies assist in dealing with uncertainty, stress, and loss.

Education

As mentioned above, there has been tremendous progress in the medical education of physicians in medical school and residency program with regard to training doctors how to address spiritual issues and sufferings with cancer patients. In these courses, medical students and residents learn:

- The data indicating spirituality are important to cancer patients in coping and about outcomes.
- Role of cultural and spiritual ritual.
- How to create trusting environments where cancer patients can share spiritual issues if they chose.
- How to do a spiritual assessment with a cancer patient and their caregiver.
- How to work with interdisciplinary teams, including chaplains, clergy, and culturally based healers.
- How to address and respond to cancer patient's spiritual needs.
- How to recognize spiritual distress and pain in cancer patients and their caregivers.
- How to recognize the cancer patient's inner resources of strength, such as hope.
- How to integrate spirituality into the cancer treatment plan, as appropriate.
- Ethical boundaries and issues related to spirituality.
- Case formulation with regard to spirituality as part of whole patient care (Association of American Medical Colleges 1999).

Many medical schools and residency programs are also focused on self-care of the professional caregiver, looking at the physician's own spiritual beliefs and values and how that affects the physician and those for whom the physician cares. This curriculum is being expanded to all the different specialties, including oncology. Elements of this curriculum are being expanded and should include not just the cancer patient, but also the family and friends of cancer patients (Puchalski 2006).

Social work has also developed curricula in religion, spirituality, and health, which are offered in some training programs. Most of these courses are taught in the context of cultural competency and holistic care (Sheridan and Hemert 1999). A survey of 132 baccalaureate nursing programs in the United States revealed that few schools had a defined curriculum in spiritual care (Callister et al. 2004; Purnell et al. 2004). Although most nurses believe spiritual care is important, most feel unprepared because there is little in their curricula on spiritual interventions (McEwen 2004). Topics to include in the curriculum include establishing a trusting relationship, providing a supportive spiritual environment, responding to patient's spiritual needs, and integrating spirituality into the care plan, as well as specific topics related to illnesses or life situation, such as cancer or crisis (Callister et al. 2004).

There needs to be standardized and tested training programs for all professions, including physicians, nurses, social workers, home health nurses and aids, physical and occupational therapists, and psychologists as well as family caregivers. In addition, an increased recognition of the role of spiritual care providers, such as chaplains, pastoral counselors, spiritual directors, and clergy and ways in which the healthcare teams can include the spiritual care providers for both cancer patients and their families, should be emphasized. Education of clergy and religious leaders on the specific needs of cancer caregivers is important. As more research is done on spiritual interventions, professionals can be educated about these interventions and how to use them to better help cancer patients and caregivers.

There are several training programs including Stephen's Ministry and Zen Buddhist Hospice in San Francisco, California, that train lay volunteers on being spiritual companions to the dying and seriously ill, including patients who have cancer. One of these is being studied by our group and Last Acts (Puchalski 2003). While most of these address patients and families secondary to family, it would be important to develop training programs specifically for a companion to the family caregiver. In this way, the family caregiver is recognized as the person in need of spiritual support for themselves and not just as extensions of the patient. Hospice is an excellent model of integrated care for patients and families. Many hospices have family support groups and bereavement follow-up care. However, there is still a need in hospices for specific training programs in spirituality (Larson 1997). Support groups for family in faith-based, community cancer centers and hospitals would be beneficial.

Finally, there need to be workshops, literature, and resources developed for family cancer caregivers with regard to spirituality in their lives, how their spirituality affects them, and their stress, their ability to cope with caregiving, and, ultimately, with uncertainty. Examples of helpful resources include specific counseling sessions dealing with spiritual issues, retreats for caregivers, pamphlets, Web-based courses, and self-spiritual assessment tools (Puchalski 2002; see Table 11.7). Education on pastoral care providers and what they do to help cancer caregivers with their spiritual issues would be important since many people do not know what these professionals do.

Table 11.7 FICA for self-assessment. (© 1996 Christina Puchalski, MD)

FICA: A spiritual self-assessment tool. The acronym FICA can help structure questions in taking a personal spiritual history
F: Do I have a spiritual belief that helps me cope with stress? With illness? What gives my life meaning?
I: Is this belief important to me? Does it influence how I think about my health and illness? Does it influence my healthcare decisions?
C: Do I belong to a spiritual community (church, temple, mosque, or other group)? Am I happy there? Do I need to do more with the community? Do I need to search for another community? If I don't have a community, would it help me if I found one?
A: What should be my action plan? What changes do I need to make? Are there spiritual practices I want to develop? Would it help me to see a chaplain, spiritual director, or pastoral counselor?

As all these programs are being developed, it is important to conduct ongoing evaluation to ensure the training programs are effective and long-lasting.

Clinical Practice and Policy

Hospitals, hospices, long-term care facilities, and outpatient clinical sites need to endorse the integration of spirituality, not only for cancer patient care, but also for family and professional caregivers. This means endorsing and offering training courses, sponsoring research, scheduling retreats and discussion groups, and providing pastoral care services. Families and friends of cancer patients need to be recognized as persons in need of attention and care separate from the patient. Therefore, funding needs to be allocated to ensure a strong, fully staffed pastoral care department in all sites, including home-based programs that serve not only the patients, but also the family and staff/professional cancer caregivers. Spiritual care in the broad sense of compassionate presence, caring, taking a spiritual assessment, listening to patient's and caregiver's spiritual concerns, and helping implement intervention that might be helpful should be done by all professional and personal caregivers. However, more in-depth spiritual care needs to be done by trained spiritual care providers, i.e., the pastoral care team. In the ideal setting, all interdisciplinary teams should include a chaplain so that spiritual care is coordinated. There also need to be spiritual care competencies to which all healthcare professionals adhere to ensure optimum patient care.

Funding should be directed at training programs and resources for cancer staff and family caregivers. Caregivers need to be supported in their caring of others, whether in the personal or professional role. Professional cancer caregivers are under tremendous stress and face many of the same issues with which family caregivers deal. All clinical sites should recognize that our work is essentially spiritual: We are all in service to others and, as such, in the unique professions of walking with others in the midst of their suffering. We have the professional obligation to put other's needs ahead of our own and be fully present to our patients and their families. This is particularly challenging given that healthcare systems today are being ravaged

Table 11.8 Resources. (© Puchalski 2002)

George Washington Institute for Spirituality and Health, George Washington University
  (www.gwish.org)
Center for the Study of Religion/Spirituality and Health, Duke University
  (www.dukespiritualityandhealth.org)
Conversations in Care (www.conversationsincare.org)
Partners in Care Foundation (www.picf.org)
Partnership for Caring, Inc. (www.partnershipforcaring.org)

by the turbulent times of economic pressures and change. For the most part, the
healthcare system is being driven by economic concerns rather than or in addition to
values-centered concerns. Thus, it is often a struggle for healthcare professionals to
take the time to be fully present to cancer patients and their families.

It is critical that we return medicine to its spiritual roots and develop systems that
are caring for others, including staff, and that place priority on values and mission.
This can be manifested by cancer care systems that create an atmosphere where
money is not the bottom line, however, patient, family, and staff satisfaction is what
is measured and honored. Some ways of beginning the process of change include:

- Support from top administrators.
- Retreats and education programs for families and staff.
- Pastoral care services for patients, families and staff.
- Funding directed at spiritual services.
- Support for research projects in spirituality.
- Enabling rituals to take place that help families, patients, and staff.
- Providing rooms for meditation and ritual.
- Education of hospital administrators, government officials, and religious leaders
  so that they can recognize the needs of family and professional cancer caregivers.

Conclusion

Spirituality can be an important dimension in the lives of cancer patients and their
family and professional caregivers, particularly when dealing with the chronicity,
stress, and suffering frequently associated with a cancer diagnosis. Spirituality is
an aspect of all human beings that seeks to find meaning in life and, hence, a way
that people may heal. All care providers—doctors, nurses, chaplains, psychologists,
social workers, therapists, family, and faith communities—can participate in this
dimension of patient and caregiver life. Cancer care providers should learn to use appropriate assessment tools and interventions in care plans. Personal and professional
cancer caregivers should reflect on their own spirituality and how their beliefs and
values affect their life, their coping with stress, and their relationship with others,
especially those for whom they care. Each professional and family caregiver deals
with spiritual issues in a different way. By working together as a team, we can ensure
that cancer patients, our loved ones with cancer, family caregivers who give so much

of themselves, and professional caregivers who specialize in oncology participate and create the best possible compassionate, caring healthcare system to support the needs of all cancer caregivers and patients. In order to do this, it is important that we develop research and education agendas that can support the changes needed in both the healthcare system and society, thus ensuring that care is optimal for families touched by cancer (Table 11.8).

References

Alcoholics Anonymous World Services, Inc. (1976). *Alcoholics anonymous.* New York: Alcoholics Anonymous World Services, Inc.

American Nurse Association. (2001). *Code for nursing.* Washington: American Nurse Publishing.

Anderson, B., Kiecolt-Glaser, J., & Glaser, R. (1994). A biobehavioral model of cancer stress and disease course. *American Psychologist, 49,* 389–405.

Association of American Medical Colleges. (1999). *Contemporary issues in medicine: Communication in medicine: Medical school objectives project* (Report III). Washington: Association of American Medical Colleges.

Astrow, A., Puchalski, C., & Sulmasy, D. (2001). Religion, spirituality, and health care: Social, ethical, and practical considerations. *American Journal of Medicine, 110,* 283–287.

Baines, E. (1984). Caregiver stress in the older adult. *Journal of Community Health Nursing, 4,* 257–263.

Beck-Friis, B., & Stang, P. (1993). The family in hospital-based home care with special reference to terminally ill cancer patients. *Journal of Palliative Care, 9*(1), 5–13.

Benson, H. (1996). *Timeless healing.* New York: Scribner.

Benson, H., & Stuart, E. (1992). The wellness book: The comprehensive guide to maintaining health and treating stress-related illness. New York: Simon & Schuster.

Blank, J., Clark, L., Longman, A., & Atwood, J. (1991). Perceived home care needs of cancer patients and their caregivers. *Cancer Nursing, 12*(2), 78–84.

Block, S. (2001). Psychological considerations, growth, and transcendence at the end of life: The art of the possible. *Journal of the American Medical Association, 285*(22), 2898–2906.

Borneman, T. Ferrell, B., & Puchalski, C. (2010). Evaluation of the FICA Tool for Spiritual Assessment. *Journal of Pain and Symptom Management, 40*(2), 163–173.

Brakman, Sarah-Vaughan (1994). Adult Daughter Caregivers. *The Hastings Center Report, 24*(5), 26–28.

Brady, M. J., Peterman, A. H., Fichett, G., & Cella, D. (1999). A case for including spirituality in quality of life measurement in oncology. *Psycho-oncology, 8,* 417–428.

Breitbart, W. (2000). Depression, hopelessness and desire for hastened death in terminally ill patients with cancer. *Journal of the American Medical Association, 284*(22), 2907–2911.

Brody, E. (1981). "Women in the middle" and family help to older people. *Gerontologist, 21*(5), 471–479.

Brown, M., & Powell-Cope, G. (1991). AIDS family caregiving: Transitions through uncertainty. *Nursing Research, 40*(6), 338–345.

Bullis, R. K. (1996). *Spirituality in social work practice.* Washington: Taylor and Francis.

Burton, L. (1998). The spiritual dimension of palliative care. *Seminars in Oncology Nursing, 14*(2), 121–128.

Callister, L. C., Bond, A. E., Matsumura, G., & Mangura, S. (2004). Threading spirituality throughout nursing education. *Holistic Nursing Practice, 18*(3), 1606.

Carson, V., Soeken, K., Shanty, J., & Terry, L. (1990). Hope and spiritual well-being: Essentials for living with AIDS. *Perspectives in Psychiatric Care, 26*(2), 28–34.

Chang, L. C., & Ji, H. C. (2002). The correlation between perceptions of control and hope status in home based cancer patients. *Nursing Research, 10,* 73–82.

Chang, B. H., Noonan, A., & Tennstedt, S. (1998). The role of religion/spirituality in coping with caregiving for disabled elders. *Gerontologist, 38*(4), 463–470.

Cohen, S., Mount, B., Strobel, M., & Bui, F. (1995). The McGill quality of life questionnaire: A measure of quality of life appropriate for people with advanced disease: A preliminary study of validity and acceptability. *Palliative Medicine, 9,* 207–219.

Cohen, C., Wheeler, S., Scott, D., Edwards, B., & Lusk, P. (2000). Prayer as therapy: A challenge to both religious belief and professional ethics (Report by the Anglican Working Group in Bioethics). *Hastings Center Report, 30*(3), 40–47.

Conrad, N. (1985). Spiritual support for the dying. *Nursing Clinics of North America, 20,* 415–426.

Cook, J., & Wimberly, D. (1983). If I should die before I wake: Religious commitment and adjustment to death of a child. *Journal for the Scientific Study of Religion, 22,* 222–238.

Craigie, F., Liu, I., Larson, D., & Lyons, J. (1988). A systematic analysis of religious variables in the Journal of Family Practice, 1976–1986. *Journal of Family Practice, 27,* 509–513.

Cupertino, A.-P., Aldwin, C., & Schulz, R. (1998). *Religiosity, emotional strain, and health: The caregiver health effects study.* San Francisco: American Psychiatric Association.

Doyle, D. (1992). Have we looked beyond the physical and psychosocial? *Journal of Pain and Symptom Management, 7,* 302–311.

Ehman, J. W., Ott, B. B., Short, T. H., Ciampa, R. C., & Hansen-Flaschen, J. (1999). Do patients want physicians to inquire about their spiritual or religious beliefs if they become gravely ill? *Archives of Internal Medicine, 159,* 1803–1806.

Ellison, G., & Levin, J. (1998). The religion-health connections: Evidence, theory, and future direction. *Health Education and Behavior, 25,* 700–720.

Ferrans, C., & Powers, M. (1993). Quality of life of hemodialysis patients. *American Nephrology Nurse's Association Journal, 18,* 173–181.

Fetzer Institute/National Institute on Aging Working Group. (1999). *Multidimensional measurement of religiousness/spirituality for use in health research.* Kalamazoo: Fetzer Institute. Retrieved from http://www.fetzer.org/research/248-dses. Accessed 16 Feb 2012.

Foglio, J., & Brody, H. (1988). Religion, faith, and family medicine. *Journal of Family Practice, 27,* 473–474.

Folkman, S, Chesney, M, Cooke, M, Boccellari, A, & Collette, L. (1994). Caregiving burden in HIV-positive and HIV-negative partners of men with AIDS. *Journal of Consulting and Clinical Psychology, 62,* 746–756.

Forbes, E. (1994). Spirituality, aging, and the community-dwelling caregiver and care recipient. *Geriatric Nursing, 15*(6), 297–302.

Frankl, V. (1984). *Man's search for meaning.* New York: Simon & Schuster.

Funk, J. (1995). Burnout among "healers." *American Journal of Hospice & Palliative Care, 12*(3), 27–30.

Gallup, G. (1990). *Religion in America.* Princeton: Princeton Religion and Research Center.

The George H. Gallup International Institute. (1997). *Spiritual beliefs and the dying process: A report on a national survey.* Conducted for the Nathan Cummings Foundation and the Fetzer Institute. Retrieved from http://www.ncf.org/reports/rpt_fetzer_contents.html.

Gill, S., & Gilbar, O. (2001). Hopelessness among cancer patients. *Journal of Psychosocial Oncology, 19*(1), 21–32.

Glaser, R., Rabin, B., Chesney, M., Cohen, S., & Natelson, B. (1999). Stress-induced immunomodulation: Implication for infectious disease? *Journal of the American Medical Association, 281,* 2268–2270.

Greenberg, J. (1993). *Comprehensive stress management* (4th ed). Dubuque: WCB Brown and Benchmark.

Ham, R., & Sloane, P. (1992). *Primary care geriatrics.* St. Louis: Mosby-Year Book.

Handzo, G. (1990). Psychological stress on clergy. In J. Holland & J. Rowland (Eds), *Handbook of psychooncology: Psychological care of the patient with cancer* (pp. 683–687). New York: Oxford University Press.

Herth, K. (1989). The relationship between level of hope and level of coping response and other variables in patients with cancer. *Oncology Nursing Forum, 16,* 67–72.

Herth, K. (1995). Engendering hope in the chronically and terminally ill: Nursing interventions. *American Journal of Hospice and Palliative Care, 12*(5), 31–39.

Hockley, J. (1993). The concept of hope and the will to live. *Palliative Medicine, 7,* 181–186.

Holland, J. C., Passik, S., Kash, K. M., Russak, S. M., Gronert, M. K., Sison, A., et al. (1999). The role of religions and spiritual beliefs in coping with malignant melanoma. *Psycho-Oncology, 8,* 14–26.

Institute for Alternative Futures. (2004) *Patient-centered care 2015: Scenarios, vision, goals & next steps.* Alexandria: Picker Institute.

Jenkins, R., & Pargament, K. (1995). Religion and spirituality as resources for coping with cancer. *Journal of Psychosocial Oncology, 13,* 51–74.

Jivanjee, P. (1994). Enhancing the well-being of family caregivers to patients with Alzheimer's disease. *Journal of Gerontological Social Work, 23*(1/2), 31–48.

Jones, R., Hansford, J., & Fiske, J. (1993). Death from cancer at home: The carer's perspective. *British Medical Journal, 306,* 249–251.

Jones, P., Zhang, X., Jaceldo-Siegl, K., & Meleis, A. (2002). Caregiving between two cultures: An integrative experience. *Journal of Transcultural Nursing, 13*(3), 202–209.

Joslyn, H. (2002, March 8). How compassion fatigue can overwhelm charity workers and what to do about it. *Chronicle of Philanthropy's Philanthropy Careers.* Retrieved from http://philanthropy.com/article/How-Compassion-Fatigue-Can/52422/. Accessed 14 Feb 2012.

Kagawa-Singer, M. (1998). A multicultural perspective on death and dying. *Oncology Nursing Forum, 25,* 1983–1690.

Kavanaugh, K. (1996). The importance of spirituality. *Journal of Long Term Care Administration, 24*(4), 29–31.

Kaye, J., & Robinson, K. (1994, Fall). Spirituality among caregivers. *Image: Journal of Nursing Scholarship, 26*(3), 218–221.

Kloosterhouse, V., & Ames, B. (2002). Families use of religion/spirituality as a psychosocial resource. *Holistic Nursing Practice, 16*(5), 61–76.

Kuhlman, G., Wilson, H., Hutchinson, S., & Wallhagen, M. (1991). Alzheimer's disease and family caregiving: Critical synthesis of the literature and research agenda. *Nursing Research, 40,* 331–337.

Larson, T. (1997). Resuscitating and transforming hospice volunteer services. *American Journal of Hospice & Palliative Care, 14*(6), 308–310.

Larson, D., & Larson, S. (Eds) (1994). *The forgotten factor in physical and mental health: What does the research show?* Rockville: National Institute for Healthcare Research.

Larson, D. B., Pattison, E. M., Blazer, D. G., Omran, A. R., & Kaplan, B. H. (1986). Systematic analysis of research on religious variables in four major psychiatric journals, 1978–1982. *American Journal of Psychiatry, 143,* 329–334.

Levin, J., & Schiller, P. (1987). Is there a religions factor in health? *Journal of Religion and Health, 26,* 9–36.

Levin, J., Larson, D., & Puchalski, C. (1997). Religion and spirituality in medicine: Research and education. *Journal of the American Medical Association, 278,* 792–793.

Lindgren, C. (1993). The caregiver career. *Image: Journal of Nursing Scholarship, 25*(3), 214–219.

Lo, B., Quill, T., & Tulsky, J. (1999). Discussing palliative care with patients: ACP-ASIM End-of-Life Care Consensus Panel. *Annals of Internal Medicine, 130,* 744–749.

Lo, B., Ruston, D., Kates, L., Arnold, R., Cohen, C., Faber-Langendoen, K., et al. (2002). Discussing religious and spiritual issues at the end of life: A practical guide for physicians. *Journal of the American Medical Association, 287*(6), 749–754.

Loewenberg, F. M. (1988). *Religion and social work practice in contemporary American society.* New York: Columbia University Press.

Lukoff, D., Lu, F., & Turner, R. (1995). Cultural considerations in the assessment and treatment of religious and spiritual problems. *Psychiatric Clinics of North America, 18,* 467–485.

Matthew, D., Larson, D., & Barry, C. (1993). *The faith factor: An annotated bibliography of clinical research on spiritual subjects.* Rockville: National Institute for Healthcare Research.

McCord, G., Gilchrist, V. J., Grossman, S. D., King, B. D., McCormick, K. F., Oprandi, A. M., et al. (2004). Discussing spirituality with patients: A rational and ethical approach. *Annals of Family Medicine, 2*(4), 356–361.

McCubbin, H. I., & Patterson, J. M. (1983). The family stress process: The double ABCX model of adjustment and adaptation. In H. I. McCubbin, M. B. Sussman, & J. M. Patterson (Eds), *Social stress and the family: Advances and developments in family stress therapy* (pp. 7–38). New York: Haworth Press.

McEwen, M. (2004). Analysis of spirituality content in nursing textbooks. *Journal of Nursing Education, 43*(1), 20–30.

McKee, D., & Chappel, J. (1992). Spirituality and medical practice. *Journal of Family Practice, 35,* 201–208.

McNeill, J. A., Sherwood, G. D., Starck, P. L., & Thompson, C. J. (1998). Assessing clinical outcomes: Patient satisfaction with pain management. *Journal of Pain and Symptom Management, 16,* 29–40.

Melynk, B., & Alpert-Gillis, L. (1998). The COPE program: A strategy to improve outcomes of critically young children and their parents. *Pediatric Nursing, 24,* 521–527.

Miaskowski, C., Kragness, L., Dibble, S., & Wallhagen, M. (1997). Differences in mood states, health status, and caregiver strain between family caregivers of oncology outpatients with and without cancer-related pain. *Journal of Pain and Symptom Management, 13*(3), 138–147.

Mickley, J., Pargament, K., Brant, C., & Hipp, K. (1998). God and the search for meaning among hospice caregivers. *Hospice Journal, 13*(4), 1–17.

Miller, B., McFall, S., & Montgomery, A. (1991). The impact of elder health, caregiver involvement, and global stress on two dimensions of caregiver burden. *Journal of Gerontology, 46*(1), S9–S19.

Moberg, D. (1971). *Spiritual well-being: Background issues.* Washington: White House Conference on Aging.

Moberg, D. (1982). Spiritual well-being of the dying. In G. Lesnoff-Caravaglia (Ed), *Aging and the human condition* (pp. 139–155). New York: Human Sciences Press.

Moloney, M. (1995). A Heideggerian hermeneutical analysis of older women's stories of being strong. *Image: Journal of Nursing Scholarship, 27*(2), 104–109.

Montgomery, C. (1997). Coping with the emotional demands of caring. *Advanced Practice Nursing Quarterly, 3*(1), 76–84.

Montgomery, R., Gonyea, J., & Hooyman, N. (1985). Caregiving and the experience of subjective and objective burden. *Research on Aging, 7*(1), 137–152.

Murray, S. A., Kendal, M., Boyd, K., Worth, A., & Benton, T. I. (2004). Exploring the spiritual need of people dying of lung cancer or heart failure: A prospective qualitative interview study of patients and their carers. *Palliative Medicine, 18,* 39–45.

Neubauer, B., & Hamilton, C. (1990). Racial differences in attitudes toward hospice care. *Hospice Journal, 6*(1), 37–48.

Nyamathi, A. (1987). Coping responses of spouses of MI patients and of hemodialysis patients as measured by the Jalowiec coping scale. *Journal of Cardiovascular Nursing, 2*(1), 67–74.

O'Connell, L. J. (1996). Changing the culture of dying: A new awakening of spirituality in American heightens sensitivity to dying persons. *Health Progress, 77*(6), 16–20.

O'Gorman, M. (2002). Spiritual care at the end of life. *Critical Care Nursing Clinics of North America, 14,* 171–176.

Osler, W. (1910). The faith that heals. *British Medical Journal, 1,* 1470–1472.

Pauling-Kaplan, M., & O'Connor, P. (1989). Hospice care for minorities: An analysis of a hospital-based inner city palliative care service. *American Journal of Hospice Care, 6*(4), 13–21.

Pelletier-Hibbert, M., & Sohi, P. (2001). Sources of uncertainty and coping strategies used by family members of individuals living with end stage renal disease. *Nephrology Nursing Journal, 28*(4), 411–417, 419.

Petry, L., Weems, L., & Livingstone, J. (1991). Relationship of stress, distress, and immunological response to a recombinant Hepatitis B vaccine. *Journal of Family Practice, 32,* 481–487.

Pfifferling, J.-H., & Gulley, K. (2000). Overcoming compassion fatigue. *Family Practice Management, 7*(4), 39. Retrieved from http://www.aafp.org/fpm/20000400/39over.html. Accessed 16 Feb 2012.

Pierce, L. (2001). Caring and expressions of spirituality by urban caregivers of people with stroke in African American families. *Qualitative Health Research, 11*(3), 339–352.

Post, S., Puchalski, C., & Larson, D. (2000). Physicians and patient spirituality: Professional boundaries, competency, and ethics. *Annals of Internal Medicine, 132*(7), 578–583.

Pruchno, J. R., & Resch, N. (1989). Husbands and wives as caregivers: Antecedents of depression and burden. *Gerontologist, 29*(2), 159–165.

Puchalski, C. M. (1999). Touching the spirit: The essence of healing. *Spiritual Life, 45*(3), 154–159.

Puchalski, C. M. (2000). Spirituality and end-of-life care: A time for listening and caring. *Journal of Palliative Medicine, 5*(2), 289–294.

Puchalski, C. M. (2001). Spirituality and health: The art of compassionate medicine. *Hospital Physician, 37*(3), 30–36.

Puchalski, C. M. (2002). Spirituality and end of life care. In A. Berger, R. Portenoy, & D. Weissman (Eds), *Principles and practice of palliative care and supportive oncology* (2nd ed., pp. 799–812). Philadelphia: Lippincott Williams & Wilkins.

Puchalski, C. M. (2006). Spirituality and medicine: Curricula in medical education. *Journal of Cancer Education, 21*(1), 14–18.

Puchalski, C. M., & Romer, A. (2000). Taking a spiritual history allows clinicians to understand patients more fully. *Journal of Palliative Medicine, 3*(1), 129–137.

Puchalski, C., & Sandoval, C. (2003). Spiritual care. In J. O'Neill, P. Selwyn, & H. Schietinger (Eds), *A clinical guide to supportive & palliative care for HIV/AIDS*. Washington: HIV/AIDS Bureau, Health Resources and Services Administration.

Purnell, M. J., Walsh, S. M., & Milone, M. A. (2004). Oncology nursing education: Teaching strategies that work. *Nursing Education Perspective, 25*(6), 304–308.

Reed, P. (1987). Spirituality and well being in terminally ill hospitalized adults. *Research in Nursing and Health, 10,* 335–344.

Reed, P. (1994). Response to "The relationship between spiritual perspective, social support, and depression in caregiving and non-caregiving wives." *Scholarly Inquiry for Nursing Practice, 8*(4), 391–397.

Remen, R. (1977, November). "Professionalism". *The New Physician, 26*(11), 45–46.

Richardson, R., & Sistler, A. (1999). The well-being of elderly black caregivers and noncaregivers: A preliminary study. *Journal of Gerontological Social Work, 31*(1/2), 109–117.

Roberts, J. A., Brown, D., Elkins, T., & Larson, D. B. (1997). Factors influencing views of patients with gynecologic cancer about end-of-life decisions. *American Journal of Obstetrics and Gynecology, 176*(1), 166–172.

Robinson, K. (1990). The relationship between social skills, social support, self-esteem, and burden in adult caregivers. *Journal of Advanced Nursing, 15,* 788–795.

Rustoen, T. (1995). Hope and quality of life, two central issues for cancer patients: A theoretical analysis. *Cancer Nursing, 18*(5), 355–361.

Saudia, T., Kinney, M., Brown, K., & Young-Ward, L. (1991). Health locus of control and helpfulness of prayer. *Heart Lung, 120,* 60-65.

Schott-Baer, D. (1993). Dependent care, caregiver burden, and self-care agency of spouse caregivers. *Cancer Nursing, 16*(3), 230–236.

Segall, M., & Wykle, M. (1989). The black family's experience with dementia. *Journal of Applied Social Sciences, 13,* 171–191.

Selye, H. (1978). *The stress of life.* New York: McGraw-Hill.

Sheridan, M., & Hemert, K. (1999). The role of religions and spirituality in social work education and practice: A survey of student views and experiences. *Journal of Social Work Education, 35*(10), 125.

Srivastava, R. (1988). Coping strategies used by spouses of CAPD patients. *American Nephrology Nurses Association Journal, 15*(3), 174–178.

Sullivan, L. (Ed). (1989). *Healing and restoring.* New York: MacMillan.

Sulmasy, D. (1997). *The healer's calling.* Mahwah: Paulist Press.

Sulmasy, D. (2002). A biopsychosocial-spiritual model for the care of patients at the end of life. *Gerontologist, 42*(III), 24–33.

Sumner, C. (1998). Recognizing and responding to spiritual distress. *American Journal of Nursing, 98,* 26–31.

Talamantes, M., Lawler, W., & Espino, D. (1995). Hispanic American elders: Caregiving norms surrounding dying and the use of hospice services. In D. Infeld, A. Gordon, & B. Harper (Eds), *Hospice care and cultural diversity* (pp. 35–49). Binghamton: Haworth Press.

Taylor, E. J. (2003). Spiritual needs of patients with cancer and family caregivers. *Cancer Nursing, 26*(4), 260–266.

Taylor, E. J. (2006). Prevalence and associated factors of spiritual needs among patients with cancer and family caregivers. *Oncology Nursing Forum, 33*(4), 729–735.

Tsevat, J., Puchalski, C. M., Sherman, S. N., Holmes, W. C., Feinberg, J., Leonard, A. C., et al. (2003a). *Spirituality and religion in patients with HIV/AIDS.* Paper presented at the annual meeting of the Society of General Internal Medicine, Vancouver.

Tsevat, J., Sherman, S., Feinberg, J., Mrus, J., Leonard, A., Mandell, K., et al. (2003b). *Can life improve after developing HIV/AIDS?* Paper presented at the annual meeting of the Society of General Internal Medicine, Vancouver.

Udelman, D., & Udelman, M. (1991). Affects, neurotransmitters, and immunocompetence. *Stress Medicine, 7,* 159–162.

United States Conference of Catholic Bishops. (2001). *Ethical and religious directives for catholic health care services* (4th ed). Washington: United States Conference of Catholic Bishops.

University of Virginia Health Science Center. (1997). *Religious beliefs and practices affecting health care.* Charlottesville: Chaplaincy Services and Pastoral Education.

Vachon, M., Kristjanson, L., & Higginson, I. (1995). Psychosocial issues in palliative care: The patient, the family, and the process and outcome of care. *Journal of Pain and Symptom Management, 10*(2), 142–150.

VandeCreek, L., & Burton, L. (2001). Professional chaplaincy: Its role and importance in healthcare. *Journal of Pastoral Care, 55*(1), 81–97.

Waters, C. M., Stewart, B. J., Archibold, P. G., Miller, F. C., & Li, H. C. (2005). Global strain and the influence of spirituality in white and black family caregivers. *Journal of National Black Nurses Association* (in press).

Wyatt, G., Friedman, L., Given, C., & Given, B. (1999). A profile of bereaved caregivers following provision of terminal care. *Journal of Palliative Care, 15*(1), 13–25.

Yates, J., Chalmer, B. J., James, P. St., Follansbee, M., & McKegney, F. P. (1981). Religion in patients with advanced cancer. *Medical and Pediatric Oncology, 9,* 121–128.

Zarit, S., Todd, P., & Zarit, J. (1986). Subjective burden of husbands and wives as caregivers: A longitudinal study. *Gerontologist, 26*(3), 260–266.

Chapter 12
The Economics of Cancer Care: Implications for Family Caregivers

Dee Baldwin

Evidence is mounting on the escalating costs of cancer care associated with family members who provide care to their loved one with cancer (Grunfeld et al. 2004; Moore 1999; Muurinen 1986). With a few exceptions, past research on the cost of cancer has been restricted to studying treatment, screening, or prevention costs (Sherman et al. 2001; Stommel et al. 1993). The majority of research related to the costs of cancer care for family caregivers has been associated with direct medical costs, and data from insurance companies, hospitals, and Medicare files have yielded significant findings. However, these same data sources have not been useful for determining the indirect costs borne by patients and their families. As a result, there is a growing need to capture the comprehensiveness of nonmedical costs associated with cancer care (Moore 1999; Sherman et al. 2001; Stommel et al. 1993).

According to Stommel et al. (1993), "a more comprehensive view of the costs of cancer care would include the financial impact on the family of the patient and go beyond the costs of medical treatment, screening or prevention" (p. 1867). They suggest that there are three important components of family costs that are frequently subjected to neglect: (1) direct costs such as out-of-pocket cash expenditures for services not covered by third-party payers; (2) indirect costs associated with forgone earning opportunities resulting from the illness; and (3) indirect costs associated with foregone household production and/or leisure time. Estimates of these costs are greatly needed given the current trends in health care and rising cancer costs (Sherman et al. 2001; Stommel et al. 1993). According to Sherman et al., out-of-pocket expenses engender significant financial concerns to patients with cancer and their family caregivers.

This chapter focuses on the cancer costs associated with family caregiving. The chapter: (a) describes current trends impacting the economics of cancer care, (b) discuss existing direct and indirect costs associated with cancer care, (c) delineates

D. Baldwin (✉)
Georgia State University, Downtown Atlanta, GA, USA
e-mail: dbaldwi5@uncc.edu

University of North Carolina at Charlotte, 9201 University City Blvd., CHHS 449B, Charlotte, NC 28223-0001, USA

R. C. Talley et al. (eds.), *Cancer Caregiving in the United States,*
Caregiving: Research, Practice, Policy
DOI 10.1007/978-1-4614-3154-1_12, © Springer Science+Business Media, LLC 2012

costs issues identified by family caregivers as patients with cancer live beyond the initial diagnosis and treatment, and (d) provide strategies and solutions to assist family caregivers with payment issues. The chapter concludes with recommendations for future study including research, education, and policy development.

Background

Family members and other relatives play a significant role in the cancer patient's overall well-being and quality of life through social and financial support. Family members are irrevocably changed by the individual's illness while experiencing a concomitant financial challenge (Moore 1999; Sherman et al. 2001; Wein 2000). While the role that family caregivers play in supporting their family members diagnosed with cancer is well documented in the literature, the financial burden and impact is less clearly understood (Grunfeld et al. 2004). Health care is expensive and money can serve as a metaphor for value, control, and power (Wein 2000). At the outset, money can be viewed as no object and no cost is too great. However, as the disease progresses, financial resources may dwindle and the lack of money can come to be seen as a metaphor for anger, loss of hope, and exhaustion (Sherman et al. 2001; Wein 2000). Resources beyond health insurance, which help to defray the indirect costs associated with cancer care, become critical as cancer costs rise for these patients (Moore 1999; Sherman et al. 2001; Wein 2000).

Another reality for the family caregiver is that providing care to the family member with cancer is time consuming, demanding, and many times frustrating, leaving little opportunity for other household and leisure activities (Grunfeld et al. 2004; Stommel et al. 1993). Role fatigue, often associated with confinement within the home and restriction on activities outside the home, missed days from work, and mental and physical illness as a result of being a caregiver are a few of the issues experienced by family caregivers. It is well documented that the caregivers often get ill as a result of providing care to their terminally ill loved one (Grunfeld et al. 2004; Payne et al. 1999). However, the costs of the labor associated with this care and the financial burden for the family are frequently not calculated. If the cost of family labor input is considered at all, it usually is evaluated in terms of market earnings. Costs incurred by the relative who leaves or misses work to care for the patient, family members' transportation to the doctor or hospital, and the frequent necessity for household help are examples of the cancer family's uncounted costs.

Many families work through the illness without adequate financial resources. To illustrate this point, Grunfeld et al. (2004), in a longitudinal study, found that burden was the most important predictor of both anxiety and depression in family caregivers caring for family members with breast cancer. They also found that among employed caregivers, 69% reported an adverse impact related to work, while 77% of family caregivers missed work during the terminal stage of their loved one's cancer.

Hayman et al. (2001) argue that controversy continues to exist regarding how best to value the opportunity cost of caregiver's time. They suggest using the average hourly wage of working individuals with similar characteristics as an approach to measure caregiver time. They also add that since there are no appropriate wage data for some groups of caregivers, such as the retired elderly, measuring caregiving time is difficult. Hayman et al. conclude that health care expenditures for family caregiving are growing and predict they will continue to increase.

Current Status and Trends

Emerging health care trends have the potential for affecting the economics of cancer care for family caregivers (Brown et al. 2001; Mortenson 1996; National Cancer Institute [NCI], 2009). Significant gains in fighting the war on cancer were made in the 1990s (Fleck 1993; Moore 1999; NCI 2009). The cancer death rate in the United States decreased 2.6% between 1991 and 1995. This decrease in cancer deaths was the first of its kind since record keeping began in the 1930s (Fleck 1993). While cancer death rates were declining during the 1990s, health care expenditures were soaring. In 1960, health care expenditures grew from 4.5% of the U.S. Gross National Product (GNP) to 14% of the GNP in the 1990s. Health care expenditures broke the 1 trillion mark in 1996. The national cost for cancer care in 1997 was approximately $ 50 billion. According to the NCI, cancer care treatment accounted for an estimated $ 104.1 billion in 2006. As a result of these soaring prices, politicians and health care agencies are looking for ways to trim health care costs at a time when cancer research is at its most promising.

The emergence of managed care organizations was one response to these escalating costs. Managed care organizations were created to help contain and control rising costs. This meant that many employers were allowed to change their traditional health plan insurance benefits to plans in which workers no longer choose their own physicians, thus restricting and limiting coverage and benefits. For some cancer patients, this meant that coverage for cancer treatment changed to limited coverage, and choosing a health care provider became no longer an option. Due to the lower premiums, many cancer patients were forced to select a physician who was associated with a preferred provider organization (Fishman et al. 1997).

Other current societal forces that impact the economics of cancer care include oncology as a specialty area, clinical trials, use of U.S. Food and Drug Administration (FDA)-approved chemotherapy drugs, outpatient cancer care, prescription drug costs, and the provision of services for minorities, the elderly, and the poor. These trends are briefly described next.

Oncology as a Specialty Area From a cost perspective, cancer patients are not viewed as winners by some hospitals (Du et al. 2000). The specific details of the problems change frequently, however, the overall picture of cancer care is that it is expensive and can be long-term. Oncology as a specialty is experiencing several unfavorable economic conditions: increasing patient volume, growing numbers of socioeconomically disadvantaged patients needing care, hospital-intensive monitoring throughout treatment, escalating high-tech care costs, and the abundant need for psychological interventions (Brown et al. 2001). While there are many cancer-specific diagnostic-related groups (DRGs) for reimbursement, high reimbursement DRGs do not necessarily translate into profit for hospitals. For example, the DRG related to lung cancer is a high-reimbursement DRG, however, the care required for these patients is long and extensive, causing the hospital to lose money because of the complexity of the illness (Brown et al. 2001; Fleck 1993). Hospitals are given incentives to shorten the length of stay to minimize utilization, attempt to attract patients who are economic winners, and avoid attracting patients who are unable to pay for care. For the cancer patient who is hospitalized, this could mean early discharge from the hospital facility, thus transferring care to the family caregiver in the home environment (O'Mara 2005).

Clinical Trials To advance cancer care, a large number of patients are annually enrolled in clinical trials for research. Clinical trials are very costly to the hospital or clinical facility due to increased laboratory and radiology tests, a need for specialization and/or a highly educated interdisciplinary team, and higher staff/patient ratios. There is still much debate over reimbursement for clinical trials and treating cancer patients with stage III or stage IV disease (Fireman et al. 2000). These patients are viewed by some as high-risk for financial support and use of health care resources. According to Rutledge and Stair (1997), "a major barrier for both patients and institutions to participating in national studies is that third-party payers do not cover experimental treatment, which includes all research trials" (p. 1598). For cancer patients and their families, understanding if their insurance plan covers clinical trial participation is critical. Participation in a clinical trial could help to minimize the cost of treatment associated with the cancer care.

FDA-Approved Drug Use of Chemotherapy Drugs Cost drivers for the use of chemotherapy drugs include two major concerns. The first is whether or not new drug research will be slowed as the snowballing influence of managed care intensifies. The second is the long-standing need for approval of off-label usage of chemotherapeutic agents. In terms of research and under new FDA rules, anticancer drugs may be given early, market approval before their effectiveness is conclusively proven if drug companies can show that the drugs shrink tumors. In addition, the FDA has agreed to attempt to speed approval of drugs that have already been approved in other countries (FDA 2009; Fireman et al. 2000).

Off-label usage of chemotherapy drugs is becoming less of an issue as legislation has been approved across the country to address this problem (FDA 2009; Fleck 1993; Rutledge and Stair 1997). In the 1980s, the government and insurance companies began to deny reimbursement for drugs used for indications outside of the package-insert indications approved by the FDA. In practice, once a drug has received FDA approval, the pharmaceutical company does not necessarily have to reapply to the FDA when additional indications for the drug's use are identified. In the 1990s, the Association of Community Cancer Centers led an effort to introduce model legislation requiring insurance companies to use the drug compendia and the peer-reviewed medical literature in making coverage determinations rather than using the FDA-labeled indication (Fleck 1993; Rutledge and Stair 1997; FDA 2009). Many insurance companies will not pay for drugs used for indications that do not fall within the drug-package insert guidelines (Fleck 1993; Guidry et al. 1998). Cancer patients on chemotherapy may not be reimbursed for drug coverage if not indicated in their policies, leaving families to assume medication-related costs that are not covered by the insurance plan.

Outpatient Cancer Care Outpatient cancer care is another economic issue. The DRG limits for reimbursement, pressure for early patient discharge, and patient preference have been strong incentives for the accelerated growth of outpatient cancer care facilities. The delivery of quality outpatient care has quickly become possible through advanced technologic support (e.g., vascular access, ambulatory infusion pumps, etc.; Mortenson 1996).

Management of toxic effects of drugs has become possible on an outpatient basis by increasing the education and responsibility of patients and their families. This shift to outpatient care has impacted family caregivers who are providing the majority of cancer care in outpatient settings. This results in an increase in home health care costs (Arno et al. 1999; Given et al. 2001; Mortenson 1996) and a shift of more care responsibilities from the hospital to the family (Hayman et al. 2001; O'Mara 2005). Patients receiving treatment for cancer, especially chemotherapy, have felt the impact most heavily. While the shift to outpatient care has increased the need for home health care, funding for home health care has decreased, making this trend a future crisis for family caregivers. Administering oral and parenteral medications, performing wound care, and monitoring signs and symptoms are a few of the more demanding, yet routine tasks that family caregivers are expected to perform (O'Mara). Family caregivers not only have to provide more follow-up care in the home, but also worry about other cost-related issues associated with care, such as transportation to and from the outpatient setting and job absence (Guidry et al. 1998; Hayman et al. 2001).

Prescription Drug Costs Prescription drug spending is escalating at four times the rate of overall medical cost inflation (Reed and Hargraves 2003). Reasons for this increase are numerous, including the production of more sophisticated drugs by pharmaceutical companies resulting in higher prescription costs, an aging population with increased drug usage, aggressive drug marketing to consumers and providers, and the use of drug therapy prior to surgery. It is well recognized that cancer chemotherapy treatment can last several months, and much longer for patients who respond favorably. This cumulative cost of treatment can be astronomical for the patient and family caregiver (Wittes 2004).

A looming issue in cancer care is the exorbitant costs of new cancer drugs. While some family caregivers will be able to afford these new costs, others will not. According to Reed and Hargraves, working-age African Americans and Latinos are much more likely than their White counterparts to report they cannot afford all of their prescription drugs. Uninsured working-age people with chronic conditions are at particular risk for not being able to afford all of their prescriptions. These vulnerable groups will be at high risk for problems in paying for their cancer medications as out-of-pocket drugs costs escalate. The Center for Studying Health System Change

(Reed and Hargraves 2003) suggests consumers and governmental health plans will not be able to afford these new cancer drugs given their excessive costs. Several studies are beginning to show that with the new Medicare law (the government paying for senior citizens' drug costs), seniors will have to "foot the bill" for the high costs of prescription drugs (Connolly and Allen 2005).

Cancer and the Poor Cancer and the poor remain an ongoing economic issue that impacts the cost of cancer care. Problems of early cancer detection, treatment and survival, unemployment, inadequate education, substandard housing, chronic malnutrition, and diminished access to medical care disproportionately effect the poor (Fleck 1993). The expanding number of legal and illegal immigrants entering the United States is another major factor contributing to the increased number of people living below the poverty line.

In the well-known study, *Cancerin the Economically Disadvantaged*, Harold Freeman (1989), concludes that both cancer incidence and survival are related to socioeconomic status and that at least 50% of the survival difference is due to late diagnosis of the economically disadvantaged. Other studies have linked low income with the low utilization of cancer screenings services (Baldwin 1996; Phillips et al. 1999). According to Schulmeister (1999), the most serious effect of low-socioeconomic status is the delay in seeking early detection, which results in late diagnosis and delayed treatment. Late diagnosis usually is related to limited treatment options, resulting in a poorer overall prognosis. For the low-income cancer patient, the problem is due in part to a low awareness of cancer warning signs and the inability to pay for recommended preventive health care. Also, some patients first use nontraditional treatment methods for symptoms, thus delaying formal medical treatment of their cancer. Explanations for this delay have been associated with feelings of pessimism and fatalism, and a negative belief system (Phillips et al. 1999; Schulmeister 1999).

While little research is written about family caregivers of cancer patients who are at the poverty and low-income levels, it is believed that these patients and their family caregivers will experience the same economic and social pressures as most other groups, excluding the very wealthy. Money problems for the family and person experiencing cancer cut across most socioeconomic boundaries, affecting the middle class as well as the poor. According to Germino and O'Rourke (1996), "regardless of socioeconomic status, almost all families experiencing cancer and cancer treatment have financial problems" (p. 86). Nevertheless, cancer care is most burdensome to those with low incomes, especially if they experience increased out-of-pocket expenses (Given and Given 1997).

Direct and Indirect Cost Associated with Cancer

Most of the research related to cancer costs for family caregivers has been associated with direct medical costs. Direct cost is measured by expenditures for medical procedures and services associated with treatment and care. Medical costs related to cancer care are widely cited and discussed in the literature (Brown et al. 2001; Muurinen 1986; Sherman et al. 2001). Cancers of the lung, prostate, breast, and colon/rectum are responsible for a disproportionate share of burden in terms of both cancer incidence and mortality (Brown et al. 2002). These cancer sites accounted for 52% of estimated new cancer cases in 1999 and 55% of estimated deaths in 1999, and their treatment has driven up medical costs. Cancer care continues to use more hospital dollars than any other diseases, accounting for hospital expenditures of 60–75% of the total direct cost of cancer treatment compared to 35–50% for all other illnesses (Brown et al. 2002).

Cost of illness (COI) estimates typically include three main elements: direct cost, morbidity cost, and mortality cost (Brown et al. 2001). Direct costs are derived from sources such as the National Medical Expenditure Survey, which provides disease-specific data on cost per hospital day combined with data on the proportion of hospital days related to each disease entity from the National Hospital Discharge data (Cassileth 1979). Recent studies, however, describe other data sources, such as claims data related to Surveillance, Epidemiology, and End Results (SEER) and Medicare data sets. According to Chang et al. (2004), "these estimates have limitations primarily related to the source databases" (p. 3524). Morbidity costs are measured by lost income due to work disability and absenteeism associated with the disease entity (Brown et al. 2002). In other words, these are wages lost that would have been earned by patients had they not missed work because of diagnostic procedures, treatment, or prolonged disability (Cassileth 1979). Morbidity costs are estimated based on disease-specific work disability as reported to the National Health Interview Survey.

Mortality cost is measured as lost income associated with premature death (Brown et al. 2001). That is, they are wages that the person would have earned if not for premature death. These costs are estimated using the human capital approach. According to Brown and colleagues, "this approach imputes economic value to years of life lost attributable to the disease category by assigning average age-specific, gender-specific earnings to the lost years, including the value of household work for individuals not employed in the formal labor market" (p. 98). The source used to obtain information about earnings comes from the U.S. Bureau of Labor Statistics.

Indirect costs, typically not measured, are those costs associated with the work time and output lost by the patient, family, friends, and caring others (Brown and Fintor 1995). According to Sherman et al. (2001), "by definition, direct nonmedical costs are expenditures as the result of an illness but are not involved in the direct purchasing of medical services" (p. 842). These costs are rarely covered by insurance plans. Services may include travel, lodging, payment for home health aides, and equipment purchase for items such as support bars in the bathtub (Sherman et al. 2001). The time the patient and/or family members spend visiting the physician, other health professionals, and hospitalized persons are frequently not included in the overall cost estimates of the family. Special diets (dietary supplements), equipment, clothing, and family counseling are a few of the unmeasured cost areas where families incur out-of-pocket costs associated with care of the cancer patient. Hired labor and labor provided by family members are also frequently uncounted. Giving up employment to provide care, transportation related to the distance that a family caregiver travels from their residence to a treatment center, and time costs are only a few costs that are not included in the budget of the family caregiver.

To support this point, Moore (1999), in a study that analyzed breast cancer patients' out-of-pocket expenses, noted that 60% of the patients and families experienced lost income associated with a diagnosis of breast cancer. These losses included decreased monthly wages, use of sick and vacation time, and time without pay. In addition, women who were self-employed or part of a family business had to rearrange their time and the time of others to make up for the absence. Moore warns that while loss of income is not considered an out-of-pocket expense; it does engender a reduction in liquid assets.

Moreover, Gould (2002) found that returning to work following treatment was a physical and/or emotional struggle for most low-income women diagnosed with breast cancer. Following adjuvant treatment, many of these women left their paid workplaces because of debilitating side effects. Chang et al. (2004), in their study that estimated the direct and indirect costs of cancer care, found that cancer patients in the study had notably higher absenteeism than the control (noncancer) group and cancer caregivers had a mean of 2.2 absence days per month versus a mean for the controls of 1.4 days per month. These data translate into out-of-pocket expenses and lost income for family members.

While there is a growing need to accurately capture the indirect costs of cancer care, major issues surround the assessment of these types of data. For example, a major problem in assessing indirect costs rests with the use of restricted convenience samples (Hayman et al. 2001) and methods of data collection (Chang et al. 2004). Issues related to data collection include comprehensive data bases (Chang et al. 2004), the availability of tools to examine indirect costs (Moore 1999; Sherman et al. 2001), variability in individuals' response to cancer and treatment protocols (Moore 1999), reliable self-report information from patients (Moore 1999; Stommel et al. 1993), and costs associated with conducting a cost-effectiveness analysis (Du et al. 2000; Sherman et al. 2001).

Another issue surrounding the economics of cancer care is capturing the costs of illnesses experienced by family caregivers as a result of caring for their loved one with cancer. According to O'Mara (2005), becoming a family caregiver is a random event, with few training programs to help with this endeavor. Many family caregivers experience physical conditions and psychological illnesses associated with stress, coping, and depression as they provide care to their family member with cancer. Other concerns are a lack of leisure time and emotional support as the family member with cancer deteriorates. Grunfeld et al. (2004) add that "caregivers experience substantial psychological morbidity (anxiety and depression) at the onset of the patient's palliative illness and a substantial increase in caregiver burden and depression when the patient reaches a terminal state of the illness" (p. 1797).

Understanding family caregivers and how caregiving affects the family caregiver remains a critical area for research (Grunfeld et al. 2004; O'Mara 2005). More importantly, as family caregivers experience emotional and psychological disorders as a result of the cancer care they provide to their loved one with cancer, incorporating these care costs will yield a more accurate and comprehensive picture of the overall cost of cancer care (Vanderwerker et al. 2005). It is both direct and indirect cost issues that typically contribute to the overall financial burden of the family caregiver.

Cost Issues Identified by Family Caregivers

The diagnosis of cancer in one family member affects all other members of that family and frequently requires the designation of one member to serve as primary caregiver (Stommel et al. 1993). Four areas of cost have been cited in the literature related to costs experienced by family caregivers: patients' loss of income due to loss of employment, out-of-pocket expenditures for services, caregiver labor costs (lost earnings), family labor costs and total costs to family. A brief explanation of these costs is described next.

Patients' Loss of Income Cancer survivors many times want and need to work and to perform in their customary roles after the cancer diagnoses (Bradley et al. 2001). Returning to work serves as a means for coping, better recovery, and returning to normalcy. However, according to Bradley and colleagues, the ability to return to work can vary by cancer site, treatment modality, and characteristics inherent to patients and their jobs. In general, cancer patients employed in physically demanding jobs are more likely to quit their employment in comparison to those with sedentary jobs (Given and Given 1997).

For the family caregiver who belongs to the workforce, a decision to terminate their employment may occur in order to provide care for the cancer patient. The caregiver's age and own health are both likely to play a part in the caregiver's decision to remain employed (Muurinen 1986). Increases in care can raise the cost of dropping out of the labor force for those caregivers who are the sole or major income earners for their families. According to Muurinen, working caregivers may find it difficult to maintain both high levels of informal care supply and the supply of normal working hours. Therefore, many caregivers leave the labor force at the onset of the care episode. Those who choose to remain employed tend to experience reductions in working hours, sometimes with consequent income losses. Out of those caregivers who continued to work 60% report losses of income because of increased absences from work (Hayman et al. 2001; Muurinen 1986).

Out-of-Pocket Expenditures for Services Mounting research is beginning to expose the alarming cost of out-of-pocket expenses associated with cancer care. Expenses incurred by family caregivers for which they have not been reimbursed include purchases of special equipment and supplies, home health aides, medications, hospital and physician services, and special foods. Additional costs are incurred by the caregiver who leaves work to care for the patient and to transport the family member to the doctor or hospital. The frequent necessity for household help is also an example of the family caregiver's expenses that are not reflected in their overall care budget for the cancer patient. Many times the family caregiver cannot always place a dollar amount to these expenses. In a study conducted by Stommel et al. (1993), higher home care costs to families were not attributed to the result of larger cash expenditures. Rather, the largest cost component was viewed as the labor cost associated with providing the care to the cancer patient, those costs that were attributed to loss of employment. Chang et al. (2004) add that out-of-pocket costs related to deductible and copayments paid by caregivers were comparable to wages lost and should be considered in the overall burden of cancer. Moreover, Hayman et al. (2001) argue that "the frequency and intensity with which elderly cancer patients undergoing treatment rely on their families for caregiving is substantial" (p. 3223).

Caregiver Labor Costs (Lost Earnings) Costs associated with caregiver labor involves hours spent in caring for the family member with cancer, sacrificed employment, and lost earnings due to missed days at work. Most studies reveal that it is difficult to evaluate the cost of care that family members provide to patients (Chang et al. 2004; Stommel et al. 1993). This is due in part because family caregivers do not attach a market value to the services that they are providing. Moreover, for those who are not employed, they do not necessarily associate a monetary or wage value to the service they are providing. Therefore, estimates have to be used in determining caregiver labor costs. For example, Stommel et al. suggest that when there is an absence of data on usual activities of family members, then the cost of a provider, such as a home health aid, may be considered a reasonable approximation of the wage that one could charge to provide cancer care.

Family Labor Costs Frequently, family caregivers, other than the primary caregiver, are not factored into the costs of services provided to the family member with cancer. These caregivers include someone other than the spouse, such as the children, cousins, other relatives (aunts and uncles), and friends. One of the issues that often occur with family caregivers is how knowledgeable they are in caring for the cancer patient. Frequently, these caregivers are not trained in providing direct patient care. Therefore, training costs (time away from job or leisure activities) are infrequently included in the estimates of cancer care. Also, promotions denied, reduced work effort, and decline in productivity in the home not related to patient care can be experienced by family caregivers who are not the primary caregiver. These caregivers need to be included in the overall payment strategies as cancer care is evaluated.

Payment Strategies and Solutions for Family Caregivers

Cancer is an expensive illness. For the ill-prepared family, it can be disastrous and catastrophic. Families can pay for cancer treatment and care through various payment options, including Medicare, Medicaid, private insurance, and other commercial payers. Different regulations govern care and reimbursement under each of these models. It is important that families understand their insurance coverage since benefits may vary at different stages in the disease process (American Cancer Society [ACS] 2003; Cassileth 1979). Even those who are well insured can be financially devastated with gaps in coverage (Germino and O'Rourke 1996).

Medicare is the federal health insurance program that provides hospital and medical insurance for persons 65 years of age and older, and for those who receive disability payments from Social Security or railroad retirement. Medicare was established by Title XVIII of the Social Security Act in 1965. It is a two-part program, commonly known and referred to as Part A and Part B. Part A pays for inpatient hospital services for up to 90 days in a benefit period, plus a lifetime reserve of 60 additional days of hospital care, posthospital care in a skilled nursing facility for up to 100 days per benefit period so long as the skilled nursing facility follows a hospitalization of at least 3 days and the patient is admitted to the skilled nursing facility within days of the discharge from the hospital. Patients may receive up to 100 home health visits in a benefit period so long as the home visits follow hospitalization. Part A also includes home health services, hospice care, and care in Medicare-certified nursing facilities. Part B of Medicare provides for physicians' services, diagnostic services such as laboratory and radiological tests, hospital equipment for use at home, ambulance services, and outpatient physical therapy (ACS 2003; Cassileth 1979).

Title XIX of the Social Security Act established the Medicaid program. While Medicare is administered as part of the Social Security System, Medicaid is administered by the states and is optional. To receive Medicaid, the cancer patient's income and assets must be below a certain level. Under Medicaid, federal assistance is offered to states that provide medical care coverage for a minimum of specified basic services for at least everyone receiving federally aided money payments under any one of the categorical public assistance programs. Federal funds are available to match state expenditures according to a formula that considers a state's relative wealth (ACS 2003; Cassileth 1979). In addition to coverage for categorical public assistance recipients, the state may choose to cover individuals who are medically needy. This coverage includes, among others, persons whose income exceeds public assistance levels but who otherwise would be eligible for public assistance programs because they are aged, blind, disabled or members of families eligible for aid to dependent children, and children of families with incomes too low to be eligible for categorical assistance (ACS 2003; Cassileth 1979).

It should be noted that both Medicaid and Medicare are experiencing severe cuts (Connolly and Allen 2005; Mortenson 1996). These cuts have the potential to affect the future of cancer care and increase the financial burden of the family caregivers if they receive coverage under these plans.

Private insurance organizations provide health care benefits through various plans. These organizations are typically associated with an individual's employer who along with the employee makes contributions to the health insurance plan. These plans cover hospital services, physicians' services, diagnostic services, and other benefits. However, the recent increase in premiums and employees having to share more of the cost for health care could make it difficult for family caregivers to maintain their health insurance coverage. Many commercial insurance companies offer health insurance coverage. Their policies often take the form of major medical insurance plans and may vary widely in their coverage (ACS 2003; Cassileth 1979; Eisenberg 1979).

Other solutions for family caregivers include being adequately prepared financially for a major illness like cancer. This means having knowledge about one's insurance plan to ensure adequate health coverage, possessing disability insurance, and knowing about cancer centers and other community resources. Financial preparation for a major illness should be a part of every family's plans. Adequate insurance coverage includes coverage for hospitalization, outpatient services, radiation and chemotherapy, and home health services. Some insurance plans even have coverage for a catastrophic illness. Family caregivers should explore their policy to determine if they have adequate coverage. Most insurance policies, however, have poor coverage for home health care expenses (Stommel et al. 1993), in a time when home health care abounds. The insurance policy should also be noncancelable, which means that the insurance cannot be discontinued unless the individual fails to make payments (Fleck 1993).

For those who cannot afford to pay for cancer costs, the Hill-Burton program is available. The program was established by Congress in 1946 to provide grants and loans for construction and modernization to hospitals, nursing homes, and other health facilities. In return, these facilities agreed to provide treatment to a "reasonable volume" of persons unable to pay, and to all persons living in the facility's catchment area. Eligibility is based on family size and income (ACS 2003). While the program stopped providing funds in 1997, about 300 health care facilities nationwide are still obligated to provide free or reduced-cost care. Hill-Burton may cover services not provided by other governmental programs.

Disability insurance can help protect the family's income as well as protect the individual if unable to work. Disability insurance provides the individual with income at a flat rate and does not take into consideration inflation. Therefore, it is important that the cancer patient and family caregiver examine their policy to ensure that the plan will meet household expenses (ACS 2003).

Community resources are available to assist the cancer patient and family caregiver to help defray the cost of cancer care. While these resources may vary from community to community, they may also vary in the resources they provide. Many community groups will have emergency funds to help pay medical bills. Cancer centers such as the American Cancer Society, National Cancer Institute, and the Leukemia Society of America may offer free cancer treatment, transportation, and support programs. Churches and synagogues may also be able to provide cost assistance with such activities as baby-sitting, home care services, and purchasing of home equipment. Many churches and synagogues will also offer cancer support groups for the patient and family caregivers (ACS 2003).

While a wealth of support programs exists for the patient and caregiver, few economic and financial programs are available to help family members manage and disclose their illness-related financial pressures. Without disclosure, these illnesses-related demands could cause disharmony in the family leading to negative consequences for the cancer patient and the caregiver. Family caregivers can potentially benefit from having a training forum whereby they have an opportunity to express and share how they manage their finances as one of the illness-related demands.

Recommendations for the Future

Research

Research in indirect costs associated with cancer care and how these costs impact family caregivers is a major area for continued research. Most of the research related to the costs of cancer care for family caregivers has been associated with direct medical costs, which includes mostly hospital cost and doctor bills (Hayman et al. 2001). However, more research is needed to address the out-of-pocket expenses incurred by family caregivers as they care for the cancer patient. This research should focus on elderly patients with cancer (Hayman et al. 2001) and female caregivers. Evidence is mounting that as the population ages, caregivers of the future will continue to be female who are caring for elderly relatives. Studies that continue to focus on the financial impact of female caregivers as they support the cancer patient will strengthen this area of research.

Moreover, more longitudinal studies focusing on the economic burden of family caregivers are needed to better understand the out-of-pocket expenses incurred by family caregivers. Many studies on the cost burden to caregivers are based on the surveys of small convenience samples (Chang et al. 2004). Intervention studies with large randomized sample sizes will expand the research on cost burden to family members.

Cancer caregivers' knowledge of providing direct care is also an area of continued research. According to O'Mara (2005), informal caregiving is an intricate part of health care and will become a larger factor in the world of decreasing resources. Unfortunately, the selection of an informal caregiver, like the diagnosis of cancer itself, is a random event, and no education programs exist to prepare individuals to be one (O'Mara 2005). Therefore, more research is needed on the development of educational programs that will assist the informal caregiver in providing direct care. These educational programs should also include information on identifying resources (beyond insurance coverage) to support caring for the patient diagnosed with cancer.

Equally important, research is needed on family labor costs associated with not only the primary caregiver, however, with all caregivers who provide care to the cancer patient. Caregivers of adult patients undergoing cancer treatment are usually spouses, sons and daughters, or sons- and daughters-in-laws, cousins, and friends who are rarely paid (Hayman et al. 2001). The social and economic burden that these individuals encounter when caring for the cancer patient is rarely included in the overall treatment costs of the cancer patient. More research will strengthen this area of cost analysis.

In addition, little research is written about family caregivers of cancer patients who are at the poverty and low-income levels. The majority of studies with families experiencing cancer have been conducted on educated middle-class families. More studies are needed on the economic issues of cancer and the poor and with different ethnic/racial groups.

   Furthermore, research related to data sources used to calculate the economic burden on cancer is greatly needed. The economic burden of cancer is usually measured by cost-of-illness methods developed in the late 1960s and early 1970s (Chang et al. 2004). The primary data source has been national survey information, combined with claims data. Indirect measures have relied on self-report data related to work disability obtained from the National Health Interview Survey (Chang et al. 2004). More studies using additional data sources to measure indirect costs are greatly needed to capture a more comprehensive picture that family caregivers portray in care of the cancer patient. Last, little data exist on the employment experience of people with cancer who are able to work. More research is needed in this area.

Education

According to the American Association of Caregiver Education (AACE 2005), family caregiving is more prevalent than actually documented and growing faster than anticipated, adding that most Americans will be caregivers for more than one individual and more than once before or during their lifetime. AACE points out that these caregivers may not have accessed the needed information to make wise decisions about treatment options and cancer care (CancerCare 2012; Tamblyn et al. 2001). Family caregivers who provide cancer care to their loved one are typically, spouses, daughters, sons, friends, and other relatives.

   While it is well recognized that cancer caregiving places an increased burden on family caregivers, more national family caregiver education programs are greatly needed (O'Mara 2005; Pasacreta et al. 2000). Given et al. (2001) suggest that a major concern expressed by family caregivers is their need for information. Family caregivers have a need to know more about the signs and symptoms of the cancer disease, comfort measures, physical care, treatment regimens, household management procedures, and finances (Given et al. 1994). They also report needing additional information about how to arrange for activities such as transportation, nutritional support, coordination of care, and financial activities (Guidry et al. 1998; Given et al. 1994).

   Pasacreta et al. agree that family caregivers need educational programs to help with the management of their loved one with cancer. To support this notion, they conducted a study to determine caregiver characteristics before and after attendance at a family caregiver cancer education program. Upon completion of their education program, which included psychosocial support, resource identification, and symptom management for caregivers, participants believed that they were much better well informed and confident about completing caregiving tasks. Caregivers also believed that their burden did not worsen as the caretaking tasks increased in intensity because of the education program.

   Bulsa et al. (2004) agree that patients and their family members desire to remain in control and feel empowered in the management of their cancer care. They suggest that health care providers work with caregivers in terms of how best to move forward once the initial diagnosis and shock is over. Given et al. (1994) suggest that positive outcomes can be achieved for family caregivers if they are embraced as a partner of the health care team, a team that provides instruction, guidance, and information in evaluating the home care situation. The health care provider can provide information, clarify terminology, and help patients understand their treatment options.

Rabow et al. (2004) add that "family caregiving is typically at the core of what sustains patients at the end of life" (p. 483). They offer several recommendations for conducting a family meeting when the patient is unable to participate. This information includes providing family caregivers with medical updates on the patient's condition, dealing with decisions that need to be made, and education about palliative care. Rabow et al. suggest that physicians, as members of the interdisciplinary home care team, can play a key role in the multidisciplinary referrals and training family caregivers may require. They call for a national education and compensation reform to enhance physician services to family caregivers.

In its strategic plan, the NCI (2003) suggests that the quality of cancer communications need to be enhanced, including gaining a better understanding of the information needs of patients, families, and other decision makers involved in the choice of cancer interventions. Equally important, research is needed that investigates the relationship between the time that professional caregivers provide information and improved patient outcomes (Given et al. 2001). Last, economic seminars need to be sponsored to assist family caregivers with the financial realities of the cost of cancer care.

Public Policy

Given existing trends, it is likely that the cost of treating cancer will continue to escalate. Increasing costs are attributable to the aging of large numbers of our nation's citizens, improved cancer survivorship, better early detection strategies, and enhanced treatment modalities (Eisenberg 1979; Harper 2000). Increasingly large numbers of people are achieving old age, thus expanding the population of persons susceptible to develop cancer (Harper 2000). If true estimates of cancer care for the family caregiver are to be determined, then public policy that addresses both indirect and directs costs must continually be assessed. Specifically, those polices related to unpaid family care, paid home care, and out-of-pocket costs associated with skilled nursing facility placement need to be continually monitored (Hayman et al. 2001).

Navaie-Waliser et al. (2002) assert that family caregivers and their advocates have generated "a new awareness of the challenges of caregiving in the current healthcare system" (p. 411). In their study, they found that vulnerable caregivers, those 65 and over, were more likely than nonvulnerable caregivers to be providing care to their loved one with cancer. Yet, they were providing this assistance without paid compensation. Navaie-Waliser et al. suggest that pressures on unpaid caregivers are likely to increase, with Medicare "as a dependable supplement to family caregiving" dramatically reduced (p. 411). They call for the development of a broader array of accessible, affordable, and innovative services and programs to support family caregivers. Guidry et al. (1998) call for insurance programs to be broadened and include diagnostic procedures and treatments which help prevent recurrence and ease survivor anxiety and pain. Insurance programs should also eliminate the barriers imposed by those who lack means to pay for adequate health insurance coverage, including groups such as minorities, the elderly, and the poor.

According to Lukemeyer et al. (2000), family-friendly workplace policies are now being advocated by family caregivers and other consumers. They suggest that employers are beginning to respond to the costs of cancer care being shifted from the public to the private sector by helping employees meet paid work and caregiving demands. Yet, the extent to which these policies offset the cost to employers of higher absenteeism and turnover rates need to be researched. Workplace policies that help employed caregivers meet work and family demands while reducing the family caregiver's cancer care burden are beneficial to employers (Lukemeyer et al. 2000).

Promotion of increased access to cancer clinical trials is another area where policy changes are needed. According to the FDA (2009), one of the most common methods to gain access to unapproved drugs in the use of cancer care is to enroll into a clinical trial. However, studies have shown that most insurance plans do not cover the cost of participation in clinical trials (Fleck 1993). Fireman et al. (2000), in their study on the cost of care for patients in clinical trials, found that "participation in cancer clinical trials at a large HMO did not result in substantial increases in the direct costs of medical care" (p. 136). More studies exploring the cost of participation in clinical trials need to be conducted.

Another policy issue relates to insurance coverage. According to Guidry et al. (1998), insurance coverage is of utmost importance to ensure access to needed medical services. However, some employers are no longer providing complete insurance coverage for their employees due to the rising cost of private insurance premiums. Consequently, for cancer caregivers, a loss in coverage could increase their financial burden. Moreover, individuals with low or no income depend on the public insurance plan of Medicaid to provide access to health care. With recent cuts in Medicaid at the national and state levels, patients and family caregivers may experience increased out-of-pocket expenses associated with cancer care. Advocates are encouraged to petition policy makers and stakeholders to support Medicaid funding for the poor and indigent at its existing rates. Other policy areas that need to be explored include psychological stress and distress, and shortened survival as a result of caring for a loved one with cancer.

Summary

Mounting evidence on the escalating cancer costs associated with family caregiving is emerging. While most research has been conducted on direct medical care costs, significant gains in examining indirect costs have been made. Current research on family caregiving confirms the significant financial burden that cancer care places on both the family and society. A more comprehensive view of the costs of cancer care is needed—one that focuses on the financial impact of cancer care on the family as well as the patient with cancer, and goes beyond medical treatment, screening, and prevention.

References

American Association of Caregiver Education (AACE). (2005). *Medicare prescription coverage*. Family caregiver alliance, caregiver information and advice, hot topics. Retrieved from http://www.caregiver.org/caregiver/jsp/content_node.jsp?nodeid=1459. Accessed 25 March 2012.

American Cancer Society (ACS). (2003). *Medical insurance and financial assistance for the cancer patient*. Retrieved from http://www.cancer.org/Search/index?q=medical+assistance+and+financial+assistance+for+the+cancer+patient+2003&all=1&x=37&y=22. Accessed 25 March 2012.

Arno, P., Levine, C., & Memmott, M. (1999). The economic value of informal caregiving. *Health Affairs, 18*(2), 182–187.

Baldwin, D. (1996). A model for describing low-income African American women's participation in breast and cervical caner early detection and screening. *Advances in Nursing Science, 19*, 27–42.

Bradley, C. J., Given, B., Given, C., & Kozachik, S. (2001). Physical, economic and social issues confronting patients and families. In C. Yarbro, M. Frogge, & M. Goodman (Eds.), *Cancer nursing: Principles and practice* (5th ed., pp. 1550–1564). Boston: Jones & Bartlett.

Brown, M. L., & Fintor, L. (1995). The economic burden of cancer. In P. Greenwald, B. S. Kramer, & D. L. Weed (Eds.), *Cancer prevention and control* (pp. 69–81). New York: Dekker.

Brown, M. L., Lipscomb, J., & Snyder, C. (2001). The burden of illness of cancer: Economic cost and quality of life. *Annual Review of Public Health, 22*, 91–113.

Brown, M. L., Riley, G. F., Schussler, N., & Etzioni, R. (2002). Estimating health care costs related to cancer treatment from SEER-Medicare data. *Medical Care, 40*(8), 104–117 (Supplement IV).

Bulsa, C., Ward, A., & Joske, D. (2004). Haematological cancer patients: Achieving a sense of empowerment by use of strategies to control illness. *Journal of Clinical Nursing, 13*, 251–258.

CancerCare. (2012). *General caregiver resources*. Retrieved from http://www.cancercare.org/search?q=general+caregiver+resource. Accessed 26 March 2012.

Cassileth, B. (1979). *The cancer patient: Social and medical aspects of care*. Philadelphia: Lea and Febiger.

Chang, S., Long, S., Kutikova, L., Bowman, L., Finely, D., Crown, W., et al. (2004). Estimating the cost of cancer: Results on the basis of claims data analyses for cancer patients diagnosed with seven types of cancer during 1999–2000. *Journal of Clinical Oncology, 22*(17), 3524–3529.

Connolly, C., & Allen, M. (2005, 9 February). Medicare drug benefit may cost $ 1.2 trillion, *Washington Post*, p. 1.

Du, W., Touchette, D., Vaitkevicius, V., Peters, W., & Shields, A. (2000). Cost analysis of pancreatic carcinoma treatment. *American Cancer Society, 89*(9), 1917–1924.

Eisenberg, J. M. (1979). Economics of cancer and its treatment. In B. Cassileth (Ed.), *The cancer patient: Social and medical aspects of care* (pp. 45–57). Philadelphia: Leas and Febiger.

Fireman, B., Quesenberry, C., Somkin, C., Jacobson, A., Baer, D., West, D., et al. (2000). Cost of care for cancer in a health maintenance organization. *Health Care Finance Review, 18*, 51–76.

Fishman, P., VonKorff, M., Lozano, P., & Hect, J. (1997). Chronic costs in managed care. *Health Affairs, 16*(3), 239–247.

Fleck, A. (1993). Cancer economics. In S. Groenwald, M. Hansen, M. Goodman, & C. Yarbro (Eds.), *Cancer nursing: Principles and practice* (3rd ed., pp. 1485–1516). Boston: Jones & Bartlett.

Freeman, H. (1989). Cancer and the economically disadvantaged. *Cancer, 64*(1 Suppl.), 324–334.

Germino, B. A., & O'Rourke, M. (1996). Cancer and the family. In R. McCorkle, M. Grant, M. Frank-Stromborg, & S. Baird (Eds.), *Cancer nursing: A comprehensive* textbook (2nd ed., pp. 81–92). Philadelphia: Saunders.

Given, B. A., & Given, C. W. (1997). Family caregiver burden from cancer care. In R. McCorkle, M. Grant, M. Frank-Stromborg, & S. Baird (Eds.), *Cancer nursing: A comprehensive textbook* (2nd ed., pp. 93–109). Philadelphia: Saunders.

Given, B. A., Given, C. W., & Stommel, M. (1994). Family and out-of-pocket costs for women with breast cancer. *Cancer Practice, 2,* 187–193.

Given, B. A., Given, C. W., & Kozzchik, S. (2001). Family support in advanced cancer. *CA: A Cancer Journal for Clinicians, 51*(4), 213–231.

Gould, J. (2002). Lower-income women with breast cancer: Interacting with cancer treatment and income security systems. *Canadian Woman Studies, 24*(1), 31–36.

Grunfeld, E., Coyle, D., Whelan, T., Clinch, J., Renyo, L., Earle, C., et al. (2004). Family caregiver burden: Results of a longitudinal study of breast cancer patients and their principal caregivers. *Canadian Medical Association Journal, 170*(12), 1811–1812.

Guidry, J. J., Aday, L., Zhang, D., & Winn, R. J. (1998). Cost considerations as potential barriers to cancer treatment. *Cancer Practice, 6*(3), 182–187.

Harper, M. S. (2000). Health policy issues and cancer in the elderly in the 21st century. In C. P. Hunter, K. A. Johnson, & H. B. Muss (Eds.), *Cancer in the elderly* (pp. 573–584). New York: Dekker.

Hayman, J., Langa, K., Kabeto, M., Katz, S., DeMonner, S., Chernew, M., et al. (2001). Estimating the cost of informal caregiving for elderly patients with cancer. *Journal of Clinical Oncology, 19*(13), 3219–3225.

Lukemeyer, A., Myers, M., & Smeeding, T. (2000). Expensive children in poor families: Out-of-pocket expenditures for the care of disabled and chronically ill children in welfare families. *Journal of Marriage and the Family, 62,* 399–415.

Moore, K. (1999). Breast cancer patients' out-of-pocket expenses. *Cancer Nursing, 22*(5), 389–396.

Mortenson, L. (1996). Understanding cancer. In R. McCorkle, M. Grant, M. Frank-Stromborg, & S. Baird (Eds.), *Cancer nursing: A comprehensive textbook* (2nd ed., pp. 1345–1355). Philadelphia: Saunders.

Muurinen, J. (1986). The economics of informal care: Labor market effects in the national hospice study. *Medical Care, 24*(11), 1007–1017.

National Cancer Institute (NCI). (2003). *Infrastructure needed for cancer research: NCI's challenge: Quality of cancer care.* Washington: National Cancer Institute. Retrieved from http://plan2003.cancer.gov/infra/quality.htm. Accessed 26 March 2012.

National Cancer Institute (NCI). (2009). Cancer trends progress report—2009 update: Costs of cancer care. Retrieved from http://progressreport.cancer.gov/doc_detail.asp?pid=1&did=2009&chid=95&coid=926&mid=25k. Accessed 26 March 2012.

Navaie-Waliser, M., Feldman, P., Gould, D., Levine, C., Kuerbis, A., & Donelan, K. (2002). When the caregiver needs care: The plight of vulnerable caregivers. *American Journal of Public Health, 92*(3), 409–413.

O'Mara, A. (2005). Who's taking care of the caregiver? *Journal of Clinical Oncology, 23*(28), 1–2.

Payne, D., Hoffman, G., Theodoulou, M., Dosik, M., & Massie, M. (1999). Screening for anxiety and depression in women with breast cancer. *Psychosomatics, 40,* 64–69.

Pasacreta, J. V., Barg, F., Nuamah, I., & McCorkle, R. (2000). Participant characteristics before and 4 months after attendance at a family caregiver cancer education program. *Cancer Nursing, 23*(4), 295–303.

Phillips, J. M., Cohen, M. Z., & Moses, G. (1999). Breast cancer screening and African American women: Fear, fatalism and silence. *Oncology Nursing Forum, 22,* 1383–1391.

Rabow, M., Hauser, J., & Adams, J. (2004). Supporting family caregivers at the end of life. *Journal of the American Medical Association, 291*(4), 483–492.

Reed, M. C., & Hargraves, J. L. (2003). *Prescription drug access disparities among working-age Americans* (Issues Brief No. 73). Washington: Center for Studying Health System Change. Retrieved from http://www.hschange.com/CONTENT/637/. Accessed 26 March 2012.

Rutledge, V., & Stair, J. (1997). Impact of changing health care economics on cancer nursing practice. In S. Groenwald, M. Frogge, M. Goodman, & C. Yarbro (Eds.), *Cancer nursing: Principles and practice* (4th ed., pp. 1589–1607). Boston: Jones and Bartlett.

Schulmeister, L. K. (1999). Cultural issues in cancer care. In C. Miaskowski & P. Buchsel (Eds.), *Oncology nursing: Assessment and clinical care* (pp. 383–399). St. Louis: Mosby.

Sherman, E., Pfister, D., Ruchlin, H., Rubin, D., Radzyner, M., Kelleher, G., et al. (2001). The collection of indirect and nonmedical direct costs (COIN) form. *Cancer, 91*(4), 841–851.

Stommel, M., Given, C., & Given, B. A. (1993). The cost of cancer home care to families. *Cancer, 71*(5), 1867–1874.

Tamblyn, R., Laprise, R., Hanley, J., Abrahamowicz, M., Scott, S., Mayo, N., et al. (2001). Adverse events associated with prescription drug cost-sharing among poor and elderly persons. *Journal of the American Medical Association, 285*(4), 421–429.

U.S. Food and Drug Administration (FDA). (2009). *FDA center for drug evaluation and research: Access to unapproved drugs.* Retrieved from http://www.fda.gov/AboutFDA/Transparency/Basics/ucm194958.htm-13k-2009-12-23. Accessed 26 March 2012.

Vanderwerker, L. C., Laff, R. E., Kadan-lottick, N. S., McColl, S., & Prigerson, H. (2005). Psychiatric disorders and mental health service use among caregivers of advanced cancer patients. *Journal of Clinical Oncology, 23*(28), 6899–6907.

Wein, S. (2000). The family in terminal illness. In L. Baider, C. L. Cooper, & K. De-Nour (Eds.), *Cancer and the family* (pp. 427–441). New York: Wiley.

Wittes, R. (2004, 15 June). Cancer weapons out of reach. *The Washington Post*, p. A23.

Chapter 13
Legal Issues in Cancer Caregiving

Marilyn Frank-Stromborg and Kenneth R. Burns

The importance of looking at the legal issues of being a caregiver of a cancer patient is underscored by the number of people diagnosed with cancer and the number of individuals who serve as caregivers. A total of 1,399,790 new cancer cases and 564,830 deaths from cancer are expected in the United States in 2006 (Jemal et al. 2006).

> Cancer patients used to spend long periods of time in the hospital, but they are much less likely to do so now. So, that person and whoever is the significant caregiver are often called upon to manage complex treatment, understand what is going on in terms of side effects, and incorporate this diagnosis and treatment into their everyday lives. (*Caregiving Challenges* 2006, p. 1)

There are 52 million informal or family caregivers who provide care to someone aged 20 years or older who is ill or disabled (Family Caregiver Alliance 2005), and 8% report providing care to someone with cancer (Northouse 2005).

Current Status of Legal Issues in Caregiving

One of the first legal issues encountered in any discussion of family caregivers is whether or not a legally enforceable obligation exists to provide caregiving assistance to the individual. A nonfamily member would have no obligation to provide care unless they agreed to be a caregiver. This is especially true when active family involvement is essential to the implementation of the individual's desired care plan, for instance, when the individual prefers to remain in her/his own home rather than entering a nursing home. While it might be argued that there is a moral duty to care for one's family, no law compels family members to personally provide direct,

M. Frank-Stromborg (✉)
DeKalb County Courthouse, 133 West State Street, Sycamore, IL 60178, USA
e-mail: mstromborg@dekalbcounty.org

K. R. Burns
Division of Nursing, Martin Methodist College, 433 West Madison Street, Pulaski, TN 38478, USA
e-mail: kburns@martinmethodist.edu

R. C. Talley et al. (eds.), *Cancer Caregiving in the United States,*
Caregiving: Research, Practice, Policy,
DOI 10.1007/978-1-4614-3154-1_13, © Springer Science+Business Media, LLC 2012

hands-on care to dependent relatives (Kapp 2003). The same is true for the situation in which a family insists on participating in the caregiving for an ill relative who objects to such care. "Families have neither a duty nor a right to be involved, as long as the individual who objects to the family providing direct services to them is capable of making and expressing their own autonomous decision" (Kapp 2003, p. 50). However, once a family member enters into the role of caregiver, every state has a statute that makes it illegal for the caregiver to willfully ignore the basic needs of, or otherwise through acts or omissions, endanger the dependent person. The basis of these statues resides in elder abuse. In the overwhelming majority of states, when health and human-service professionals suspect cases of abuse or neglect, they have a legal obligation to report their suspicions to local Adult Protective Services agencies (Kapp 1995). In the remaining states, health and human-service professionals have immunity against any liability if it is a good faith report.

Kapp (2003) addresses the issue of whether or not the caregiver needs a professional license to take care of the family member. If there is a willing family member, it is commonplace for home health agencies, hospital, and nursing facility discharge planners to train the willing family member in how to care for the cancer patient (e.g., change dressings, suction tubes, administer medications). While no state empowers family caregivers to administer medications and other medical treatments, no state expressly prohibits their administering medications and treatments when caring for a family member. The reality is that throughout this country, caregivers are delivering every conceivable type of physical care to family members hundreds of times a day without any reported criminal prosecutions for practicing nursing without a license (Kapp 2003).

While there is not a duty to provide physical care for a parent, there are family or filial responsibility statutes in 26 states. These statutes impose a duty on adult children, if they are able, to provide financial assistance to indigent parents (Jacobson 1995; Lee 1995). For example, in the *Americana Healthcare Center v. Randall* (1995), the South Dakota Supreme Court held that an adult child with financial ability is liable for the support of an indigent parent. The court also upheld the constitutionality of a statute requiring such support (Jacobson 1995). Filial responsibility laws are rarely enforced, and when they are, the enforcement has sometimes led to the law's repeal (Lee 1995).

The statute in Illinois defining a caregiver is typical of that found throughout the country in state statutes on this subject. The applicable statute in Illinois (IL St Ch 320 § 65/15, 1993) defines a caregiver as an adult family member, or another individual, who is an informal provider (not compensated for the care he or she provides) of in-home and community care to an older individual, or a grandparent or older individual who is a relative caregiver.

In general, the following facts are known about caregivers: (a) More than one-third of caregivers spend a minimum of 40 hours per week providing care to the family member; (b) Almost half (44%) of caregivers are male (*Did you know?* 2005); (c) The majority of caregivers are middle-aged (35–64 years old; Family Caregiver Alliance 2005); and (d) Most caregivers are employed (Bond et al. 1998). Research has documented that psychological health appears to be the aspect of the family caregiver's life that is most affected by providing care, with depression the most common mental health alteration (Given et al. 2004; Schulz et al. 1995).

Research has documented the differences in caregivers of patients with cancer. Comparison between caregivers providing care for patients with cancer versus those without cancer showed that "a greater percentage of cancer caregivers reported taking time off from work, having less time to socialize with family and friends, and wanting help managing stress than non-cancer caregivers" (Northouse 2005, p. 2). Cancer caregivers also are more likely to provide care in situations with higher levels of burden. In one study, more than half of cancer caregivers (56%) provide care at the two highest levels of burden in contrast to less than one-third of noncancer caregivers (31%; Northouse 2005).

Caregiving of cancer patients presents considerable challenges: physical, emotional, economic, and legal. The nature and extent of home care have changed markedly over the past decade. Technological advancements permit sophisticated services that previously were limited to use within health care institutions, however, can be rendered today with the usually preferred location of the patient's own home. Virtually every diagnostic and treatment modality that can be made portable can be provided in the home (Kapp 1995). Because of the multiple issues and challenges (e.g., physical, emotional, economic, and legal) involved with caregiving for cancer patients, the legal issues encountered by caregivers can seem confusing and complicated. This is especially true if the care recipient is impaired or facing end-of-life issues. Four major legal issues faced by caregivers include: (1) caregiver employment issues, (2) care recipient health insurance, (3) legal issues encountered by the caregiver when planning for the incapacity of the care recipient, and (4) legal issues surrounding advance directives.

Employment

Caregiving itself can have financial consequences for the caregiver. One study found that caregivers lose an average US$ 659,130 over their lifetimes as result of reductions in their salaries and retirement benefits (National Alliance for Caregiving 2005). Six in ten employed caregivers reported that caregiving forced them to make changes at work, such as going in late, leaving early, taking time off, or leaving their jobs altogether (National Alliance for Caregiving 2005).

Caregivers need to be made aware of the 1993 Federal Family and Medical Leave Act (FMLA; 29 U.S.C. 2654). The FMLA entitles most workers to unpaid leaves of absence for up to 3 months to care for a family member. Unfortunately, because it is an unpaid leave, more than three in four employees need but do not take family and medical leave because they cannot afford the loss of income (National Center on Women & Aging at Brandeis University & the National Alliance for Caregiving 1999). Caregivers are entitled to take a total of 12 weeks of unpaid leave during any 12-month period to provide care to an immediate family member (spouse, child, or parent) with a serious health condition, including cancer. To be eligible for FMLA, the employee must have been employed for at least 12 months, worked at least 1,250 hours during the 12 months immediately preceding the requested leave, and either works in the home office of the employer or at a satellite office that has 50 or more employees and is located within 75 miles of the home office (Gelak 2005). Caregivers have the right to return to their job or an equivalent job. An equivalent job is defined as one with the same pay, benefits, and responsibilities (National Partnership for Women & Families 2005). More than 35 million Americans have taken leave under this law since it was passed in 1993 (U.S. Department of Labor 2000). The problem with a nonpaid leave from work is that some cancer diagnoses span a lengthy period of time of alternating remissions and physical crises as well as coexist with diseases which require the caregiver to have multiple employment absences.

Depending on where the caregivers live, they could be afforded more help under state laws. Only one state, California, has created a comprehensive paid family and medical leave insurance program in the nation. Through the California paid family leave insurance program most employees, over 13 million, can receive 55–60% of their salary up to a cap of US$ 728 per week for up to 6 weeks of leave per year to care for a seriously ill family member or a new baby (Bell and Newman 2003). The program is funded by the employees themselves, at an estimated cost of US$ 27 per worker per year. While California has an explicit paid *family leave law*, other states have enacted provisions that provide at least some assistance to working caregivers.

There are at least 26 states that have regulations or laws that permit caregivers, if they are public employees, to use their sick leave to provide care for certain sick family members. These states include: Arizona, California, Colorado, Connecticut, Florida, Hawaii, Idaho, Indiana, Iowa, Kansas, Kentucky, Maryland, Minnesota, Montana, Nebraska, Nevada, New Hampshire, North Carolina, North Dakota, Oklahoma, South Carolina, South Dakota, Tennessee, Texas, Utah, and Washington. In five states, private employers are required to allow caregivers to use their sick leave to care for certain sick family members. These states include: California, Connecticut, Hawaii, Minnesota, and Washington (Bell and Newman 2003).

In addition to federal and state laws, caregivers have other avenues to explore that may help provide paid time off, partial paid time off, or a guarantee that their job or an equivalent will be available when they return to work. Caregivers need to investigate their employer's company policies, know their state's laws pertaining to caregiving leaves and schedule a meeting with their employer's human resource representative to request an extended leave.

Considering the success of the FMLA, it is recommended that the federal government takes steps to make FMLA a more viable option for families who cannot afford to take the leave as it currently stands. Enacting a federal paid family leave bill is not a politically viable option at this time with a nation coping with a war, the aftermath of Hurricane Katrina, and a growing budget deficit. The climate simply does not support a broad federal initiative; rather it is recommended that incremental steps be taken, such as: (1) commissioning a Department of Labor report on the cost implications of various workplace-friendly programs, including California's paid family leave bill and (2) creating a tax credit for companies which voluntarily provide some measure of paid family leave, or create greater flexibility in the workplace for employee caregivers (Bell and Newman 2003).

With a significantly increasing aged population, the need to develop a more viable option for families who cannot afford to take a nonpaid leave of absence from work is becoming more urgent. Managed care and state and federal health benefits have shortened hospital stays. Shortened stays have resulted in more families spending a greater amount of time providing intensive, ongoing care to a family member with cancer. Unfortunately, the pool of family caregivers will dwindle in the coming years. By 2050, the ratio of caregivers to each person needing care will be 4 to 1 compared to 11 to 1 in 1990 (Institute for Health and Aging as cited in National Family Caregivers Association 2003).

The time required and the amount of care the family member needs may be so significant that the person providing the care and services must take considerable time off work or find it necessary to stop working. The time frame for such extensive care may last from a few weeks to several years (Warren et al. 2004). Based on the negative financial impact on family caregivers, arguments have been put forth regarding the need to pay caregivers as one method of addressing the issue of nonpaid leaves of absence. However, the practice of paying relatives as caregivers remains controversial. A research study conducted in Arkansas found that family members who hired family versus nonfamily workers received more service and had equal or superior satisfaction and health outcomes as compared to those who hired nonrelatives (Simon-Rusinowitz et al. 2005). Several countries do have policies for caregiver payment. Australia, Norway, Sweden, and the United Kingdom are examples of countries that offer a care wage to caregivers of severely disabled and elderly persons (White and Keefe 2005).

Reimbursement for Caregiver Services

If a family caregiver is not paid while he or she is delivering care, can they recover payment from the estate once the sick family member dies? Unfortunately, after the death of the family member, it is common for such a care provider to face obstacles when attempting to recover from the estate. Other relatives may refuse to allow compensation, and the care provider may be forced to litigate his or her claim against the estate. "Many states have an evidentiary rebuttable presumption that services rendered to a family member are gratuitous in nature, so the caregiver cannot recover. However, in states with such a presumption, these are not always hard and fast rules" (Simon-Rusinowitz et al. 2005, p. 96). It should be noted that the presumption of gratuity is applied only in the absence of a contract between the parties, which can be either an express contract, a written contract between the two parties, or an implied contract made through statements or impressions imparted by the care recipient to the caregiver that he or she will be rewarded from the estate for their caregiving services. The courts will take into account multiple factors in deciding whether to award payment for caregiving services upon the death of the family member. Evidence provided by the caregiver for payment must demonstrate that the expectation of payment was reasonable, given the extraordinary nature of the services provided and the nature of the relationship of the parties.

Health Insurance and Disability Benefits

Nearly one in every four Americans is enrolled in Medicare or Medicaid. These programs provide health care for the aged, disabled, and indigent populations and are administered by the Centers for Medicare and Medicaid Services (CMS; formerly HCFA, the Health Care Financing Administration). Medicare is the federal health insurance program for people aged 65 or older. It also covers certain younger people with disabilities and people with End-Stage Renal Disease. Medicaid is a joint federal and state program that helps with medical costs for some people with limited income and resources. Coverage varies from state to state, and a person may be covered by both Medicaid and Medicare.

Medicare covers hospitalization, skilled nursing, home health and hospice care, however, requires certain deductibles, premiums and copayments. For patients receiving outpatient care, Medicare will cover 80% of *allowable* outpatient medical services after a US$ 100 deductible. The patient is responsible for 20% of the charge, regardless of the cost. If the health care provider or supplier accepts "assignment" the patient does not have to pay anything since "assignment" is an agreement between Medicare and the health care providers to accept the Medicare-approved amount as payment in full. On January 1, 2006, Medicare began offering a new program of prescription drug coverage. This new coverage can provide help with drug costs, no matter how the person pays for drugs today, and everyone with Medicare can join a drug plan to get this coverage. The Medicare prescription drug coverage is insurance, in that insurance companies and other private companies approved by Medicare provide the coverage. The patient chooses a drug plan and pays a monthly premium (*Medicare Basics* 2005). To date, significant problems with this program have been reported in the very low-income Medicare beneficiaries who also qualify for Medicaid.

Out of approximately 7.2 million low-income seniors who are eligible for the low-income subsidies that were designed to help make medicines affordable, only about 1.7 million, or 24%, are actually receiving those subsidies. The poorest of the poor—those very low-income Medicare beneficiaries who also qualify for Medicaid—have worse drug coverage today than they had before the new Medicare Part D program began in January. These so-called "dual eligibles," approximately 6.3 million needy seniors, had good drug coverage through Medicaid before Part D began. This group now has drug coverage through private Medicare plans that, in several respects, is not as good as the Medicaid coverage they used to have (Steinberg 2006).

Medicare also offers home health care benefits if the patient meets four conditions: (1) the attending physician must identify and prescribe the need for in-home medical care; (2) the patient must need intermittent skilled nursing care, physical therapy, speech or occupational therapy; (3) the patient must be homebound; and (4) the home health agency providing care must be approved by the Medicare Program. The skilled nursing care must be at a level requiring a registered nurse or licensed practical nurse to provide the essential care. Medicare does not pay for full-time personal care, 24-hour/day care at home, and homemaker services such as shopping and cleaning. In addition, home meal delivery is not covered.

There are multiple issues associated with Medicare, including problems with accessing the health care system and physician specialists (Trude and Ginsburg 2002). In one community survey, the percentage of Medicare seniors reporting delays in or not receiving needed care rose from 9.1% in 1997 to 11.0% in 2001. In addition, Medicare seniors and older privately insured people are also waiting longer for appointments with their physicians. By 2001, more than a third of Medicare seniors waited more than 3 weeks for a checkup and a similar percentage waited a week or more for an appointment for a specific illness (Trude and Ginsburg 2002). At the same time, the proportion of physicians accepting all new Medicare patients fell from 74.6% in 1997 to 71.1% in 2001. These health care access problems are the result of the changes in Medicare payments for specialist physicians made in the Balanced Budget Act of 1997.

In general, Medicare needs to be revised to reflect the fact that people no longer die within a few years after reaching the age of 62 or 65. Increasingly, life expectancy may be to the mid-1980s. There are several major problems with Medicare, including inadequate program funding, program rigidity, and the impact it has had on accessibility to health care for the elderly. In addition, the current Medicare system attempts to place all seniors into a centrally planned system. As the senior population becomes more diverse and medical care changes and advances, the more outdated and unfair this system becomes to seniors (Beckner 2003). The financial stability of Medicare is another significant issue. As the baby boom population begins to reach Medicare-eligible age in 2010, the costs to both Part A and Part B will begin to sky-rocket and force Congress to attempt to impose cost controls on a system already beginning to deliver inadequate care to a diverse senior population (Beckner 2003). The Trustees of the Federal Hospital Insurance (HI) and the Supplementary Medical Insurance Trust Funds (SMI) report annually to Congress on these trust funds' short- and long-term financial health. The 2005 report estimates that Medicare will remain solvent until 2020. Policy reforms that enable Medicare to continue, albeit with different rules on eligibility and coverage, are urgently required.

Caregivers frequently want to know how the care recipient may qualify for Medicaid coverage for nursing home services or home- and community-based long-term-care services. Medicaid is embodied in 42 U.S.C. § 1396 et seq. (http://www.law.cornell.edu/uscode/42/ch7schXIX.html). Medicaid was first enacted in 1965 as an amendment to the Social Security Act of 1935. Medicaid pays health care providers for rendering specified health-related services to specified groups of people who satisfy a financial means test. If seniors and disabled people have incomes and assets low enough to qualify them for the federal Supplemental Security Income (SSI) cash assistance program, they most likely qualify for Medicaid benefits (Kapp 2003).

Many states allow people to become eligible under a "medically needy" category if they "spend down" their income and assets on care. Since its inception, the program has been plagued by fraud from both health care providers and patients. To curb these abuses, Congress passed a law in 1996 making persons criminally liable for committing fraud in order to become eligible for medical assistance.

When the Health Insurance Portability and Accountability Act (HIPAA) of 1996 (Public Law No. 104–191), came into effect, it exposed to criminal punishment for fraud and abuse anyone who "knowingly and willfully disposes of assets (including by any transfer in trust) in order for an individual to become eligible for medical assistance under Medicaid, if disposing of the assets results in the imposition of a period of ineligibility for such assistance." President Bush signed a law making it more difficult to give away assets and then qualify for nursing home care under Medicaid. Previously, if applicants transferred assets within 3 years of applying for Medicaid long-term care, they faced a delay in becoming eligible. The new law lengthens the period for most asset transfers to 5 years. It also states you may not qualify for Medicaid if you have home equity of more than US\$ 500,000. These measures were instituted because Medicaid is a very costly program. In addition, the goal of the new legislation is cost containment as well as preserving the original purpose of Medicaid to help the truly needy or poor (Miller 2006). These recent laws have significant implications for caregivers, especially in terms of caregiver burden, as they may result in the patient not being able to qualify for Medicaid nursing home services, home- and community-based long-term-care services. All of these services are frequently needed when people have a cancer diagnosis. Another change of which caregivers should be aware concerns the requirement that care recipients provide satisfactory documentary evidence of citizenship or nationality when initially applying for Medicaid or upon a recipient's first Medicaid redetermination. The requirement to provide proof of citizenship to be eligible for Medicaid was instituted on July 1, 2006 (Public Law No. 109–171, Deficit Reduction Act of 2005, Section 6036; CMS 2006).

While many laws may have a daunting impact on recipients as well as caregivers, several recent laws promise to increase funding for support services for family caregivers and for stimulating state innovations in long-term care. The key development is the enactment of the National Family Caregiver Support Program (NFCSP) in 2000, an amendment of the Older Americans Act (OAA; Fox-Grage et al. 2001). This bill was codified as Title III-E of the OAA. The NFCSP signifies national recognition of and commitment to providing direct support services to caregivers. It is the first major nationwide program initiative under the Older Americans Act since the 1970s. Under broad federal guidelines, the NFCSP calls for states, working in partnership with area agencies on aging and local service providers, to develop multifaceted systems of support for family and informal caregivers within five basic categories by offering: (1) information to caregivers about available services; (2) assistance to caregivers in gaining access to available services; (3) individual counseling and training to help caregivers in making decisions; (4) respite care to temporarily relieve caregivers; and 5) supplemental services, on a limited basis, to complement the care given by caregivers (Feinberg et al. 2004). The importance of the support offered by the NFCSP is underscored by the research on the cost of caregiving for the terminally ill by Aoun et al. (2005). Aoun et al. report that caregivers providing support to individuals receiving palliative care identified unmet needs for information, communication, service provision, and support from health and community services.

Under the NFCSP, states use federal funds to offer direct support services to family caregivers of persons aged 60 and older. All income groups are eligible for services. However, states must give priority to those providing care to older individuals in the greatest social or economic need with particular attention to low-income individuals (Feinberg et al. 2004). While the NFCSP is emerging both as a key program to enhance the scope of services available to caregivers and as fuel for innovation in this area, it is inadequately funded. The level of funding to states in 2003 was US$ 138.7 million, which left gaps in caregiver support services and varied substantially from state to state.

Feinberg et al. (2004) conducted a 50-state study on caregiver support with the passage of NFCSP. They made five recommendations for achieving a better caregiver support system across the United States. The five recommendations include: (1) raise the funding level of NFCSP to reduce gaps in caregiver support; (2) improve data collection and reporting under the NFCSP; (3) conduct a national public awareness campaign on family caregiving; (4) invest in innovation and promising practices; and (5) strengthen and expand uniform assessment of caregiver needs in all Medicaid home- and community-based services programs that provide some component of caregiver support.

Planning for Incapacity

Caregivers should begin making legal preparations when the family member has been diagnosed with cancer. Cancer creates strain on the family's physical, psychological, and financial resources. People with cancer may have the capacity to manage their own legal and financial affairs when diagnosed, however, as the disease advances, they will need to rely on others to act in their best interests. The transition may occur rapidly or gradually over a long period of time. However, no matter how rapid or prolonged, this transition is never easy. Advance planning allows people with a long-term disease and their families to make decisions together for future events.

The legal issues that must be considered when a person is (or may become) incapacitated include: (a) management of the person's financial affairs during his lifetime; (b) the management of the person's personal care such as medical decisions, residence, and placement in a nursing facility; (c) arranging for payment of long-term health care; (d) preserving the family assets; and (e) the distribution of the person's assets on his or her death.

Financial and Health Care Management Issues

Health care information is considered confidential, and there has always been reluctance on the part of health care providers to share private information with family unless directed to do so by the patient. Complicating confidentiality issues is the set of federal regulations (45 Code of Federal Regulations Parts 160 and 164) that became effective on April 14, 2003, to implement the medical privacy provisions of Health Insurance Portability and Accountability Act (HIPAA). These health care privacy laws require written documentation that the health care provider is authorized to discuss a family member's care with the caregiver. These regulations impose significant restrictions and documentation requirements on health care providers, among others, regarding the release of identifiable medical information to persons other than the patient. Therefore, it is essential that as soon as possible after a diagnosis of cancer is confirmed that the caregiver secures the necessary paperwork to have access to health care information about their family member (Kapp 2003).

How can a family make financial/legal decisions on behalf of the cancer patient? A Durable Power of Attorney (DPA) for Property is a document that allows the cancer patient to give authority to another person to make financial/legal decisions and financial transactions on their behalf. It is called "durable" when, by its terms, it remains effective even if the principle becomes mentally incompetent (Sabatino 2001). The powers given to the attorney-in-fact can be as limited or as broad as the patient wants, and can include the power to buy property, to invest, to contract, to engage in tax planning, to make gifts, and to plan for government benefits such as Supplemental Security Income. A DPA usually becomes effective as of the day it is signed and executed. However, a "springing" DPA becomes effective at a later date when the patient becomes mentally incompetent. It "springs" into effect at the point the patient is certified by a physician as having lost capacity.

If decisions have not been made regarding durable or springing power of attorney prior to the cancer patient becoming incapacitated, the Court can appoint an individual or professional to act on the care recipient's behalf. The terms used for these protective proceedings vary by state, however, in general are called: (a) a "guardianship" in which control is given over the incapacitated person's financial affairs and (b) a "conservatorship" to describe a proceeding giving control over the person's personal affairs (Prensky 2004). Family members and interested parties may petition the court to become either a guardian or conservator.

Most states have three documents that help ensure that even if patients cannot speak for themselves, they will get only the care they desire when gravely ill. These documents are a living will, a Durable Power of Attorney for Health Care (DPAHC), and a do-not-resuscitate order. The first two are legal documents that are administered according to a state's laws; the third is a medical directive, like a prescription order, that is filed with the patient's medical chart (AARP 2006). The DPAHC is an advance directive that allows the patient to appoint a health care "agent" or "proxy" to make health care decisions in the event that they can no longer speak for themselves. Every state recognizes a DPAHC, however, laws governing directives vary from state to state. While state laws may vary, the powers the patient gives to the caregiver usually include: (a) the right to select or discharge care providers and institutions; (b) the right to refuse or consent to treatment; (c) the right to access medical records; (d) the right to withdraw or withhold life-sustaining treatment; and (e) the power to make anatomical gifts (Sabatino 2001). A DPAHC is executed when it is signed by the patient, witness, or notary public verifying that the patient is competent and acting under his or her own volition.

Though the name of living wills varies by state, this document, also known as a declaration, instruction directive, or wishes for terminal illness, outlines the type of treatment the patient would or would not like in the event that they have been given a terminal diagnosis or are in a terminally unconscious state (Villet-Lagomarsino 2000). Most living wills direct that only "life-sustaining" or "life-prolonging" treatments should be withdrawn. These are generally defined as treatments used to artificially prolong the dying process but which will not ultimately prevent someone from dying. Most states accept the validity of living wills, and some states impose penalties on health care providers who do not comply with the patient's instructions. Some states have living will statutes that provide protections for life insurance benefits that might otherwise be jeopardized. The patient's rights to advance medical directives are protected by the Federal Patient Self-Determination Act. This federal law requires all health care agencies and managed care plans to give their patients covered by Medicare or Medicaid information about advanced directives. Before the document can become active, though, most states require that two doctors record a terminal diagnosis on the individual's medical records.

Since end-stage cancer patients will generally not benefit from cardiopulmonary resuscitation (CPR), it is not unusual for the patient to fill out a Do-Not-Resuscitate Order (DNR). The DNR is placed directly into the patient's medical file or chart so that medical staff will be on notice not to attempt CPR. The DNR should be filed with every physician and care institution that the patient will use, as it is not transferable between institutions.

There are special issues that arise when the caregiver is in a lesbian, gay, bisexual, or transgender (LGBT) committed relationship, typically referred to as same-sex relationships or domestic partnerships. Without legal protections in place, these relationships might not be legally recognized and could be questioned or contested by a biological family member. When the LGBT caregiver and care recipient first learn of the cancer diagnosis, there should be discussion of the possible financial and legal decisions that need to be made in the event of incapacity, and the couple should investigate local and state laws related to LGBT relationships. Currently, some states have laws granting legal rights to same-sex couples and define these relationships as marriages, civil unions, domestic partnerships, or reciprocal beneficiaries (Wenzel 2005). These states are California, Connecticut, Hawaii, Maine, Massachusetts, New Jersey, Vermont, and Washington (Human Rights Campaign 2006). California's Domestic Partnership Law (AB205) went into effect on January 1, 2005 but does not affect federal benefits (such as Social Security survival benefits), because the federal government currently does not recognize domestic partnerships (Wenzel 2005).

When cancer has been diagnosed in one of the partners, the LGBT caregiver should do estate planning either with a Will or a Living Trust, a Durable Power of Attorney for Finances and Property and for Health Care. The LGBT persons receiving and giving care may also want to consider a Revocable Trust, which provides for an orderly distribution to beneficiaries of a person's assets upon death. A trust also has incapacity language in it, which may become effective before death. The Durable Power of Attorney for Property/Finances and the Durable Power of Attorney for Health Care functions for LGBT persons in the same manner it does for other people. The Durable Power of Attorney for Health Care is known in California as an Advance Health Care Directive and ensures that all health care needs and desires of the LGBT person are carried out and monitored by a trusted person when the principal can no longer make or communicate health care decisions.

Proactive Planning by Care Recipients and Care Providers

Caregivers form the foundation of ever-expanding home-based long-term care for individuals experiencing altering life illnesses or disabilities that interfere with their ability to perform activities of daily living. Both caregivers and care recipients need to collaboratively work through multiple issues to ensure a satisfying experience. While potential filial caregivers may feel obligated to provide care to a family member, it is important to first consider the financial impact of accepting such responsibility as the level of care may require the arrangement of unpaid leaves of absences. Another consideration is to determine the ramifications that an unpaid leave or cessation of work to provide full-time care will have on maintaining personal health insurance. While it may be difficult, discussions concerning reimbursement and reaching a form of agreement for caregiver services can avoid costly legal expenses as well as long-term family disagreements and dissention.

Caregivers of cancer patients need to be aware of the stress associated with care-giving, potential social isolation, time commitment, potential for alterations in their own physical and emotional health, and the high level of burden that is associated with the role of caregiver. Therefore, it is important to be proactive to insure "time-off" from caregiving responsibilities, as well as time to take care of personal needs such as clinic visits, financial/banking, and other family responsibilities. Such arrangements can be made during discussions with family members, through exploring what is available through state and federal programs, by examining the care recipient's health, disability, and long-term care insurance policies for respite care, as well as seeking assistance in caring for the individual.

To assure that the plan of care is followed and both the care recipient and care-giver have a satisfying experience, care recipients should ensure that the caregiver has access to his or her health care information. The caregiver should be enabled to discuss the treatment plan with the physician or other health care staff members to guarantee an understanding and accurate implementation of the plan. The care recipient needs to sign the appropriate release forms for all clinics, outpatient services, and hospitals. These forms should be placed in the patient's chart within each service delivery agency. Care recipients should establish with their caregivers that access to this information obligates them to maintain confidentiality unless expressly granted permission to disclose. Early on, it is beneficial for care recipients to plan for incapacity by establishing Durable Power of Attorney for Health Care (DPAHC), Finances and Property (DPAFP), and a Living Will, as well as their decision regarding resuscitation. Not all familial caregivers are named as holding DPA. Early identification of the individual or individuals holding the DPA provides the caregiver with the necessary information to assure that the care recipient's instructions and desires are fulfilled, assets are protected, and the financial obligations are discharged.

While the role of caregiver may seem overwhelming, federal and state statutes and regulations are changing to alleviate this based on: (a) the increasing number of individuals desiring to remain in the comfort of their homes versus admission to long-term care facilities; (b) shortened hospital stays; and (c) the recognition of the challenges and burdens experienced by caregivers, as well as the lack of information and services available to them. In addition, as ongoing research continues to demonstrate the positive outcomes of homecare and the challenges, barriers and economic burdens experienced in attempting to fulfill the role of caregiver, more attention will be given to changing laws at the federal and state levels to lessen family economic burdens and to assure ready access to information and resources essential to this role.

References

American Association for Retired Persons (AARP). (2006). Legal tips and resources legal glossary. Retrieved from http://www.aarp.org/families/legal_issues/tips_resources/a20040324-li_legalglossary.html?print=yes.

Jacobson, R. M. (1995). Americana Healthcare Center v. Randall: the renaissance of filial responsibility. 40 S.D.L. Rev. 518.

Aoun, S., Kristjanson, L. J., Currow, D. C., & Hudson, P. L. (2005). Caregiving for the terminally ill: At what cost? *Palliative Medicine, 19,* 551–555.

Beckner, P. (2003). Medicare's two fundamental problems. Letter to Congressional leaders on Medicare reform. FreedomWorks. Citizens for a Sound Economy. Retrieved from http://www.freedomworks.org/informed/issues_template.php?issue_id=1486.

Bell, L., & Newman, S. (2003). *Paid family and medical leave: Why we need it, how we can get it.* San Francisco: Family Caregiver Alliance, National Center on Caregiving.

Bond, J. T., Galinsky, E., & Swanberg, J. E. (1998). *The 1997 national study of the changing workforce.* New York: Families and Work Institute.

Caregiving challenges. (2006). Retrieved from http://www.cancerandcareers.org/coworkers/what-to-say(2012)/.

Centers for Medicare & Medicaid Services (CMS). (2006). Proof of citizenship. Retrieved from http://www.cms.hhs.gov/MedicaidEligibility/05_ProofofCitizenship.asp.

Did you know? (2005). Retrieved from www.caregivers4cancer.com/articles.html(2012).

Family Caregiver Alliance. (2005). *Selected caregiver statistics.* San Francisco: Family Caregiver Alliance. Retrieved from http://www.caregiver.org/caregiver/jsp/publications.jsp?nodeid=345.

Feinberg, L. F., Newman, S. L., Gray, L., & Kolb, K. N. (2004). *The state of the states in family caregiver support: A 50-state study*. San Francisco: Family Caregiver Alliance.

Fox-Grage, W., Coleman, B., & Blancato, R. (2001). *Federal and state policy in family caregiving: Recent victories but uncertain future* (Policy Brief No. 2). San Francisco: Family Caregiver Alliance.

Gelak, D. (2005). How FMLA and other laws apply to caregivers. National partnership for women & families. Retrieved from www.nationalpartnership.org.

Given, B., Wyatt, G., Given, C., Sherwood, P., Gift, A., DeVoss, D., et al. (2004). Burden and depression among caregivers of patients with cancer at the end of life. *Oncology Nursing Forum, 31*(6), 1105–1117.

Human Rights Campaign. (2006). *Relationship recognition in the U.S.* Washington: Human Rights Campaign. Retrieved from www.hrc.org.

Jacobson, R. M. (1995). American Healthcare Center v. Randall: The renaissance of filial responsibility. *South Dakota Law Review, 40*(3), 518–545.

Jemal, A., Siegel, R., Ward, E., Murray, T., Xu, J., Smigal, C., et al. (2006). Cancer statistics, 2006. *CA: A Cancer Journal for Clinicians, 56,* 106–130.

Kapp, M. B. (1995). Family caregiving for older persons in the home: Medical-legal implications. *Journal of Legal Medicine, 16*(1), 1–31.

Kapp, M. B. (2003). Family caregivers' legal concerns. *Generations, 27*(4), 49–55.

Lee, A. (1995). Singapore's maintenance of Parents Act and U.S. filial responsibility laws. *Loyola: International & Comparative Law Journal, 17*(3), 671–699.

Medicare basics: A guide for families and friends of people with Medicare. (2005). Washington: Center for Medicare and Medicaid Services. Retrieved from http://www.medicare.gov/Publications/Pubs/pdf/11034.pdf(2012).

Miller, A. (2006, March 12). Medicaid will go after assets; Homes may be sold to reimburse the state. *The Atlanta Journal-Constitution*. Retrieved from http://www.alanpowell.net/?go=viewnews&newsid=1639.

National Alliance for Caregiving. (2005). *Care for the family caregiver: A place to start*. San Francisco: Family Caregiver Alliance, National Center for Caregiving. Retrieved from www.caregiving.org.

National Center on Women & Aging at Brandeis University & the National Alliance for Caregiving. (1999). The Metlife juggling act study: Balancing caregiving with work and the costs involved. Retrieved from http://www.metlife.com/WPSAssets/28510693001172586490V1FJugglingStudy2007.pdf (For a copy of the study, contact the MetLife Mature Market Institute, MMI_Metlife@metlife.com).

National Family Caregivers Association (NFCA). (2003). *Family caregiver statistics*. Kensington: National Family Caregivers Association. Retrieved from www.nfcacares.org.

National Partnership for Women & Families (U.S.) (2005). Expecting better: A state-by-state analysis of parental leave programs. Retrieved from www.Nationalpartnership.org/site/DocServer/ParentalLeaveReport May05.pdf?docID=1052(2012).

Northouse, L. (2005). Helping families of patients with cancer. *Oncology Nursing Forum, 32,* 743–750.

Prensky, H. (2004). *Fact sheet: Protective proceedings: Guardianships and conservatorships*. San Francisco: Family Caregiver Alliance. Retrieved from www.caregiver.org/caregiver/jsp/print_friendly.jsp?nodeid=436.

Sabatino, C. P. (2001). *Fact sheet: Durable powers of attorney and revocable living trusts*. San Francisco: Family Caregiver Alliance/National Center on Caregiving. Retrieved from http://www.caregiver.org/caregiver/jsp/content_node.jsp?nodeid=434.

Schulz, R., O-Brien, A. T., Bookwaise, J., & Fleissner, K. (1995). Psychiatric and physical morbidity effects of dementia caregiving: Prevalence, correlates, and causes. *Gerontologist, 35,* 771–791.

Simon-Rusinowitz, L., Mahoney, K., Loughlin, D., & Sadler, M. (2005). Paying family caregivers: An effective policy option in the Arkansas cash and counseling demonstration and evaluation.

In R. K. Caputo (Ed.), *Challenges of aging on U.S. families: Policy and practice implications* (pp. 83–105). Binghamton: Haworth Press.

Steinberg, M. (2006). *The Medicare drug program fails to reach low-income senior: More than three out of every four low-income seniors eligible for special subsidies are still without drug coverage* (Families USA Publication No. 06–103). Washington: Families USA. Retrieved from http://www.familiesusa.org/assets/pdfs/Medicare-Enrollment-report-May-2006.pdf.

Trude, S., & Ginsburg, P. B. (2002). *Growing physician access problem: Complicate Medicare payment debate* (Issue Brief No. 55). Washington: Center for Studying Health System Change. Retrieved from http:// www.hschange.org/ CONTENT/ 466/?PRINT=1.

U.S. Department of Labor. (2000, October). *Balancing the needs of families and employers: Family and medical leave surveys.* Washington: U.S. Department of Labor. Retrieved from http://www.dol.gov/dol/topic/benefits-leave/fmla.html.

Villet-Lagomarsino, A. (2000). *A guide to advance directives.* Arlington: Educational Broadcasting Corporation, Public Affairs Television, Inc. Retrieved from http://www.pbs.org/wnet/onourownterms/articles/advance.html.

Warren, L., Kirch, D., & Anderson, D. (2004, November). Claims against an estate for care rendered to a decedent. *Colorado Law, 93*(11), 93–99.

Wenzel, H. V. (2005). *Fact sheet: Legal issues for LGBT caregivers.* San Francisco: Family Caregiver Alliance. Retrieved from www.caregiver.org/caregiver/jsp/print_friendly.jsp?nodeid=436.

White, S., & Keefe, J. (2005, June). *Paying caregivers: A briefing paper.* Halifax: Maritime Data Centre for Aging Research & Policy Analysis, Mount Saint Vincent University, in partnership with the Canadian Caregiver Coalition. Retrieved from http://www.ccc-ccan.ca/pdf/caregiverCompensationEng2005.pdf.

Chapter 14
Cancer Caregiving: Policy and Advocacy

Dale L. Kaufman, Ann O'Mara and Christine M. Schrauf

In almost every way, cancer care in the United States today reflects brilliant advances in research, education, and training. Patients receive sophisticated treatments that have become so routine family members can provide them at home. When they want to be involved in treatment decisions, these same patients and families can turn to the Internet and learn about clinical trials and recommendations from the best medical facilities throughout the world. As patients receive chemotherapy and other treatments at home, medical professionals are turning over care to families and other nonprofessional caregivers. However, while cancer diagnosis and treatment explode with promise for the future, policies that support families providing care lag far behind.

A step back in time provides important insight on what it will take for policies to change. At the turn of the twentieth century, for instance, cancer inevitably was a death sentence. Scientific and technical discoveries changed that automatic prognosis—however, something else allowed our health system to progress, at each step of the way. And, that was shared outrage by the American community of health professionals and consumers, men and women, young and old, at the unfair fate of people with cancer and the need to launch a "war on cancer." At each step of the way, outrage at this fate led to a commitment on the part of political leaders and the health system to change the future of people with cancer.

D. L. Kaufman (✉)
U.S. Department of Veteran's Administration, Washington, DC, USA
e-mail: Dale.Kaufman@cms.hhs.gov

U.S. Department of Health and Human Services, Centers for Medicare and Medicaid Services, 200 Independence Avenue S.W., 309D-02, Washington, DC 20201, USA

A. O'Mara
Center for Medical Health Services/SAMHSA, Rockville, MD, USA
e-mail: omaraa@mail.nih.gov

DHHS/NIH/NCI/DCP, MS-7340, Rockville, MD 20892, USA

C. M. Schrauf
Division of Nursing, Elms College, 291 Springfield St. BH 431, Chicopee, MA 01030, USA
e-mail: schraufc@elms.edu

R. C. Talley et al. (eds.), *Cancer Caregiving in the United States,*
Caregiving: Research, Practice, Policy,
DOI 10.1007/978-1-4614-3154-1_14, © Springer Science+Business Media, LLC 2012

It will take similar outrage to find a solution to the unfairness that exists today for the families and other nonprofessional caregivers who care for loved ones with cancer. It will take determined advocacy, strong policies, and the unyielding conviction that society must address the needs of caregivers along with those of the patients.

The statistics reveal that a movement to support the needs of caregivers for persons with cancer has never been more important. If current cancer incidence rates were applied to U.S. Census Bureau projections for the next five decades, due to population growth and aging the number of cancer patients is expected to double from 1.3 to 2.6 million between 2000 and 2050. In addition, the number and proportion of older persons with cancer are expected to increase dramatically. In the next 30 years, the absolute number of cancers in persons 65 years and older is expected to double (Edwards et al. 2002).

And, there are other changes that have implications for people with cancer and their caregivers—from dependence on two incomes to sending patients home from the hospital more quickly, and from smaller family size to greater geographic mobility, limiting family availability. As the need grows while the pool of potential caregivers shrinks, we must ask, "How will we fill the need for care?" Families and community groups simply would not be able to fill all the needs without the support of good state and national policies.

Current Issues

The challenges of caring for the elderly, especially those suffering from cognitive impairment such as Alzheimer's disease, have propelled caregiving to a subject of national attention. Former and current caregivers for elderly family members have been leaders in forming advocacy groups and working toward measures such as respite care. However, although caregivers for cancer patients have benefited from the groundbreaking activism of caregivers for aging family members, cancer brings different caregiving issues. Alzheimer's and other diseases of aging are usually chronic and long-term illnesses, while cancer often is an acute illness that often brings with it an avalanche of crises. For all caregivers there may be a change in family roles, however, cancer can telescope the experience. Suddenly, a wife is taking physical care of her husband, while independence, emotional and physical, is thrust prematurely on their children. And, caregiver needs do not end when the patient is in remission or dies. Issues, from survivorship to bereavement, not only stress families—they can rewrite their future. Like most illnesses that involve expensive treatments, which may or may not be covered by insurance, cancer can impoverish a family. The quicker move to outpatient care may reduce expenditures by the healthcare system, however, savings are exacted in terms of psychological, physical, and financial burdens at home. And, often, a cancer patient may become debilitated or die in the prime wage-earning years, leaving a legacy of lost income.

Another key issue, both for cancer care and other illnesses, is that caregiving is a woman's issue. Most studies show that the number of women caregivers far surpasses the number of men caregivers. According to a recent report from the

Foundation for Accountability and The Robert Wood Johnson Foundation (2001), 68% of caregivers are women. The Family Caregiver Alliance (FCA 2006) reports that estimates of the percentages of family or informal caregivers who are women range from 59 to 75%.

In addition, by all accounts, women unequivocally are the ones who quit their jobs or take leave as well as provide more physical and nursing care than men. As Carol Levine, from the United Hospital Fund (UHF), observed, "The AIDS epidemic has lessons for caregivers. The male caregivers expected more and they got it" (Giorgianni 1997). Men expected more and asserted themselves, and that is what cancer caregiving advocacy needs.

Advocacy

Greta Greer, a social worker for the American Cancer Society (ACS), effectively summarized the challenge to cancer care advocacy when she said: When you ask a caregiver what she needs, you get a horrified look, like addressing her needs will take away from the patient's care (Greer 2002, Personal communication). Because of the relatively acute nature of cancer, as well as the fact that it can strike people in their prime, cancer caregivers are transformed into acute care nurses who barely can see beyond their responsibility to the patient.

Advocacy and consumer organizations have largely provided cancer-related information and referral to information resources (Shelby et al. 2002). However, the changing trajectory of cancer to a more chronic condition, as well issues surrounding survivorship, may change the cancer caregiver's exclusive focus on patient suffering. Online support groups for cancer caregivers, including one from the ACS at http://www.acscsn.org, are providing ways for cancer caregivers to share their difficulties—psychological, physical, and financial. At the same time, they are helping cancer caregivers recognize common difficulties in cancer care—from costs of care to need for information to help caregivers. In addition to numerous resources to help caregivers cope with the demands of being a caregiver, the ACS website also provides a link to the American Cancer Society Cancer Action Network (ASCAN). As a nonprofit, nonpartisan advocacy affiliate, this organization assists interested individuals to participate in political activism on the national or state level to make the fight against cancer a priority agenda item (ACS 2012a). Strategies to make one's voice heard through written messages or face-to-face meetings with legislators are also clearly described on the ACS website (ACS 2012b).

While caregiving advocacy initially grew out of efforts on behalf of caregivers for the aged, these efforts now are providing momentum for cancer caregiving advocacy. In July 2001, The National Alliance for Caregiving (NAC), in collaboration with the Partnership for Caring, convened a Caregiver Empowerment Summit to create a movement for caregivers. In the proceedings of the Summit, it was observed that, "Large-scale change to help family caregivers—through public laws, healthcare benefits, and workplace policies—is needed, however, cannot happen without a unified political voice. Despite their huge numbers, at present, American caregivers have none" (NAC 2001). Meeting participants called for a collaboration among all family caregivers to impact public policy, develop public awareness about caregiving, and create a grassroots plan to promote activism.

Two caregiving organizations originally started for caregivers for aging persons, The NFCA and NAC took on "The Family Caregiver Self-Awareness and Empowerment Project" to bring together family caregivers for persons with mental illness to mental retardation, and from cancer to AIDS. The goal is to develop "self awareness as a potential trigger to empowerment and action" (Hoffman 2002). The project started with a literature review and communications audit on self-awareness and empowerment, which it published online in February 2002. According to the report, the review confirms "that millions are taking on the heavy burdens of caregiving without acknowledging the magnitude of those burdens on every aspect of their lives. Even those organizations and individuals who seek either to serve caregivers or to capitalize upon the existence of this new population are slow to recognize the inherent conflict so many caregivers face." The project is identifying these caregivers who think of themselves as wife, husband, or daughter of the patient without recognizing their need for support as caregivers. Once it is clear where and who the caregivers are, the project will develop a communications campaign to reach them and help them take actions to gain assistance they need.

At the same time, as part of its series on Strengthening Families and Communities for Caregiving, the NFCA conducted Town Hall Meetings in five cities (Philadelphia, Washington, DC, Chicago, Boston, and San Francisco) in 2002–2003 to encourage dialogue on the needs of family caregivers. Again, although the NFCA was created for caregivers of elderly persons, the goal—and effect—is to focus attention on needs of all caregivers.

At the end of the twentieth century, the Rosalynn Carter Institute for Caregiving (RCI) ushered in a new era for caregiving advocacy when it adopted caregiving as its priority. Through partnerships with professionals, groups, and individuals, the RCI is stimulating and supporting public awareness activities and advocacy for better caregiving practices. To strengthen the impact of these efforts, the RCI established the National Quality Caregiving Network in 2007, which supersedes the RCI's sponsorship of the National Quality Caregiving Coalition (NQCC), which was founded in 1990.

Current Status

Federal Legislation, Regulations, and Initiatives

Support of Federal policies to improve the well-being of caregivers has been limited and incremental. In 1993, the Family Medical Leave Act (FMLA) was passed into law, requiring that employers covered by the Act grant employees up to 12 work weeks of unpaid leave during a 12-month period to care for an immediate family member with a serious health problem. Although this was a landmark law, it leaves out many caregivers. For one thing, the law applies only to employers of 50 or more employees, so small businesses are excluded. And, for another, many caregivers simply cannot afford to take leave without pay for 3 months. Efforts to expand provisions within the FMLA during the 108th and 109th Congressional sessions have been unsuccessful, however, have included attempts to both increase the eligible employee base as well as provide some paid leave within the allotted time away from work (National Center on Caregiving [NCC] 2006).

The National Partnership for Women and Families has made family leave policies an important piece of their policy agenda. In addition to grassroots lobbying efforts to expand FMLA provisions, they have produced a detailed guide to the FMLA. This document explains provisions in the law addressing specific individual and family situations requiring a work leave. A comprehensive 2006 publication, *Where Families Matter: State Progress Toward Valuing America's Families*, provides an overview of the paid family and medical leave initiatives that were introduced in state legislatures during 2005.

Another milestone for caregiving came in the year 2000, when the Older Americans Act was amended to include the National Family Caregiver Support Program (NFCSP), which provides funding for states to work in partnership with area agencies on aging and local community service providers on providing basic services for family caregivers. The five services for caregivers identified in the program include: information about available services, assistance in gaining access to support services, individual counseling and caregiver training to assist caregivers in solving problems related to their caregiving roles, respite care, and limited supplemental services to complement care provided by caregivers. However, this program also comes with significant limitations for cancer caregivers of younger patients. As it is part of the Older Americans Act, it applied only to family caregivers of adults over 60 years or to grandparents or other relatives of children 18 years or younger.

Several caregiving-related bills received the attention of the 109th Congress. H.R. 6197, the Older Americans Act Amendments of 2006, was passed by the 109th Congress and signed into law on October 17, 2006. As Public Law 109–365, the Act amends the Older American Act of 1965 to authorize aging appropriations for fiscal years 2007 through 2011. The Act also lowers the age from 60 to 55 years for grandparents and other relatives caring for children 18 years or younger (Administration on Aging 2012a).

The Caregiver Assistance and Relief Effort (CARE) Act of 2005 was introduced again in 2006 with the aim of providing funding and incentives for caregiver support and long-term care assistance. It would also amend the Internal Revenue Code, allowing a tax credit to caregivers assisting family members to meet care needs. Also introduced in the 109th Congress was the Re-Entry Enhancement Act, which included a provision to totally eliminate the age requirement for relative caregivers under the NFCSP. Neither of these bills made it out of committee (NAC 2004).

A highlight of 2006 was passage of the Lifespan Respite Care *Act* of 2006 (HR 3248). The legislation, originally introduced in 2002, was signed into law by the President on December 21, 2006. The Act authorizes US$ 289 million over 5 years for state grants to develop Lifespan Respite Programs. Programs are to provide assistance to families in obtaining quality, affordable respite care. The Act defines lifespan respite programs "as coordinated systems of accessible, community-based respite care services for family caregivers of children and adults with special needs." The law authorizes funding in four areas: (a) development of state and local lifespan respite programs based on models and best practices; (b) planned or emergency respite care services; (c) training and recruitment of respite care workers and volunteers; and (d) caregiver training (Administration on Aging, 2012b).

Although targeted primarily toward caregivers of the elderly, the Administration on Aging (AoA) has developed the NFCSP, mentioned earlier, with a focus on consumer education. Information about program eligibility and services is provided through written information, televised public service announcements, and other information accessed through their website. Especially useful for caregivers and care recipients of all ages is a link on the home page to a document produced by the National Conference of State Legislatures, *Family Caregiver Support—State Facts at a Glance,* providing detailed information about programs and services available in every state (Link et al. 2006). Another link on the AoA website is to the *Compendium of Department of Health and Human Services (HHS) Caregiver Support Activities,* which reflects several programs that add to our understanding of caregiving prevalence and to our awareness about caregivers in the workplace (HHS New Freedom Initiative Caregiver Support Workgroup 2006). The projects and services, however, focus on caregivers for elderly people or children with disabilities and not on caregivers for people with cancer.

Similarly, the Center for Medicaid and Medicare (CMS) has developed a project that targets caregivers for elderly people, however, is breaking ground by exploring issues that often affect caregivers for people with cancer: caregivers in the workplace. The CMS Caregiver/Employer Project provides tools and information for caregivers of seniors on Medicare, and it is conducted through employers with caregiver employees. The materials, *Medicare and Eldercare Essentials: A Toolkit for Employers,* has several components: *Medicare Basics,* for caregiver decisions; *When Employees Become Caregivers: A Manager's Workbook,* for employers to assist employee caregivers; and *New Medicare Prescription Drug Coverage: A Message for people Who Care for Someone with Medicare* (Centers for Medicaid and Medicare Services 2006).

Another issue, the major role of women as caregivers, was addressed in the context of aging at a hearing sponsored by Senators John Breaux and Barbara Mikulski in February 2002. Although the hearing was part of an effort to encourage legislative changes in the long-term care system that would acknowledge the role of women as caregivers, the concerns explored touched on the realities of cancer caregivers. Experts testified on the disproportionate share of caregiving assumed by women and the effects on their health, as well as additional costs related to caregiving expenses such as transportation, utilities, and dietary needs.

Accrediting agencies potentially can play a powerful role in requiring healthcare agencies, such as home healthcare facilities, to standardize its support and training of family and informal caregivers of chronically ill cancer patients. To date, however, that role is more of an implicit than explicit one. Two major players responsible for accrediting healthcare agencies are the Joint Commission on Accreditation of Healthcare Agencies (JCAHO) and The National Commission for Quality Assurance (NCQA). As of April 2007, minimal information related to family caregiving was available on either the JCAHO (five articles, primarily from other sources) or NCQA (one article related to professional caregiving) websites.

Accrediting Organizations

The National Committee for Quality Assurance (NCQA) is a nonprofit organization that sets standards for the quality of care and service that health plans provide to their members (NCQA 2011a). Three different tools are used to evaluate healthcare: accreditation (a rigorous on-site review of key clinical and administrative processes), the Health Plan Employer Data and Information Set, and a comprehensive member satisfaction survey. Of the three activities, NCQA's accreditation of organizations from HMOs and PPOs to Managed Behavioral Healthcare Organizations (MB-HOs) could have significant impact on informal caregivers. However, review of the standards used to evaluate and accredit these organizations reveals no reference to informal caregiving. One category NCQA uses in its accreditation process is "Living with Illness," and a key question is, "How well does the health plan care for people with chronic conditions (NCQA 2011b)." Without question, assessments could be included that focus on support and education of family caregivers.

The Home Care Accreditation section of the JCAHO website (http://www.jcrinc. com/HC-Resources) identifies the types of programs that are part of JCAHO's accreditation process, most of which are clearly relevant to cancer caregiving. They are Home Health, Personal Care and/or Support, Home Medical Equipment, and Hospice (JCAHO 2012). Although the standards primarily relate to services provided by healthcare professionals, several of the National Patient Safety Goals used in the accreditation process specify involvement of patients and families. They are Goal 2: Improve the effectiveness of communication among caregivers, Goal 7: Reduce the risk of healthcare-associated infections, Goal 8: Accurately and completely reconcile medications across the continuum of care, Goal 9: Reduce the risk of patient harm resulting from falls, and Goal 15: Identify safety risks inherent in the patient population (JCAHO 2010).

State Policies

Activities on the federal level, from the NFCSP to the New Freedom Initiative, increasingly have handed states considerable responsibility for providing community services for the elderly and for persons with cognitive impairments and developmental disabilities, as well as for their caregivers. The federal government has handed states responsibility for services for the frail elderly and persons with disabilities, and the high cost of this care, along with a consumer movement to help family members live at home, fuel a growing trend for state policies that support family caregiving. Lynn Friss Feinberg, Deputy Director of the NCC of the FCA, comments on another motivation, "Family caregiving is a growing issue for states rising societal value placed on caregiving as more women and caregivers now hold elective offices" (National Health Council [NHC]and National Quality Caregiving Coalition [NQCC] 2002, p. 14).

Services are largely targeted to caregivers of elderly persons and the cognitively impaired, however, they support growing acknowledgment caregiver needs in general. Given the dismal financial climate for states, the economic benefits of supporting family caregivers have become clear to most state governments. Although funds may be far from adequate, the incentives for state policies on caregiving are enormous. State funding is pieced together from a variety of sources. The NFCSP, which the U.S. Administration on Aging administers for elderly recipients care, provides limited funding. General revenues and the US\$ 286 billion, 25-year settlements in the late 1990s between states and the tobacco industry provide a major source of funding. Medicaid waivers, specifically for home- and community-based services (HCBS) for frail elderly, provide services that indirectly benefit caregivers by enhancing recipient care, such as training and respite services. However, for the most part, this funding does not benefit caregivers of persons with cancer.

As previously referenced, the National Conference of State Legislatures, in association with the National Association of State Units on Aging, has developed a document detailing a state-by-state description of programs for caregivers of the elderly. An additional resource developed by the Family Caregiver Alliance (FCA) in 2004, *The State of the States in Family Caregiver Support: A 50 State Study*, provides a broader and more detailed review of state programs available to patients and their families of all ages (Feinberg et al. 2004). Available in PDF format through their websites, these resources can be used by caregivers of cancer patients to determine if specific programs might be applicable to them. Contact information for the state agency administrating each program is also provided.

In a policy research report, *Family Caregiver Support Services* (Feinberg et al. 2005), the AARP describes services offered by states to caregivers, primarily through NFCSP funding. These include:

- Information to caregivers about available services.
- Assistance to caregivers in gaining access to services.
- Individual counseling.
- Organization of support groups.
- Caregiver training in making decisions and solving problems relating to their roles.
- Respite care for temporary relief from caregiving responsibilities.
- Supplemental services to complement care provided by caregivers.

Through its Public Policy Institute, the American Association of Retired Persons (AARP) has produced a scorecard identifying how well individual states have done in delivering long-term services and supports to older persons, individuals with physical disabilities and family caregivers. Twenty-five individual indicators were used to assess state performance and identify characteristics of those with the highest level of supportive public policies (Reinhard et al. 2011).

The FCA seeks to advance the development of high-quality, cost-effective policies and programs for caregivers in every state through its NCC established in 2001. Its recent 50-state study of caregiver support programs, funded by the AoA, describes publicly-funded programs developed since passage of the federal act establishing the NFCSP (Feinberg et al. 2004). Through surveys and telephone interviews, detailed state information enabled the authors to key themes in state program development. Their findings show:

- Increasingly available, however, diverse and uneven, publicly-funded caregiver support services across and within states.
- Enhancement and innovation in caregiver support services due to the NFCSP, however, inadequate funding to service most caregiving families.
- Broad recognition of the value of uniformly assessing caregiver needs, and the importance of adequate training and technical assistance in this area.
- Mixed views among the states on the importance of caregiver support services, approaches to systems development, and methods to integrate family caregiving programs into existing home- and community-based care.

The 50-state study is supplemented by a web-based searchable resource map, enabling easy access to information about individual state caregiver programs. NCC web links to current state-by-state legislation offers detailed information for each state, however, is not regularly updated. However, a free electronic newsletter, *Caregiving Policy Digest*, provides semimonthly information about new state legislation and policy. The newsletter also covers federal legislation, policy and reports, as well as international news, upcoming conferences related to caregiving, and funding opportunities for caregiver research.

A more in-depth FCA report, *Family Caregiver Support: Policies, Perceptions and Practices in 10 States Since Passage of the National Family Caregiver Support Program* (Feinberg et al. 2002), identifies commonalities and differences in 10 states that represent 37% of the U.S. population. Chosen for their diversity in geography, culture and age range, the states (Alabama, California, Florida, Hawaii, Indiana, Iowa, Maine, Pennsylvania, Texas, and Washington) were studied through site visits and interviews with key officials and stakeholders. They represented states with state-funded caregiver support programs already in place, as well as states that had just begun to develop programs.

This in-depth focus was intended to stimulate discussion among state leaders about ways to integrate new NFCSP funds into existing programs of caregiver support, or how to best create new programs. Although the report reflects state caregiving emphasis on caregivers for elderly persons, the themes across states provide lessons for developing cancer caregiver programs. Many of this study's findings were later corroborated in the 50-state study, however, others also emerged, including:

- Providing explicit support for caregivers represents a paradigm shift in current healthcare reimbursement philosophy.

- In addition to limited funding, workforce shortages challenge development and implementation of caregiver support services.
- Respite care and supplemental services (e.g., consumable supplies) are viewed as the top service needs of family caregivers.
- Use of consumer-directed options for respite care differs among the states, however, when available, most families choose relatives, friends or persons they already know.
- Uniform data collection on family caregivers, especially outcome data, is lacking, making it difficult to measure the impact of services and assure quality.

The FCA also issues policy briefs, funded through federal grants or nonprofit foundations, which address emerging issues and initiatives in caregiver support. The briefs addressing working caregivers highlight an important cancer caregiver advocacy issue since family members often balance work and home caregiver demands, and consumer-directed home care, which provides families direct control over scarce resources to meet their own specific needs.

Donna Wagner, in her paper on state initiatives for working caregivers, notes that state programs specifically targeted to working caregivers are extremely limited. However, she comments, in taking greater initiative to develop partnerships that address needs of working caregivers, states can work with state businesses and industry to promote economic stability and growth (Wagner 2001). One method to achieve change is through state provisions which build on the national Family and Medical Leave Act as described by Bell and Newman (2003). State-administered insurance programs to provide payments for temporary disability or family leave are offered by some states. Others require employers to allow employees to use sick leave to care for sick family members. Retention of skilled workers through these types of initiatives has been shown to benefit employers through lower hiring and training costs. Pavalko and Henderson (2006) demonstrate that women are still more likely to leave the labor force when family caregiving is needed then their male counterparts. However, workers in jobs that provide access to flexible hours, unpaid family leave, and paid sick or vacation days are more likely to remain employed and maintain work hours.

Problems related to retirement planning once family caregivers are forced to leave the workforce to care for loved ones are addressed by Young and Newman in another FCA policy brief (2003). Reduced wages and reduced job security may be experienced in the short term, however, long-term consequences can impact family caregivers as they near retirement age. Factors contributing to this problem are reduced social security benefits based on earnings, limited access to employer-sponsored pensions as work hours decrease, and limited personal savings as monies must be used on current medical expenses.

Consumer-directed home care, although successfully used by some states, continues to be controversial as it shifts the locus of decision-making and control of services from providers and payers to consumers and families. In defending the stance that an ethical imperative exists for paying caregivers, Larry Polivka also acknowledges concern about containing costs. He draws on lessons from early home- and community-based services waiver programs, and presents suggestions for keeping expenditures within budget limits, including restrictive eligibility based on functional need, financial resources, and caregiver availability and enabling nonfamily caregivers to dispense medicine, give shots, and provide other healthcare services under supervision of a nurse. Polivka also comments that available evaluations of Caregiver Pay Programs for long-term care recipients in Germany and Austria suggest that paying caregivers is a cost-effective alternative to institutionalization (Polivka 2001).

Doty (2004) describes three models of consumer direction: (1) control restricted to hiring and supervision of personal aides or assistants; (2) "cash and counseling," which increases resource use options to purchase of needed technology or home modifications; and (3) a no-strings-attached cash benefit, usually available only from private insurers. The "cash and counseling" approach was tested on a broad scale in a three-state Medicaid demonstration project, implemented in Arkansas, New Jersey, and Florida. Results among Arkansas families participating in the project showed a decrease in caregiver strain and better well-being, especially among working caregivers. The absence of serious problems with abuse, neglect, mistreatment, or financial exploitation by family members or directly hired workers has assisted to quell concerns among skeptics to these programs.

Following the early success of the "cash and counseling" model, the AoA extended this initiative to another 11 states in 2004, and the model is also being implemented in a range of federal and state-funded HCBS programs. A study to identify the role of consumer-based direction in the United States in 2003 (Feinberg and Newman 2005) found that the NFCSP appears to be speeding the adoption of consumer direction in family caregiving support programs. Although personal care and respite care are the most likely services that families can be paid to provide, spouses are not allowed to be paid to provide care in nearly two-thirds of these programs.

The reluctance to provide compensation to family members, especially spouses, reflects some policymakers' concerns about contributing to a major shift away from caring as part of normal family responsibility (Kunkel et al. 2003–2004). These authors summarized empirical evidence that demonstrates that payment to family members providing care in U.S. programs has not lessened the commitment of family members to care for their loved ones, and actually contribute to the satisfaction of both care recipients and caregivers. In a similar theme, Li (2005) demonstrated that informal caregivers do not relinquish caregiving when publicly paid home care is available, which is another concern of policymakers.

The fact that these and other caregiving initiatives across states target caregivers for the elderly or persons with mental impairment highlights the paucity of services targeting cancer care. However, these programs also serve as models for cancer caregiving advocacy. For instance, the California Caregiver Resource Center (CRC) delivers caregiver support services through 11 regional sites throughout the state. Although an important innovation of the CRC program is a statewide clearing house on caregiving and cognitive impairment, California has expanded its caregiving services to caregivers for adults with other chronic conditions. The Pennsylvania Family Caregiver Support Program provides up to US$ 200 per month in respite and chore services to caregivers of persons 60 and older, as well as funding for home modification, counseling, and caregiver training. As research continues to demonstrate the societal benefit of supporting family caregiving in states willing to test innovative models, advocacy will be critical in convincing policymakers to implement similar programs.

Education

According to a study in New York City conducted by the UHF and the Visiting Nurse Service of New York, nearly 60% of New York's family caregivers do not receive the training they need to assist in essential responsibilities. These responsibilities include medical tasks, such as managing prescription medications and providing physical assistance, such as bathing or moving a loved one. The lack of consistent policies on education and training puts both patient and caregiver at risk (Levine et al. 2000). Recent attempts to improve education of family caregivers, especially when loved ones are hospitalized, include web-based publications, such as *A Family Caregiver's Guide to Hospital Discharge Planning* (Hunt and Levine 2002).

Although nonprofit and private groups largely have assumed responsibility for conducting training for caregivers, state governments are increasingly developing caregiver support activities that include training, information, and referral services.

A policy brief from the FCA, *Federal and State Policy in Family Caregiving: Recent Victories but Uncertain Future,* reviews model state initiatives on education, many of which are targeted to caregivers of elderly persons (Fox-Grage et al. 2001). The authors identify model programs in California, Pennsylvania, Washington, and Maryland. For example, Maryland's General Assembly established the Caregiver Support Coordinating Council in the Department of Human Resources to coordinate statewide planning, development, and implementation of family caregiver support services.

The Pennsylvania Department of Health has been a leader in funding training for cancer caregivers through its support of the University of Pennsylvania's development of the Strength for Caring program. This program was designed to help caregivers understand cancer and its treatment, meet the physical and emotional needs of the patient, deal with changing family roles, improve their own mental and physical health, and find and take advantage of community resources. With funding from OrthoBiotech, Inc., the program now is available nationwide at http://www.strengthforcaring.com.

The FCA issued a report to describe five widely used caregiver education and support programs that have empirical evidence to support their effectiveness (Toseland 2004). Although requiring caregivers to commit to a series of group meetings, the programs represent diverse ways to fit attendance into the caregiving life, offering half-day and evening programs supplemented by booklets, workbooks, and videos. In addition to detailed information about the five programs, this resource provides guidance to program facilitators in selecting the appropriate program for a targeted audience, preparing to implement the program and recruiting participants.

There are numerous electronic resources available for cancer caregivers. On the NAC website, links to several publications for caregivers is provided, some with reference specifically to cancer caregivers (Met Life Mature Market Institute and NAC 2007). *Resources for Caregivers 2004,*produced by NAC and the MetLife Mature Market Institute, includes sections for caregivers of various major disease categories. Under "Cancer," there are three resources described including the *Cancer Survival Toolbox: An Online Audio Resource Program* produced by the National Coalition for Cancer Survivorship (2005). In the toolbox is an audio entitled *Caring for the Caregiver,* which was developed specifically to provide resources and support for cancer caregivers. The NAC also lists *Palliative Care: Complete Care Everyone Deserves* as a resource for caregivers who need to understand what palliative care is, who provides it, and how best to assess its quality.

Caregivers for people with cancer do not typically turn to caregiver organizations for information; they are more likely to get information from cancer groups. A 2012 search using the keyword "caregivers" within the ACS website produced over 40,000 hits, listing articles or resources either produced by the ACS or linked to other caregiver websites (ACS 2012). Offerings include a brief but supportive document, Being a Caregiver, as well as articles addressing *Concern for Families and Caregivers, Anxiety Check for Caregivers*, and *Coping Check-up for Caregivers*. These documents build on findings from professional cancer journals that describe cancer caregiver research, thus demonstrating the growing interest and concern in supporting families of cancer victims.

The National Cancer Institute (NCI) at the National Institutes of Health (NIH) has also expanded its communications efforts to caregivers. Using their website, a search using the word "caregivers" resulted in the listing of several booklets and other web resources, specific to the needs of cancer caregivers. They include information and electronic booklets such as *Caring for the Caregiver, When Someone You Love is Being Treated for cancer,* and *Family Caregivers in Cancer: Roles and Challenges* (NCI 2012). A link to the Family Care Research Program at Michigan State University also provides cancer patients and their families with general information about health management in addition to several information resources specific to family caregiver issues. NCI also funds research grants on caregiver education and training.

The Family Caregiver Self-Awareness and Empowerment Project, initiated by the NFCA in 2000 and described on their website, seeks to gain a better understanding of why so many family caregivers do not self-identify and what can be done to gain their attention (NFCA 2012). The first phase of this project consisted of market research to develop a communications strategy to reach family caregivers and resulted in five reports: A base-line survey conducted by AARP, a communications audit, an appendix of available information, a caregivers' focus group report, and a message testing report. Much of this information concludes that many caregivers are reluctant to embrace the caregiver label, that they prefer to focus on the quality of care they provide rather than their own needs, and that media messages must be crafted with these and other findings in mind. Phase II, the implementation portion of the project, is currently under development.

For caregivers who can obtain information and support from others through online exchanges, a blog is available through the WebMD site featuring guest bloggers who are experts in numerous areas of concern to family caregivers (NHC & WebMD 2012). Discussion topics include insurance issues and legal advice in addition to numerous questions relating to medical symptoms and treatment options. These personalized exchanges with numerous types of experts offer caregivers a home-based approach to troubling questions.

Practice

As Jane Ingham, Director of Palliative Care at Georgetown University's Lombardi Cancer Center, observes:

> The system does not consistently formally recognize the caregiver as either a part of the 'unit of care' or a part of the care team itself. This occurs even though the caregiver is physically and emotionally impacted by the illness and even though he or she also may become at a number of times through the course of cancer care an 'around the clock nurse.' Oncology care is commonly delivered in specialized environments, away from the 'family practice' model of care, and thus the caregiver often is not 'linked' in any structured way within the same system of medical care as the patient. Although there is an increasing recognition of caregiver needs, until a patient reaches the point where care is delivered within the context of hospice, the systems, policies, reimbursement structures, and attitudes that are commonly linked to oncology settings do not provide a consistent, supportive structure for addressing the unique and important care, support and educational needs of caregivers. This lack of formal recognition anchors the caregiver truly as an 'informal' caregiver within a system that presents significant challenges – rather than supports – to both caregivers and health professionals as they seek to foster caregiver well-being and good health. (Ingham, personal communication 2003)

Most initiatives for health professionals to partner with family caregivers are started in hospitals and hospices. A current example is the *Peer Partners Program* at Emory's Winship Cancer Institute. As one of Emory's many cancer survivorship programs, this initiative matches cancer survivors and caregivers with those currently dealing with a new diagnosis of cancer. One-to-one support is offered by survivors and their caregivers based on their own personal experiences. In order to facilitate program success, professional staff offer training and supervision to individuals who volunteer to become peer partners (Emory 2012).

A long and ongoing project to bring family caregiving to the forefront in partnering with health care professionals has also been the work of the United Hospital Fund (UHF), a research and philanthropic organization in New York City. Spearheaded by Carol Levine, director of the UHF Families and Health Care Project and a former spousal caregiver, *Next Step in Care* is a multiyear project to change usual practice in health care settings so that family caregivers are involved in planning and coordinating care for their loved one (UNF 2012).

The *Next Step in Care* campaign offers free downloadable guides for caregivers to assist them to understand and navigate complex health care systems. Transitions from one care setting to another are frequently difficult for caregivers because they are often excluded from care coordination activities. The guides and associated checklists provide assistance in ensuring that caregivers remain part of the transition planning process. Other guides written for health care professionals offer information about how to work with family caregivers more effectively.

The important practice of provider assessment of caregivers is currently identified as one of the emerging trends in addressing the needs of family caregivers (Feinberg et al. 2006). The value of identifying needs of not only the care recipient, but also their primary caregiver, is recognized as a fundamental need to sustain caregiving families and help them stay "on the job." Although caregiver assessments are used to tailor caregiver services in some states, it is widely recognized that a universal assessment tool would be beneficial for both practice and research.

In September, 2005, the FCA convened an invitational National Consensus Development Conference for Caregiver Assessment, bringing together recognized leaders in health and long-term care with two goals: to generate principles and guidelines for caregiver assessment, and to build common ground among leaders committed to innovation, experimentation, and the systematic generation of new knowledge. Reports summarizing the conference achievements include the participants' ability to form consensus on fundamental principles and practice guidelines for caregiver assessment. These are applicable to a range of practitioners, providers, and care managers in a variety of settings (FCA 2006).

Research

In an article investigating where terminally-ill patients look for assistance with nonmedical needs from personal care to transportation, Emanuel et al. found that most cancer patients rely completely on family members and friends for assistance (Emanuel et al. 1999). In a comprehensive summary of five publications that included the economic value of care provided by informal caregivers to ill and disabled adults, Gibson and Houser (2007) report that its estimated value is about $350 billion per year. This figure is more than total spending for Medicaid ($300 billion in 2005) and is more than four times the total amount spent on formal paid home care services.

Other studies stress the indirect costs of family caregiving. For example, as leading researchers Barbara and Charles Given observe, "The cost in personal, physical and mental health of caregivers has yet to be fully explored. What's known is they often give up leisure, physical exercise, and proper nutrition. Unknown are the use of medications such as tranquilizers or other medications and the number of primary care visits" (Given and Given 2002, p. 1). In another article, Given and Given identify four areas where research especially is needed: (1) symptom management strategies; (2) patient-caregiver communication to understand key elements of a productive patient caregiver relationship; (3) defining patient outcomes as a basis for developing standards of care; and (4) cost-effectiveness (Given et al. 2001).

Methodological issues have greatly limited research on caregiving. Most studies on caregivers to date have been descriptive, and there is a paucity of empirical research including controlled studies comparing caregivers with noncaregivers. There is a need for instruments specifically designed to evaluate the quality of life of caregivers of cancer patients (rather than measuring specific outcomes like distress) and to detect changes in caregiving needs over the course of illness and shifting goals. The literature reflects that caregiving studies use small samples, rather than the larger samples that are needed to adjust for different relationships among caregivers to the patient and for different needs of different cancers. Convenience samples typically have been used, especially as caregivers often are reluctant to participate in research when patients are very ill. Population-based studies are needed to explore prevalence for family-based care and variability in family variables.

In July 2001, the NIH's National Institute of Nursing Research conducted a State of the Science Workgroup Meeting on *Research in Informal Caregiving* (Grady and Armstrong 2001). The purpose was to identify research opportunities on informal caregiving, and the workgroup listed three key areas for research investment:

- Informal Caregiving Populations, including persons with cancer, diverse populations, and hard to reach groups.
- Caregiver Knowledge, Skills, Support, including developing instruments for outcome measurement.
- Impact on the Caregiver, including influence of family dynamics, evaluation of effectiveness, and financial impact.

Future Directions and Conclusion

Reflection on the advances made in policies and programs benefiting family caregivers during the early 2000s has relevance for anyone committed to improve the ability of cancer caregivers to care for themselves and their loved ones. This summary of current initiatives has relevance for further work in political and regulatory advocacy, education of both families and healthcare practitioners, professional oncology practice, and research to further identify caregiver needs and how best to meet them.

Advocacy and Policy Development

The need to support family caregivers was most prominent in the policy arena with the passage of the 2000 Older Americans Act and development of the NFCSP. Although this initiative resulted in more state caregiver programs, budgetary constraints have limited program expansions, both in terms the populations served and services available. However, efforts to educate policymakers and health professionals about the needs of specialty caregiver groups, such as cancer caregivers, must continue so that awareness of needs can precede opening of the "policy window" in the future.

Although the major caregiver groups advocate for "caregiver-friendly" policies and programs on the national level, advocacy for the specialty needs of cancer caregivers may be most effective on the state and local levels where legislators are most accessible. In addition, specific caregiver populations served by federal and state-funded programs are often determined by state agencies, based on available information. Specific actions that can be taken to advance development of beneficial policies and programs include:

- Educate state lawmakers, especially those who serve on committees which review health legislation, about the realities of care needs at home preceding, during, and after cancer therapies. Use stories of families' experience with cancer, especially families in congressional districts which these legislators represent.
- Be ready to identify specific changes in family leave policies that would alleviate both short- and long-term burden on families facing unexpected care needs. Look to states that have implemented beneficial programs as examples of change.
- Link cancer caregiver needs to the benefits that the business community realize when policies and programs support these employees through enhanced leave options, ability to use sick time, or transfer of sick time use from other willing employees.
- Investigate expansion of tax credit options for cancer caregivers with local and state governments.
- Educate payers of healthcare about the benefits of family cancer care in enhancing patient outcomes as well as maximizing scarce professional care resources.
- Utilize the media to highlight the role that family caregivers play in treatment and ongoing care and support of cancer patients undergoing active therapy as well as cancer survivors. Use existing annual timeframes which highlight cancer awareness. On a national level, efforts by professional cancer advocacy groups to quantify the contributions of cancer caregivers, both in terms of their numbers as well as care dollars saved, would increase awareness of policymakers and the general caregiving advocacy community. This strategy has been successfully used by groups representing caregivers of the elderly, especially those caring for persons with cognitive disorders such as Alzheimer's disease.

Education and Communications

The explosion of Internet-based information for caregivers, both through cancer-specific websites and general caregiver-focused sites, is of great benefit to cancer caregivers and their healthcare providers. Increasing availability of this information to all cancer caregivers is the current challenge. We also now recognize that the term "caregiver" may not be internalized by those providing care at home to their loved ones. In addition, access to cancer caregivers in the home, especially those without computer access presents a further challenge. Efforts to increase education and communication can include:

- Make caregiver information an important part of established cancer resources, including 1–800 numbers, especially to reach the large number of cancer caregivers who are more likely to seek information about cancer than about caregiving.

- Ensure that information for caregivers is linked to cancer websites, and that websites for cancer patients and their families are linked to one another. Links to the AoA and FCA sites would be particularly useful since they contain a wealth of caregiver information.
- Begin education and training of caregivers throughout the trajectory of illness, beginning with diagnosis, before caregivers become overwhelmed by the illness and responsibilities.
- Identify caregiver resources available for Hispanic and other prominent local language communities. When possible, adapt cancer-specific educational materials for use by local ethnic communities.
- Adapt proven caregiver education programs to the needs of cancer caregivers and encourage their use through local agencies serving caregiving families.
- Educate healthcare professionals (oncology practitioners, home care nurses, etc.) who are most likely to have contact with family caregivers of cancer patients about resources available.

Practice

With the beginning development of standards and guidelines for caregiver assessment, healthcare professionals in all specialty areas will benefit in adequately assessing caregiver needs. As policies develop, practitioners must also update their knowledge of laws, regulations, and emerging programs useful to the cancer caregiving community. Transfer of this knowledge to family members needs to take place wherever and whenever possible—during hospital admissions, in oncology offices and clinics, or during home visits. Specific recommendations include:

- Incorporation of standardized caregiver assessment tools at times and in settings when home caregivers are expected to participate in care and support of their loved ones.
- A shift in the care paradigm of persons with cancer to the family as the unit of care.
- Incorporation of updates about policies and programs benefiting caregivers in beginning and continuing education of oncology and home care healthcare providers.

Accreditation

- Educate accrediting agencies about the benefits of incorporating involvement of family caregivers into standards addressing hospital discharge and home care. Use research findings demonstrating caregiver well-being on patient outcomes. Use principles underlying the hospice paradigm as an example.

- Encourage development of standards addressing caregiver assessment and direction to programs which can enhance their well-being and maintain the integrity of their caregiving role.

Research

- Frame cost studies in the context of the *value* of caregiving, not as cost-effectiveness studies. In their issue brief detailing the economic value of caregiving, Gibson and Houser (2007) note '... it is essential to prevent family caregivers from being overwhelmed by the demands placed upon them. The cost of funding more services and supports for caregivers is minute compared to the value of their contributions. (p. 7)'
- Develop instruments and approaches that address current methodological limitations of caregiving research. Focus on issues such as measuring overall quality of life of caregivers, designing controlled studies, and exploring prevalence and variability of family-based care.
- Conduct studies on caregiver burden, to address the costs of not making better policies for caregivers.
- Conduct studies on costs of cancer to families, as well as on symptom management, patient outcomes and best caregiver practices, and caregiver-patient communication.
- Conduct policy evaluations of programs in countries outside the United States to pay family caregivers.

Concluding Comments

Cancer is a tragic illness that can cause tremendous suffering and cut lives short. Care also comes with huge costs to the family caregiver, who takes on tremendous responsibilities for a loved one. Cancer affects the whole family. And, as a society, we cannot afford not to support better policies for caregivers.

References

Administration on Aging, Department of Health & Human Services. (2012a). *National Family Caregiver Support Program (OAA Title IIIE)*. Retrieved February 29, 2012 from http://www.aoa.gov/AoA_programs/HCLTC/Caregiver/index.aspx.

Administration on Aging, Department of Health & Human Services. (2012b). *Lifespan respite care program*. Retrieved on February 29, 2012 from http://www.aoa.gov/AoAroot/AoA_Programs/HCLTC/LRCP/index.aspx.

American Cancer Society. (2012a). *Help laws to defeat cancer*. Retrieved on February 26, 2012 from http://www.cancer.org/Involved/Advocate/index.

American Cancer Society. (2012b). *Tops for becoming an effective cancer advocate.* Retrieved on March 3, 2012 from http://www.cancer.org/Involved/Advocate/TipsforCancerAdvocate/index.

American Cancer Society (ACS). (2012c). *Caregivers.* Retrieved on March 16, 2012 from http://www.cancer.org/Treatment/Caregivers/index.

Bell, L., & Newman, S. (2003). *Paid family and medical leave: Why we need it, how we can get it.* San Francisco: Family Caregiver Alliance. Retrieved from http://www.caregiver.org/caregiver/jsp/content_node.jsp?nodeid=1012.

Centers for Medicaid and Medicare Services. (2006). *Caregiver partnerships and caregiver workgroup.* Retrieved from http://www.cms.hhs.gov/Partnerships/12_Caregiver.asp.

Doty, P. (2004). *Consumer-directed home care: Effects on family caregivers.* Retrieved from http://www.caregiver.org/caregiver/jsp/content_node.jsp?nodeid=1193.

Edwards, B., Howe, H. L., Ries, L. A., Thum, M. J., Rosenberg, H. M., Yancik, R., et al. (2002). Annual report of the nation on the status of cancer. *Cancer, 94*(10), 2766–2792.

Emanuel, E. J., Fairclough, D. L., Slutsman, J., Alpert, H., Baldwin, D., & Emanuel, L. L. (1999). Assistance from family members, friends, paid caregivers, and volunteers in the care of terminally ill patients. *New England Journal of Medicine, 341,* 956–963.

Emory Winship Cancer Institute. (2012). *Peer partners program.* Retrieved on March 16, 2012 from http://winshipcancer.emory.edu/survivorship/WinshipContentPage.aspx?nd=910.

Family Caregiver Alliance (FCA). (2006). *Caregiver assessment: Principles, guidelines and strategies for change* (Report from a National Consensus Development Conference; Vol. 1). San Francisco: Family Caregiver Alliance.

Feinberg, L. F., & Newman, S. L. (2005). *State policy in practice: Consumer direction and family caregiving: Results from a national survey.* Retrieved from http://www.caregiver.org/caregiver/jsp/content_node.jsp?nodeid=1499.

Feinberg, L. F., Newman, S. L., & Van Steenberg, C. (2002). *Family caregiver support: Policies, perceptions and practices in 10 states since passage of the National Family Caregiver Support Program.* San Francisco: National Center on Caregiving, Family Caregiver Alliance. Retrieved from http://www.caregiver.org/caregiver/jsp/content_node.jsp?nodeid=451.

Feinberg, L. F., Newman, S. L., Gray, L., & Kolb, K. (2004). *The state of the states in family caregiver support: A 50-State study.* Retrieved from http://www.caregiver.org/caregiver/jsp/content_node.jsp?nodeid=1276.

Feinberg, L. F., Newman, S., & Fox-Grage, W. (2005). *Family caregiver support services: Sustaining unpaid family and friends in a time of public fiscal constraint.* Retrieved from http://www.aarp.org/research/housing-mobility/caregiving/fs112_hcbs.html.

Feinberg, L., Wolkwitz, K, & Goldstein, C. (2006). *Ahead of the curve: Emerging trends and practices in family caregiver support.* Retrieved from http://www.aarp.org/research/longtermcare/resources/inb120_caregiver.html.

Foundation for Accountability & The Robert Wood Johnson Foundation. (2001). *A portrait of informal caregivers in America.* Retrieved from http://www.rwjf.org/files/publications/other/CaregiverChartbook2001.pdf.

Fox-Grage, W., Coleman, B., & Blancato, R. (2001). *Federal and state policy in family caregiving: Recent victories but uncertain future.* San Francisco: National Center on Caregiving, Family Caregiver Alliance. Retrieved from http://www.caregiver.org/caregiver/jsp/content_node.jsp?nodeid=839.

Gibson, M. J., & Houser, A. (2007, June). *Valuing the invaluable: A new look at the economic value of family caregiving.* Retrieved on March 18, 2012 from the AARP Public Policy Institute at http://assets.aarp.org/rgcenter/il/ib82_caregiving.pdf.

Giorgianni, S. J. (1997). *The Pfizer journal: A profile of caregiving in America.* New York: Impact Communications, Inc.

Given, B., & Given, C. (2002). *Home health care takes toll on caregivers, patients.* Press Release on Research Grant Award. Michigan State University, East Lansing, MI.

Given, B. A., Given, C. W., & Kozachic, S. (2001). Family support in advanced cancer. *CA Cancer Journal for Clinicians, 51,* 213–231.

Grady, P. A., & Armstrong, N. (2001). *Executive summary: The National Institute of Nursing Research session on research in informal caregiving.* Bethesda: National Institutes of Health. Retrieved from http://www.ninr.nih.gov/NR/rdonlyres/5B7C2DB8-9C63-4F26-A26B-13D1F947FFCB/4868/WorkingGrouponInformalCaregiving.pdf.

Hoffman, M. K. (2002). *Self-awareness in family caregiving: A report on the communications environment.* Retrieved from http://www.nfcacares.org/pdfs/CommEnvironmentFINAL.pdf.

Hunt, G., & Levine, C. (2002). *A family caregiver's guide to hospital discharge planning.* Retrieved from http://www.uhfnyc.org/usr_doc/DischargePlan_Fam.pdf.

Joint Commission on Accreditation of Healthcare Agencies (JCAHO). (2010). *National patient safety goals.* Retrieved on March 4, 2012 from http://www.jcrinc.com/Joint-Commission-Requirements/Homecare/#NPSG.

Joint Commission on Accreditation of Healthcare Agencies (JCAHO). (2012). *Home care resources.* Retrieved on March 4, 2012 from http://www.jcrinc.com/HC-Resources.

Kunkel, S. R., Applebaum, R. A., & Nelson, I. N. (2003–2004, Winter). For love and money: Paying family caregivers. *Generations, 27,* 74–80.

Levine, C., Kuerbis, A., Gould, D., Navaie-Waliser, M., & Feldman P. (2000). *Family caregivers in New York City: Survey findings and implications for the changing health care system.* New York: United Hospital Fund and Visiting Nurse Service of New York.

Li, L. W. (2005). Longitudinal changes in the amount of informal care among publicly paid home care recipients. *Gerontologist, 45*(4), 465–473.

Link, G., Dize, V., Folkemer, D., & Curran, C. (2006). *Family caregiver support: State facts at a glance.* Washington: National Conference of State Legislatures. Retrieved from http://www.ncsl.org/programs/health/forum/caregiversupport.htm.

Met Life Mature Market Institute and National Alliance for Caregiving (NAC). (2007). *Resources for caregiving.* Retrieved on March 4, 2012 from http://www.caregiving.org/pdf/resources/resourcesforcaregivers07.pdf.

National Alliance for Caregiving (NAC). (2001). *Toward a national caregiving agenda: Empowering family caregivers in America.* Proceedings from a conference convened by the National Alliance for Caregiving, in collaboration with the Partnership for Caring. Retrieved from http://www.caregiving.org/data/summit.pdf.

National Alliance for Caregiving (NAC). (2004). *Summary of caregiving legislation in 109th congress.* Retrieved on March 4, 2012 from http://www.familycaregiving101.org/news/list.cfm.

National Center on Caregiving (NCC). (2006) NCC services. Retrieved from http://www.caregiver.org/caregiver/jsp/content_node.jsp?nodeid=368.

National Cancer Institute (NCI), National Institutes of Health. (2012). *Coping with cancer: For caregivers, family, and friends.* Retrieved on March 4, 2012 from http://cancer.gov/cancertopics/coping/familyfriends.

National Coalition for Cancer Survivorship. (2005). *Cancer survivor toolbox: Caring for the caregiver.* Retrieved from http://www.cancersurvivaltoolbox.org/.

National Committee for Quality Assurance (NCQA). (2011a). *Accreditation.* Retrieved on March 10, 2012 from http://www.ncqa.org/tabid/66/Default.aspx.

National Committee for Quality Assurance (NCQA). (2011b). *New online NCQA reports show how well health plans treat key illnesses.* Retrieved on March 10, 2012 from http://www.ncqa.org/tabid/275/Default.aspx.

National Family Caregivers Association (NFCA). (2012). *Yes, I am a family caregiver.* Retrieved on March 16, 2012 from http://www.thefamilycaregiver.org/caregiving_resources/v4_a3.cfm.

National Health Council & National Quality Caregiving Coalition (NHC and NQCC). (2002). *Family caregiving: Sharing strategies, celebrating progress* (Conference Report). Washington: National Health Council. Retrieved from http://www.nationalhealthcouncil.org/pubs/CaregivingReport123.pdf.

National Health Council and WebMD Health Network (NHC & WebMD). (2012). *A different normal.* Retrieved on March 16, 2012 from http://exchanges.webmd.com/chronic-disease-and-disability-exchange.

National Partnership for Women and Families. (2006). *Where families matter: State progress toward valuing America's families.* Washington: National Partnership for Women and Families. Retrieved from http://paidsickdays.nationalpartnership.org/site/DocServer/WhereFamilies Matter2005Report.pdf?docID=1056.

New Freedom Initiative Caregiver Support Workgroup. (2006). *Compendium of HHS caregiver support activities.* Washington: U.S. Department of Health and Human Services.

Pavalko, E., & Henderson, K. (2006). Combining care work and paid work: Do workplace policies make a difference? *Research on Aging, 28*(3), 359–374.

Polivka, L. (2001). *Paying family members to provide care: Policy considerations for states* (Policy Brief No. 7). San Francisco: National Center on Caregiving, Family Caregiver Alliance. Retrieved from http://www.caregiver.org/caregiver/jsp/content/pdfs/op_2001_10_ policybrief_7.pdf.

Reinhard, S. C., Kassner, E., Houser, A., & Mollica, R. (2011, September). *Raising expectations: A state scorecard on long-term services and supports for older adults, people with physical disabilities, and family caregivers.* Retrieved on March 10, 2012 from the AARP website at http://www.aarp.org/relationships/caregiving/info-09-2011/ltss-scorecard.html.

Shelby, R. A, Taylor, K. L., Kerner, J. F., Coleman, E., & Blum, D. (2002). The role of community-based and philanthropic organizations in meeting cancer patient and caregiver needs. *Cancer Journal for Clinicians, 52,* 229–246.

Toseland, R. W. (2004). *Caregiver education and support programs: Best practice models.* San Francisco: Family Caregiver Alliance. Retrieved from http://www.caregiver.org/ caregiver/jsp/content/pdfs/Education_Monograph_01-20-05.pdf.

United Hospital Fund (UNF). (2012). *Family caregiving.* Retrieved on March 18, 2012 from http://www.uhfnyc.org/initiatives/family-caregiving.

Wagner, D. (2001). *Enhancing state initiatives for working caregivers* (Policy Brief No. 5). San Francisco: National Center on Caregiving, Family Caregiver Alliance. Retrieved from http://www.caregiver.org/caregiver/jsp/content/pdfs/op_2001_10_policybrief_5.pdf.

Young, L., & Newman, S. (2003). *Caregiving and retirement planning: What happens to family caregivers who leave the work force* (Policy Brief). Retrieved from http://www.caregiver.org/ caregiver/jsp/content/pdfs/op_2003_retirement_planning.pdf.

Chapter 15
Caregivers of Patients with Cancer: Ethical Issues

Martin L. Smith and Mary Elizabeth Paulk

Since the 1960s, healthcare treatments, diagnostic procedures, and other interventions have become more effective and hope-filled with each new medical discovery, technological advancement, and research breakthrough. At the same time, the healthcare delivery has become a more complex, perplexing, and dilemmatic undertaking due to rising healthcare costs, shifting cultural beliefs (e.g., emphasis on individualism, freedom of choice, self-determination), disparities in access to treatments, expanded legal and regulatory oversight as well as litigation, higher expectations for what medicine can accomplish, and increased life expectancy that can be accompanied by protracted debility and dependence. Due to these and other factors, there is a growing need for both professional and family caregivers to consider the ethics of cancer care.

In this more complicated arena of healthcare provision, cancer professionals need ethically based knowledge, understanding, awareness, and skills to better provide high-quality care to cancer patients and to address the needs of caregivers. This chapter is designed to help healthcare professionals become more aware of and understand how ethical issues and decision-making involve and impact caregivers of patients with cancer, particularly when patients approach the end of life. To the extent applicable, this chapter will focus on practice, research, education/training, and policy/advocacy of the ethical elements to be reviewed. In keeping with the overall structure of this book, current status (what is known) and future directions (what is needed) will be noted. In the United States and many other parts of the world, the fields of bioethics and clinical ethics have been greatly influenced by the identification and explication of basic principles and duties of healthcare professionals,

M. E. Paulk(✉)
Division of General Internal Medicine,
University of Texas Southwestern Medical Center,
5323 Hines Boulevard, Dallas, TX 75390-8889, USA
e-mail: Elizabeth.paulk@UTSouthwestern.edu

M. D. Anderson Cancer Center, Houston, TX, USA
Center for Ethics, Humanities, and Spiritual Care,
Cleveland Clinic, 9500 Euclid Avenue, Cleveland, OH 44195, USA

R. C. Talley et al. (eds.), *Cancer Caregiving in the United States,*
Caregiving: Research, Practice, Policy,
DOI 10.1007/978-1-4614-3154-1_15, © Springer Science+Business Media, LLC 2012

therefore, some guiding and foundational principles will first be presented briefly and then used as foundational reference points for the material and information that follow.

Guiding Ethical Principles: What Is Known

Clinical ethics refer to the day-to-day moral decision-making of those caring for patients (Callahan 2004). As a precursor to concrete, practical decision-making, "Healthcare professions typically specify and enforce obligations, thereby seeking to ensure that persons who enter into relationships with their members will find them competent and trustworthy" (Beauchamp and Childress 2001). Sources for identifying such ethical obligations include the codes of ethics of the various healthcare professions, including medicine, nursing, and the multiple allied health professions. However, many of the duties and obligations asserted in such codes can be viewed as derived from an even more fundamental set of principles: respect for patient autonomy, nonmaleficence, beneficence, and justice (Beauchamp and Childress 2001). These four principles are generally regarded as important for guiding and creating a framework for treatment decisions and will be useful for discussing the ethical issues and dilemmas faced by caregivers.

Respect for Autonomy

The first bioethical guiding principle is respect for patient autonomy and for patient self-determination. Such respect includes recognizing and promoting individuals' freedom to make their own choices without the controlling influence of others. Respect for autonomy undergirds the doctrine of informed consent, which obligates healthcare professionals to provide patients all materially relevant information when treatment decisions are to be made, to involve patients as partners in their own treatment decisions, to involve family members and caregivers when patients lack decisional capacity (i.e., "competence") to make their own decisions, and ultimately to respect the wishes and choices of patients. In most situations, patients with decisional capacity must authorize medically recommended diagnostic procedures or treatments through the informed consent process. It is also the process by which they are educated, in language and concepts understandable to them, about the nature, purpose, risks, benefits, and alternatives of the proposed procedure or treatment. Life-threatening and emergency situations are exceptions to this general rule. A significant implication to the fact that patients in most situations must first authorize their own treatments is that informed patients with decisional capacity can also refuse recommended treatment at any time, including after signing informed consent forms. Respect for autonomy is also the guiding principle behind other professional duties such as veracity (i.e., truth telling) and confidentiality.

Nonmaleficence

The second bioethical principle is nonmaleficence, or the "do no harm" principle, obligating healthcare professionals not to inflict harm intentionally on patients. In the concrete reality of clinical practice and cancer care, the professionals, patients, and caregivers must understand that little is able to be done diagnostically or by way of treatment without some harm, risk of harm, or negative side effects (such as those resulting from the administration of chemotherapy). A simple surgical example is the use of intravenous (IV) fluids after tumor resection. The fluids may help to stabilize a patient's blood pressure transiently, which is the goal of the IV intervention, but they risk pain or infection at the IV site, increased urine output leading to bed sores, or pulmonary edema. In each circumstance resulting in some harm or risk of harm to patients, the anticipated burdens of the intervention must be weighed against the potential or likely benefits, with the aim of minimizing harms while maximizing benefits. From an ethical perspective, based on nonmaleficence, healthcare professionals do not have an obligation to provide treatments that they know will be excessively harmful or burdensome to patients and which will have little or no benefit. Although there has been an extensive published literature since the late 1980s about the issue of "medical futility" and patient and caregiver demands for treatments judged to be medically inappropriate, more research is needed to understand how often and why physicians and other professionals accede to such demands.

Beneficence

The companion principle of nonmaleficence is beneficence. Stated simply, beneficence obligates professionals "to do good" and to promote patient benefit, health, and well-being. This should be the goal when any treatment or diagnostic procedure is presented to patients and then initiated. Medical advice and recommendations should always be based on what physicians and the other members of the healthcare team believe to be in patients' best interests and what is medically appropriate. Professionals' efforts to achieve and maintain clinical competence and skills support the principle of beneficence. To the extent that cancer professionals have knowledge and expertise to administer up-to-date treatment regimens of chemotherapies or bioimmunotherapies, for example, and apply appropriate palliative and symptom-management agents and techniques, they are fulfilling the ethical obligations associated with beneficence. Neither beneficence nor nonmaleficence is a stand-alone principle in clinical practice; the benefits and burdens of proposed treatments or procedures must always be considered together and weighed against each other.

Justice

The fourth guiding principle of bioethics is justice. The principle of justice demands fair, equitable, nondiscriminatory, and appropriate treatment in the light of patients' medical needs. A moral maxim often associated with justice is that healthcare professionals should treat similar patients similarly. In situations where there are limited healthcare resources (e.g., ICU beds, nurses, time, money), justice obligates professionals, healthcare organizations, and society to identify fair and ethically justified criteria for the allocation and distribution of those limited resources.

Issues of justice or fairness arise in many different situations in cancer care. For example, a bedside nurse ought to provide each patient and family caregiver with the level of care and attention needed. If she spends a disproportionate amount of time with a single patient or family (perhaps because they are friends or acquaintances), she deprives other patients of their fair share of her time and attention. However, on a more macro, organizational level, if this same nurse is assigned a disproportionate number of patients because of nursing personnel cut-backs and she is unable to attend to the legitimate needs of her assigned patients and caregivers, the organization may have the greater culpability regarding the injustice and patient safety issues that have been created.

Many other issues related to justice exist on a societal level and even on the global level, such as whether indigent patients without healthcare insurance should have equal access to expensive treatments like bone marrow transplantation (BMT). Within a healthcare delivery system with limited resources, every possible treatment or intervention cannot be offered to all patients. Therefore, when making allocation decisions, healthcare professionals, organizations, and society must articulate fair criteria that will be equitably applied to all similar patient cases.

These criteria should be transparent and available publicly so that patients and caregivers can understand the bases for allocation decisions, especially if and when they are denied needed or desired treatment. National policies do not exist in the United States to guide cancer centers and professionals as well as to promote consistent and fair allocation of resources and access to cancer treatments. Although cancer centers can and do differ in expertise and specialization, development of general and agreed-upon criteria for appropriate access to cancer treatments could help to create a more just system nationally in the distribution of limited resources.

Standards for Decision-Making: What Is Known

Clinical decision-making and the clinician-patient relationship have undergone major revolutionary changes in the United States, starting in the last quarter of the twentieth century. Prior to the 1970s, the prevailing model for decision-making was *paternalism*. This model was founded on physicians' commitment to patients' well-being and the ethical principles of beneficence and nonmaleficence, and was dominated by physicians' expertise and authority. In this model, the patients played a passive, almost child-like role of obediently and unquestioningly following physicians' orders. Paternalism has been replaced now by an expectation of *partnership* between healthcare professionals (especially physicians) and patients. The partnership model continues to affirm clinical expertise but recognizes patients' expertise as well, i.e., that patients are the most knowledgeable persons about their own values, goals, and preferences, all of which should be incorporated into clinical decisions for a particular patient. A partnership model emphasizes mutuality and shared decisions between clinicians and patients. As a result of this partnership model, new standards for clinical decision-making have emerged, based on respect for patient autonomy and patients' abilities to participate in their own healthcare decisions.

The Gold Standard: Currently Competent Patients

The gold standard for clinical decision-making involves patients who currently have decisional capacity and are able to engage presently in the process of informed consent, i.e., patients' wishes are known simply by talking to them. Most adult patients receiving outpatient cancer care, and many hospitalized patients, meet the gold standard. If disagreement arises between patients and healthcare teams, other treatment goals can be negotiated or patients may choose to seek care from other physicians. Also, as some pediatricians and others have asserted, some mature adolescents may be able to meet this standard as well (Leikin 1983; Weir and Peters 1997; Weithorn and Campbell 1982).

Occasionally, questions arise about whether patients currently have sufficient cognitive skills to be able to make their own healthcare decisions. For a variety of reasons (e.g., sedating medications, side effects of chemotherapy, stroke, head trauma), the patients may experience temporary or permanent loss or diminution of their cognitive abilities. When doubts arise about a patient's mental faculties, the primary physician has the responsibility to assess the patient's decisional capacity. The input from mental health professionals (e.g., a psychiatrist, a neuropsychologist, or a mental health social worker) may be helpful and appropriate. Ultimately, the patient should be assessed for specific cognitive abilities to: (a) express a choice, (b) understand relevant information, (c) appreciate the medical situation and its consequences, and (d) reason with relevant information (Grisso and Appelbaum 1998).

The Silver Standard: Once Competent Patients

When a patient who once had decisional capacity is judged currently to lack decisional capacity, the silver (or second best) standard for decision-making is needed. The goal of those responsible for making decisions on behalf of the patient (professionals, family members, and other caregivers) is to identify, to the extent possible, the patient's values and any previously expressed preferences and wishes for the specific medical situation now being faced by the patient. Previous conversations that the patient may have had and the patient's life-style, values, and attitudes may help surrogate decision makers to discern and extrapolate to the current medical situation what the patient may have wanted. In essence, for the silver standard of decision-making, those involved should aim to make a substituted judgment on behalf of the patient in accordance with the patient's values and previously expressed wishes. The situation for surrogate decision makers can be complicated because they often make assessments of patients' preferences and quality of life that are different from either those of the patient or those of the medical team (Sulmasy et al. 1998). Substituted judgment should only be used if there is reason to believe that it can be done accurately, and that it will reflect the patient's wishes, i.e., the persons and caregivers representing the patient's views should have actual knowledge of the patient's wishes and represent them honestly.

The Bronze Standard: Never Competent Patients

Finally, if the patient has never had decisional capacity or there is no information that can give caregivers an insight into what the patient would have wanted, then the criterion for decision-making becomes the patient's best interest. Examples of patient profiles when the best interest standard is needed include pediatric patients, patients with severe mental retardation, and other patients for whom nothing is known about their life-styles, values, or previously expressed wishes. For decision-making standards that emphasize respect for patient autonomy, the best interest standard is the bronze (or third best) standard. Here, healthcare professionals and caregivers, without the assistance of patients' previously expressed directives, must weigh the burdens and benefits of treatments with the aim of making decisions that will be medically best for patients.

Cultural Cautions Regarding Standards for Decision-Making: What Is Needed

In the above discussion about the four fundamental ethical principles and the three standards for decision-making, there is a tendency in the United States and other western democratic societies to emphasize respect for patient autonomy when there is a conflict between and among autonomy and the other ethical principles and duties. This tendency is compounded (and supported) by a western rationalist U.S. cultural view of the human person as an independent decision maker whose individual freedom needs to be protected—and even isolated—from the influence of others. For example, in most situations in U.S. healthcare delivery, informed adult patients with decisional capacity have the right to refuse recommended treatments such as blood products or curative chemotherapy, regardless of the perspectives of others or the consequences of the decision for the patients' caregivers. In essence, from a U.S. cultural perspective, supported by mainstream bioethics and law, patient autonomy tends to "trump" other ethical principles and considerations, such as the patient's best interest as perceived by others around them.

Nevertheless, in the actual clinical application of the four guiding bioethical principles (with an emphasis on patient autonomy), the process of decision-making is not always so easy and straightforward. One reason for the difficulty and challenge is that the system and standards of ethical decision-making used in the predominant U.S. culture can be very different from other cultures, subcultures, and countries. For example, in some cultures that emphasize a more familial, communitarian, or human-interdependence approach to decision-making, there may be an expectation that healthcare decisions are based on the wishes and needs of the family rather than those of the individual patient. Also, patients in some cultures and subcultures (both inside and outside the United States) may not wish to receive information about terminal cancer diagnoses directly from healthcare professionals, but would prefer to have it first disclosed to close family members (Freedman 1993).

Further complicating cultural considerations for decision-making is that physicians and other healthcare professionals operate in a different culture than that inhabited by most informal or family caregivers. As Crawley et al. (2001) point out:

> The fact that medicine itself is a cultural system is often hidden from our awareness. Those of us embedded within the biomedical system learn to assume the authority of science.... Death as a medical event has its own specific language, values, and practices that must be translated, interpreted, and negotiated with patients, families, and communities who are outside of the professional domain of medicine.... Although the values held by medicine may privilege ethical notions of individual autonomy, disclosure, and informed choice, these values are not universally shared. (p. 40)

That values and the ranking of ethical principles are not universally identical may form the basis of conflict among patients, caregivers, and professionals, and even within families. It is very possible to have two or more people (or groups) promoting what they believe is in a patient's best interests and who propose very different clinical decisions and actions.

While it may not be appropriate to ask family members or caregivers to make decisions for patients unless a patient has requested that this be done, there is increasing support for an approach that incorporates family members and caregivers into the decision-making process to the fullest extent possible without compromising the interests of the patient (Kuczewski 1996). It can be argued that in many circumstances, attention to and caring for the whole family may be the best way of caring for the patient.

Advance Care Planning: What Is Known

As noted previously, substituted judgments are only as good as the knowledge that the surrogates have about patients' wishes, preferences, and values. Some patients may have had very specific discussions with family, friends, caregivers, physicians, or other healthcare professionals about their wishes and treatment preferences related to particular clinical situations. However, most adult patients have not engaged in such conversations or in what has been called "advance care planning."

Emanuel et al. (1995) describe advance care planning as a multistage process that promotes individuals stating their preferences for future medical care in the event of decisional incapacity. There are three stages to this patient-centered process: (1) thinking about preferences and proxies, (2) communicating preferences to others, and (3) documenting preferences and designated proxies. The goals and benefits of advance care planning include: (a) extending patient autonomy and control into situations when decisional capacity has been lost; (b) facilitating communication and minimizing conflict; (c) decreasing family anxiety, stress, and burden when significant decisions must be made for the patient; (d) reducing overtreatment or undertreatment; (e) saving healthcare resources and dollars because treatments the patient would not have wanted are not initiated or continued; and (f) providing legal protections for those with ultimate decision-making authority, especially when those decisions may lead to the death of the patient.

Barriers to Advance Care Planning

Multiple barriers have been identified to explain why most patients seem to avoid thinking about their preferences and communicating them to others and why many physicians fail to initiate advance care planning discussions with their patients. An overarching, cultural barrier is a general societal difficulty with thinking and talking about dying and death, whether one's own or someone else's. Metaphorically, death is like "the elephant in the room"—present and dominating, especially in situations of serious illness, yet calling attention to it or direct conversation about it is to be avoided almost at all costs. A narrower but similar cultural barrier exists within U.S. hospitals, ambulatory clinics, and other healthcare facilities where the dying and death of patients (and talk of such) may be viewed as professional medical or patient failure. The military metaphors often associated with cancer (e.g., the *war* or *battle* against cancer, the therapeutic *armamentarium* used to *counterattack* cancer, *defend* the body and *defeat* disease) seem to reinforce the courageous fight that patients and their physicians are expected to wage, subtly conveying that they have more control over illness than they actually do. Physicians sometimes fear that death-talk or death-preparation, especially early in an illness, will be interpreted as a sign of premature surrender to the assaulting disease.

Practical barriers to serious conversations about advance care planning, especially if substantive conversations between patients and physicians are envisioned, include time constraints and compensation concerns (Morrison et al. 1994). Advance care planning, by the very nature of its cognitive content and emotional evocations, can be time intensive and psychologically difficult and draining. Oncologists and other physicians who experience constant pressures to see more patients in the course of a day in order to generate more revenue could easily relegate advance care planning to the bottom of a priority list of issues to be addressed during a 10-to-20 minute office visit with a patient.

Some studies report that patients and physicians have diverse views about who should initiate advance care planning (Miles et al. 1996). The patients wait for physicians to initiate such discussions and physicians wait for patients to initiate such discussions. The result can be mutual misunderstandings and silence about the issue. A physician's reluctance to initiate the discussion may be complicated by discomfort with talking about dying and death, fear of causing patient distress, a desire to protect patients and maintain their hope, a belief that only older and seriously ill or terminal patients should be concerned about such issues, and a lack of training, skills, or knowledge about advance care planning and advance directives. The patients may be reluctant to initiate advance care planning discussions due to a fear of their own death, an overestimation of their medical prognosis, the lack of trust in the physician, a perception that such issues and decisions should remain private, and cultural standards and practices that emphasize communal or familial decision-making over the individualism, self-determination, and independence that can characterize patient autonomy.

Overcoming the Barriers to Advance Care Planning: What Is Needed

Studies have shown that regarding advance care planning, the patients prefer a realistic approach, particularly if it is individualized to the patient's situation and the physician projects confidence and competence (Hagerty et al. 2005; Pentz et al. 2002). Furthermore, as Puchalski et al. have affirmed, patients often view advance care planning as more than a tool for exercising autonomy and control over decision-making; they also can consider it as a means to prepare for death and dying, and an opportunity to strengthen personal and family relationships (Puchalski et al. 2000).

Physicians committed to empowering patients to be partners in their own health-care decisions are not without practical resources (Marquis 2001) and strategies. Back et al. (2003) note that a difficulty for physicians treating patients with life-threatening illnesses is acknowledging and supporting a patient's hopes while recognizing the possible seriousness of the patient's disease. These authors recommend that physicians engage patients in a conversation that has a dual agenda of "hoping for the best while preparing for the worst." They assert:

> Hoping for a cure and preparing for potential death need not be mutually exclusive. Both patients and physicians want to hope for the best. At the same time, some patients also want to discuss their concerns about dying, and others probably should prepare because they are likely to die sooner rather than later. Although it may seem contradictory, hoping for the best while *at the same time* preparing for the worst is a useful strategy for approaching patients with life-limiting illness. By acknowledging all the possible outcomes, patients and their physicians can expand their medical focus to include disease-modifying and symptomatic treatments, and attend to underlying psychological, spiritual, and existential issues. (p. 439)

Within this framework of a dual agenda, these authors recommend five practical considerations for physicians: (1) giving equal air time to hoping and preparing; (2) aligning patient and physician hopes, with a first step of directly inquiring from patients what they are hoping for; (3) encouraging, but not imposing the dual agenda of hoping and preparing; (4) supporting the evolution of hope and preparation over time; and (5) respecting hopes and fears, while responding to emotions.

When and with whom should physicians initiate discussions about advance care planning? One significant factor in answering these questions is the contrast that usually exists between outpatient and inpatient healthcare settings. In ambulatory clinics, the patients are often less stressed and anxious, and more likely to be able to focus on the issues, information, and recommendations associated with advance care planning.

Furthermore, if a physician incorporates advance care planning into routine clinical appointments with many or most patients, some of the patients' immediate worries and questions (such as "Why is my doctor bringing this up now? What does she know about my medical condition that I don't know?") may be quickly dispelled when the physician is able to say: "I'm not singling you out and I'm not holding back medical information about you. I have these conversations with all my patients." Intending the process of advance care planning to occur over time during multiple outpatient visits allows the physician to introduce the topic, encourage the patient to think about preferences and discuss them with close family and friends, and reinforce basic information by providing the patient with take-home materials. These may include pamphlets, copies of advance directives, videotapes, and value history worksheets aimed at reenforcing basic information (Leland 2001). Using this kind of a strategy increases the likelihood that outpatient appointments will be extended only by a few minutes.

Not all physicians will be persuaded to initiate advance care planning with all or most of their patients. Nevertheless, there can be specific clinical indicators and markers that signal a degree of urgency for physicians to initiate end-of-life discussions. Quill (2000) opines that the following situations are more urgent indicators for meaningful end-of-life discussions: the patients facing imminent death, patients who talk about wanting to die, patients or families inquiring about hospice, patients recently hospitalized for severe progressive illness, and patients suffering out of proportion to prognosis. At a minimum, physicians need to be attentive to patients manifesting such clinical "triggers" and to respond quickly by initiating advance care planning discussions with them.

Physicians, when facing the multitude of barriers to be overcome, should remember that they play a key but not an all-encompassing role in the advance care planning process. In addition to raising issues, helping the patients understand their diagnoses and prognoses, and encouraging patients to reflect on their preferences and values, physicians can and should direct patients, their families, and their caregivers to appropriate support persons and resources. These may include psychologists, social workers, chaplains, and midlevel practitioners, including physician assistants and advance practice nurses, who are knowledgeable and skilled in this area.

Documenting Preferences and Proxies: What Is Known

The third stage for advance care planning, as noted previously, is documenting preferences and designated proxies. All states in the United States now have legislatively approved advance directive forms (with individual state variations), whether for providing instructions regarding medical treatment in the event of a terminal or irreversible condition (usually called a Living Will), or for designating a surrogate or proxy decision maker when a person loses decisional capacity (a Medical Power of Attorney). Typically, Living Wills can be executed by any adult person with decisional capacity, regardless of current state of health, and are intended to provide instructions regarding care at the end of life. The more traditional purpose of a Living Will has been to direct the limitation or cessation of treatment for specified medical conditions, but some states (e.g., Texas) allow patients to request to be kept alive in a terminal or irreversible condition using available life-sustaining treatment. In either case, physicians should be open and honest with patients about their willingness and ability to honor the advance directive.

Living Wills have been criticized for failing to meet their original purposes and aims. Fagerlin and Schneider (2004) identified five failures of the living will: (1) despite their availability in most U.S. jurisdictions for at least two decades, most people have not completed one; (2) people do not know enough about illnesses and treatments to make prospective life-or-death decisions about them; (3) it is nearly impossible for persons to state accurately and lucidly their preferences, due to the use of especially using generic and vague preprinted documents; (4) the completed documents are too frequently unavailable to decision makers and caregivers; and (5) decision makers and caregivers too infrequently understand and follow the living will's instructions. The President's Council on Bioethics (2005) has echoed the same sentiment about the failure of the living will.

Many commentators acknowledge that documents designating proxy decision makers are more flexible and more useful than Living Wills. Often called a Medical Power of Attorney for Healthcare, this document allows the patient to assign responsibility for decision-making to another person (proxy or surrogate) in the event that the patient is unable to make decisions. The patients do not have to be terminally ill for this document to take effect. For example, if a patient is sedated during surgery, and a medical decision is needed, a surrogate decision maker could step in. However, in an autonomy framework for decision-making, even the more flexible Medical Power of Attorney is only useful if a patient designates a proxy decision maker who knows the patient well. It assumes that the proxy understands the patient's values, life-style, and preferences, or who has had substantive conversations with the patient about the patient's wishes for various anticipated medical circumstances.

In the absence of Medical Power of Attorney, most state laws designate a hierarchy of decision makers, usually starting with a spouse, and followed by adult children, parents, and adult siblings. Although such legally prescribed hierarchies, based on social custom, provide a reasonable default position for patients who do not complete a Medical Power of Attorney, the legally designated persons might not always be the best ethical surrogate for the patient. For instance, the person who knows the patient best (e.g., same-sex partner) could be preferable ethically to a legally recognized estranged parent. Whenever possible, the perspectives of all legitimately involved persons should be considered when the "silver standard" for decision-making is invoked.

Cautions about the Medical Power of Attorney document include: (a) it should not supersede the patient's expressed wishes, either in a previously existing document, or as directly expressed to the physician or other clinicians; (b) it does not apply if the patient has decisional capacity; and (c) it applies only to medical decisions and not to other realms of life.

Since 1991, U.S. federal law has required hospitals, health maintenance organizations, and hospices to inquire from patients, upon admission, whether they have an advance directive (Patient Self-Determination Act: Omnibus Budge Reconciliation Act (OBRA), 1990). A patient's response to this inquiry is recorded in the patient's medical record; many healthcare organizations encourage patients to provide copies to be placed in their medical records (La Puma et al. 1991). The federal law is clear that access to care is not contingent on whether a patient has completed an advance directive; that is, an advance directive cannot be used as a way for the healthcare system to limit treatment and care available at the end of life (Levinsky 1996).

Documenting Preferences and Proxies: What Is Needed

Many patients will complete advance directive documents without the participation or knowledge of their primary care physician or oncologist. In an outpatient setting, routinely asking patients whether they have completed advance directives can be an excellent entry into a discussion about advance care planning. Although the execution of legislatively approved forms is probably the most common manner for patients to document preferences and proxies, completion of these forms is not the only way to document patient wishes. When physicians engage patients in such conversations, written summaries should be documented in the progress notes of patients' medical records.

For many patients, self-determination and control may not be the only considerations that they value. Attempts to document patient preferences without exploring the diverse values that underlie them underestimate the complexity of human decision-making and are inevitably flawed. End-of-life preferences are best understood not in isolation, but within a broader context of patient values, cultural traditions, spiritual beliefs, and social relationships. Only in this way can patient autonomy be truly respected.

One caution about documenting preferences and proxies is the tendency to reduce what should be a quality conversational and educational process to the signing of documents—similar to the tendency to reduce the informed consent process to the event of getting a patient's signature on an informed consent form. An argument can be made that completing advance directives is the least important step in the process of advance care planning. The first two steps, which include reflection, education, discussion, and communication, are much more important.

If advance directives do not exist, or they are contrary to what physicians and others perceive as patients' best interests, or are in conflict with the wishes of family members or other caregivers, conflicts can arise. Armed with an understanding of the guiding principles of bioethics and the standards of decision-making, the strengths and weaknesses of advance directives, and expectations of families and caregivers regarding the decision-making process, healthcare professionals in most situations should be able to negotiate conflicts to find ethically supportable solutions that work for all participants in the process.

Decisions at the End of Life: What Is Known

Cancer patients, like most people, face significant end-of-life treatment options and choices. Their caregivers must have an adequate understanding and comfort with these choices because frequently caregivers will be participants in the end-of-life care that cancer patients receive (e.g., offering emotional support, assisting with activities of daily living, administering medications, communicating with the members of the healthcare team about the patient's condition). Five major decisions at the end of life can be distinguished. All five routinely result in the dying and death of the patient, and therefore their ethical and legal implications have great significance.

Withholding and Withdrawing Life-Sustaining Treatment

For terminally ill cancer patients, decisions are routinely made to forego (i.e., withhold or withdraw) life-sustaining treatments such as a ventilator, dialysis, artificial nutrition and hydration, blood products, and cardiopulmonary resuscitation (CPR). Decisions to forego these treatments, with the foreknowledge that death will be a likely result, usually are based on a combination of patient wishes and patient best interests. For many patients, a decision to forego life-sustaining treatments is a first step for entry into a hospice program or a hospice mode of care. Although there are many myths about whether foregoing life-sustaining treatments are ethically justified and legally permitted (Meisel et al. 2000), a general ethical and legal consensus exists, especially for terminally ill patients, that life-sustaining treatments can be foregone so that a more "natural death" can occur.

Comfort Care That Could Hasten Death

Most dying patients wish to spend their last days in as little pain as possible. For cancer patients with advanced and progressive disease, the need for symptom control and analgesia can increase as their cancer progresses or becomes metastatic.

Since some pain medications in higher doses (e.g., morphine) have the possibility of occasionally (or only even rarely, Fohr 1998) hastening death or shortening life through the suppression of respiration, some healthcare professionals, patients, and caregivers may be reluctant to provide aggressive pain management using these medications. For persons who oppose euthanasia (defined and described below) on ethical grounds or who fear legal repercussions for even the appearance of euthanasia through the administration of high doses of morphine, a conflict of duties and an ethical dilemma can arise: How is adequate comfort and pain relief for dying patients provided while not crossing an ethical, moral, and legal boundary by directly causing patients' deaths?

In contemporary bioethics, the principle of double effect has emerged as an ethical explanation and justification for providing adequate palliation for dying patients. The principle of double effect states that an action with multiple possible effects, good and bad, is morally permitted if the action: (a) is not in itself immoral, (b) is undertaken only with the intention of achieving the possible good effects, without intending the possible bad effects even though they may be foreseen, (c) does not bring about the possible good effect by means of the possible bad effect, and (d) is undertaken for a proportionally grave reason. As Sulmasy and Pelligrino (1999) note, "Treating dying patients in pain with appropriate doses of morphine is generally done in a manner that satisfies the criteria of double effect." They explain:

> The use of morphine (1) is not itself immoral; (2) it is undertaken only with the intention of relieving pain, not of causing death through respiratory depression; (3) morphine does not relieve pain only if it first kills the patient; and (4) the relief of pain is a proportionally grave reason for accepting the risk of hastening death. (p. 545)

The principle of double effect is not without its detractors (Quill et al. 1997). A central criterion of the principle is that the bad effect or consequence of the action is foreseen, but unintended. Human intentions for a single act can be multiple, ambiguous, and unclear, and even contradictory. The principle of double effect assumes almost a clearly purposeful and single-minded intention. Furthermore, in many other spheres of life, including civil and criminal law, people are held accountable for all reasonably foreseeable consequences of their actions, not just the intended consequences (e.g., the death of a pedestrian hit by an automobile driven by someone under the influence of alcohol). Why should physicians and clinicians be exempted from a similar expectation and responsibility for foreseen but unintended consequences of their actions?

Despite these criticisms, the principle of double effect remains a recognized ethical justification for providing adequate palliation that could hasten death. On a practical level, physicians and other clinicians should administer palliative medications only in response to patients' manifestations (or reasonably anticipated manifestations) of symptoms of pain and distress. Documentation in patients' medical records should include not only the medications prescribed and administered, but also the symptoms being palliated.

Palliative Sedation

An additional and similar application of the principle of double effect is the occasional practice of palliative sedation (Rousseau 2004), which is sometimes called terminal sedation (Quill et al. 2000). In rare instances, the only recourse for treating intractable pain and discomfort is to sedate a patient to unconsciousness. Palliative sedation, while providing comfort, prevents patients from interacting with family members, caregivers, and healthcare professionals, and from taking food and drink by mouth. These burdens and negative consequences may be acceptable to patients in exchange for the comfort and relief that palliative sedation will bring. Palliative sedation will, therefore, have stronger ethical justification when the patient's or surrogate's informed consent has been obtained. Even though palliative sedation could hasten the dying of patients, it can be justified through the principle of double effect as long as it is used with the intention of palliating and controlling intractable signs and symptoms of pain and discomfort.

Physician-Assisted Suicide

Primarily because of an emphasis on patients' autonomy and their right to control both their living and dying, proposals have emerged to allow physicians to assist in the suicide of terminally ill patients. Under this social policy proposal, physicians would be permitted to both prescribe medications (e.g., pentobarbital) and provide information so that patients could kill themselves. Ultimately, the actions proposed would remain suicide (i.e., self-killing), but they would be carried out with the means and knowledge provided by physicians.

Arguments and reasons for opposing physician-assisted suicide include fears that vulnerable populations (e.g., the elderly, indigent, minorities, those coping with physical or mental disabilities) will be coerced by social policy or expectations to take their own lives. They also have concerns that a "license to kill" will have negative effects on the medical profession; and there will be conflicts of interest by family members and caregivers, who frequently shoulder the burdens of caring for the terminally ill. Those who oppose physician-assisted suicide also worry that a right to die could become a duty to die (Foley and Hendin 2002). Arguments in favor of physician-assisted suicide, and that it is a necessary component of excellent hospice and palliative care, include patient autonomy and control, relief of pain and suffering, nonabandonment of patients in intractable pain, and a wider view of human suffering that can be unendurable and beyond relief (Quill and Battin 2004).

Currently, in the United States, physician-assisted suicide is clearly legal only in the state of Oregon where the majority of voters, by referendum, have supported a Death with Dignity Act in both 1994 and 1997. To request from a physician a prescription for lethal medications, the Oregon Death with Dignity Act requires that a patient must be: (a) 18 years of age or older; (b) a resident of Oregon; (c) have decisional capacity; (d) be diagnosed with a terminal illness that will lead to death within

6 months and that the diagnosis has been confirmed by the prescribing physician and a consulting physician; (e) must make two oral requests to the physician, separated by 15 days; (f) provide a written request to the physician, signed in the presence of two witnesses; (g) be referred for a psychological examination if the patient's judgment is believed to be impaired by a psychiatric or psychological disorder; (h) be informed about feasible alternatives (e.g., hospice care); and (i) be requested, but not required, to notify next of kin about the prescription request (Oregon Department of Human Services 2005). From 1998 to 2004, 208 citizens of Oregon (approximately 9.9 per 10,000 total deaths) have used physician-assisted suicide to end their lives.

Euthanasia

The word "euthanasia" literally means "a good death," and is used usually to refer to "mercy killing," i.e., the intentional and direct killing of another person, motivated by the desire to end the person's pain and suffering. Euthanasia can and should be distinguished from physician-assisted suicide in view of who does the killing. For euthanasia, the doer of the deed is someone else; for physician-assisted suicide, the doer is person or patient, with assistance of information and medication from a physician. Euthanasia can be voluntary (i.e., in accord with the patient's expressed wishes), involuntary (i.e., a patient did not request it, but was capable of doing so), or nonvoluntary (a patient is not capable of requesting it). Arguments or reasons for and against euthanasia are similar to those expressed in the debate about physician-assisted suicide.

From the point of view of public policy, euthanasia is legal only in Holland and nowhere else in the world. For a nine-month period in 1996–1997, euthanasia was a legal medical treatment within the Northern Territory of Australia where two men and two women died making use of this legislation, while three others attempted to, but died from other causes (Kissane 2002). Although the formal legalization of euthanasia in Holland did not occur until 2001, since the mid-1980s, there have been consensus guidelines permitting euthanasia that were supported by the Dutch courts, the Royal Dutch Medical Association, the Ministry of Justice, and the Dutch Health Council (Hendin 2002). The guidelines are similar to those noted above for physician-assisted suicide in Oregon and include a voluntary, well-informed, and well-considered request by the patient; intolerable and intractable pain and suffering; formal consultation with a second physician; and physicians reporting specific acts of euthanasia to designated medical and legal authorities. In 1995, there were approximately 3,000 deaths in Holland as a result of euthanasia. The total deaths in Holland in 1995 were approximately 135,000 (Groenewoud et al. 2000). Pertaining to the Dutch practice, concerns have been raised regarding clinical and technical problems (e.g., difficulty inserting an IV line, myoclonus, longer-than-expected intervals between administration of medications and death), and that in some cases "voluntariness is compromised, alternatives are not presented, and the criterion of unrelievable suffering is bypassed" (Groenewoud et al.).

Guidelines for Caregivers: What Is Needed

Three of the key decisions made at the end of life have clear and growing ethical, legal, and societal support. The first set of decisions involves foregoing life-sustaining treatment, providing comfort care that could hasten death, or dispensing palliative sedation. The other two decisions, allowing physician-assisted suicide and euthanasia, are much more controversial and continue to be debated, especially whether social policy and medical practice should be changed to allow them.

When considering the decision to forego life-sustaining treatment, specific and practical concerns and dilemmas arise regarding decisions to withhold CPR and the accompanying medical order of "do-not-resuscitate" (DNR). In general, the lay public is not well informed about realistic outcomes from CPR, especially for cancer patients with metastatic disease. One retrospective, inpatient CPR outcome study, for example, differentiated sudden, unexpected cardiac arrests versus anticipated cardiac arrests. During a five-year period that was studied (1993–1997), of the 171 cancer patients who experienced an anticipated cardiac arrest, no patients survived to hospital discharge (Ewer et al. 2001). The patients and caregivers need to understand that CPR is an intervention that is most effective after sudden and unexpected cardiac arrests secondary to such events as drowning, electrocution, suffocation, drug intoxication, or automobile accidents. CPR is generally not an effective intervention in the setting of advanced cancer and multiorgan failure, and rarely staves off death for more than a short period of time. Furthermore, although a patient has a right to refuse CPR, respect for the patient autonomy does not generate a right to demand CPR when it is medically inappropriate. The principles of nonmalfeasance and beneficence can "trump" patient or surrogate wishes in some clinical situations. From an ethical perspective, healthcare professionals do not have an obligation to provide treatments (including those that are life-sustaining) that are judged to be medically inappropriate, ineffective, or overly harmful. Furthermore, as observed by Reid and Jeffrey (2002), "it is generally accepted that doctors have no legal obligation to offer any treatment, which in their professional judgment will not be beneficial."

Caregivers should be attentive to and find appropriate ways to respond when dying patients raise any of these major decision areas. A training program called "Education in Palliative and End-of-Life Care" (EPEC 1999), originally developed by the American Medical Association, can provide guidance for appropriate responses.

The EPEC program consists of multiple educational modules on various aspects of end-of-life care, including Module 5, which focuses on physician-assisted suicide. This module presents and explains a six-step protocol for responding to requests for physician-assisted suicide and euthanasia. The six steps are:

1. *Clarify the request* by providing an immediate compassionate response, using open-ended questions, and inquiring about suicidal thoughts and plans.
2. *Determine the underlying causes of the request* by exploring with the patient the possible dimensions of suffering (psychological, social, physical, spiritual), with a particular focus on fears for the future, and depression and anxiety.

3. *Affirm a commitment to care for the patient* by listening, acknowledging fears and feelings, and assuring the patient of a commitment to help find solutions together.
4. *Address root causes of the request* by discussing with the patient goals and preferences for the end of life, and explaining palliative care approaches and services.
5. *Educate the patient and discuss legal alternatives* to physician-assisted suicide and euthanasia such as refusal of treatments, withholding and withdrawal of life-sustaining treatments, comfort care, and palliative sedation.
6. *Consult with others* by seeking support from trusted others such as nurses, social workers, and physicians who have experience in caring for dying patients.

These guidelines are founded on caregivers' willingness and ability to listen, probe for underlying issues, and commit to being present with the patient during the dying process.

Conflicts and Conflict Resolution: What Is Known

Respect for patients' autonomy includes honoring their wishes to the extent possible and when medically appropriate. Promoting patients' best interests includes making reasonable judgments about the burdens and benefits of treatments, and then acting accordingly. In most clinical situations, when patients, family members, caregivers, and the involved healthcare professionals are able to agree about the goals of treatment, and corresponding diagnostic procedures can be given, appropriate treatment plans may be developed.

A useful model for understanding the matrix of relationships in which these choices and decisions are made is outlined by Loscalzo and Zabora (1995). Basically, these stakeholders in the decisions (patients, family members, and caregivers) exist as interconnected spheres in equilibrium such that if there is stress on one party, the others will try to compensate. The greater a threat is to the patient, the more dynamic can be the response from family and caregivers, as they try to maintain the equilibrium. Furthermore, "the greater the shared sense of threat and disruption to the integrity of the family system, the more likely patients and families will act in unison toward resolution of identified problems." This model and matrix can apply to the involved healthcare professionals as well. The more they are in agreement with the patient and family, the more easily they will move toward a unified goal, and help the patient and family move in that same direction. However, to the extent that any one of the involved persons has a different perspective or a different expectation, moving toward a common goal will be more difficult. When family responses are not those expected by healthcare personnel, tension may be generated between family members and healthcare providers at a time when clarity and effective interaction are essential. If the staff is not in agreement with the family, then power struggles can take over, leading to fear, mistrust, and conflicts. Pertaining to staff challenges, Loscalzo and Zabora (1995) note:

Healthcare professionals practice in an extremely demanding environment. Although they are prepared to function well within the context of intellectual challenges and multiple technical and instrumental tasks, staff is seldom prepared for the psychological and emotional demands of patients, families, and their own idiosyncratic responses. (pp. 241–242)

Healthcare professionals ignore the psychological and emotional demands of patients, family members, and caregivers with significant peril because without understanding the equilibrium dynamic and assisting the stakeholders in addressing those issues, consensus on goals usually cannot be reached and conflicts will arise.

Reasons and Sources of Conflict

Conflicts among patients, families, caregivers, and healthcare professionals occur for a variety of reasons, but especially when there are breakdowns in communication or ethical dilemmas arise. Abbott et al. (2001) found that conflict between Intensive Care Unit (ICU) staff and families occurred in about 46% of cases, as reported by families whose loved ones did not receive life-sustaining treatment. Sixty-three percent of family members had spoken previously with the patients about their end-of-life treatment preferences, which may have lessened the burden of the treatment decision. Conflicts primarily centered on communication and perceived unprofessional or disrespectful behaviors by physicians and nurses, but conflicts were also reported concerning decisions to withdraw or withhold life-sustaining treatments, pain control, perception of quality of care, and quality of life of the patients. Discussions and decisions about withdrawing or withholding treatment were rarely an isolated source of conflict.

Conflicts may be more likely in settings of patients with agitated delirium, poor symptom control, a history of substance abuse or psychiatric illness, a family previously and significantly involved in patient care, or a history of intrafamilial conflict. Also, utilization of coping mechanisms such as displacement (transfer of emotional concerns about one issue that is too difficult to cope with, to another that is more tolerable), denial (unconscious repudiation of all or one aspect of reality), and distancing (conscious postponing, or focusing on all or one aspect of reality) may contribute to or aggravate conflicts (Dunkell-Schetter et al. 1992). Ferrell (2001) found that anxiety is prevalent in caregivers of dying patients; anxiety was present in 32% of caregivers at the time their loved ones were referred to a home care team, and persisted in 26% of caregivers during the last week of their loved ones' lives (Ferrell 2001). As Loscalzo and Zabora (1995) have observed when patients are dying of cancer:

In these circumstances, anxiety and confusion should be understood as an expression of overwhelming nature of this experience for family caregivers who are highly uncertain concerning their ability to manage. Significant anxiety will disrupt any attempt for effective communication because family members may be unable to comprehend or retain complex or technical information.... Disruption by families is a communication, a disguised and confused plea for help, which is best handled by attending to the underlying concerns of the family and not the distractions, such as imperfections in the staff. (p. 233)

Sources of conflicts can be: (a) honest disagreements about what is best for patients (e.g., family believes that a terminally ill cancer patient will improve by placement of a feeding tube while the medical team asserts that administration of hyperali-mentation will increase patient's discomfort); (b) pathological conflicts related to relational dysfunctions within families or healthcare medical teams; or (c) a combi-nation of both. Factors predisposing situations to pathological conflicts include high stress levels for family (either internal, such as guilt, or external, such as financial problems), distrust of the healthcare system, poor coping skills, and the "Daughter from California" syndrome (i.e., a family member who is emotionally and at times geographically distant from the patient, and who, in a time of crisis for the patient, strongly inserts opinions or demands into the situation, Molley et al. 1991). Staff characteristics that may predispose them to conflicts include a fractionated team, team style, personal stress, and maladaptive behaviors.

More complex and potentially explosive situations can arise when patients lack decisional capacity. In such situations, family members and caregivers are usually asked to provide substituted judgments (i.e., to make decisions in accord with the "voice" and values of the patient). However, the preferences and values of these deci-sion makers may conflict with those of each other and with those of the patient. This may be especially true if patients, when competent, did not engage in advance care planning or execute advance directives applicable to their current medical situations.

A Five-Step Model for Conflict Resolution: What Is Needed

Karlawish et al. (1999) describe a consensus-based, conflict-resolution strategy that keeps what is known about patient wishes and values in the foreground, but also expects guidance from physicians and other healthcare professionals, and elicits input from family members and caregivers who have knowledge about the patient. Their five-step process has application for many healthcare conflicts, not only for those in which the patient lacks decisional capacity:

1. *Identify the main participants in the decision-making.* Participants should include a Medical Power of Attorney if one has been designated and is needed, as well as close family members and caregivers. The most important criterion for who should be included is knowledge about the patient. It should also be noted that "the legally mandated and the ethically appropriate person are not always the same (e.g., an adult daughter may be a more ethically appropriate surrogate than an estranged wife; a homosexual partner may be a better choice than a parent)" (Faber-Langendoen and Lanken 2001).
2. *Allow participants to narrate how the patient has come to this stage of illness.* A useful technique is to ask family members and caregivers to share their per-spectives about the patient's illness up to this point. Sharing narratives can have multiple benefits, including helping to clarify differences in beliefs and under-standings of the current disease state, prognosis, quality of life, and previously

stated values. This process allows the physician and other professionals to understand the relationships within the family; it also helps the healthcare team to understand the "whole patient" and not only the clinical and physiological factors of the case.

3. *Teach the decision makers about the expected clinical course of the patient's disease.* This step should include a discussion about the general goals of treatment and care, and descriptions of how the illness will impact activities of daily living. Explanations about additional medical and nursing needs as well as the availability of palliative care and symptom management, coupled with assurances of nonabandonment, should always be included. The family's perception that they are being well informed can be a major determinant of their level of satisfaction (Kristajanson 1989).

4. *Advocate for the patient's quality of life and dignity.* In addition to asserting that all participants will want to look back on this chapter of the patient's life and know confidently that the patient was treated with dignity and respect, the physician and other healthcare team members should explore concretely what "being treated with dignity and respect" means to the family and other caregivers.

5. *Provide guidance on the basis of existing data and clinical experience.* Here, healthcare team members, patients (if able to participate), and family members and caregivers need to combine their various areas of expertise, i.e., clinical and medical knowledge (especially about likely outcomes), and patient wishes and preferences as known. Ultimately, the burdens and benefits of identified options must be weighed in the light of treatment goals and the patient's dignity and quality of life.

If this five-step strategy fails to build a consensus about a treatment plan, Karlawish et al. (1999) recommend the following: (a) postpone the decision-making and ask participants to take time to think about and discuss key issues; (b) understand and separate from each person's perspective the goals of treatment and the treatment choices to achieve these goals; (c) identify new solutions (e.g., a time-limited trial rather than an all-or-nothing solution); (d) avoid power struggles or personalizing the conflict; (e) call in a third party to help negotiate or mediate (e.g., ethics consultant (Aulisio et al. 2003), trusted clergy, palliative care consultant); and (f) do not violate fundamental values of the patient, family, caregivers, physician, or other clinicians.

If it is not possible to arrive at a consensus, the healthcare team must ultimately decide whether to make concessions or proceed without unanimity. If the issue is small and the action would not harm a patient, concessions might be appropriate. Truog et al. (2001) cite the example of a patient in the final stages of dying and exhibiting agonal respirations. While this is not likely a cause of distress to the patient, it can be very stressful for family members and caregivers. The physician could insist that additional medications are unnecessary, but he could also accede to a family request by providing a small amount of sedative or opioid to decrease the appearance of discomfort.

Caregivers' Experiences of Illness: What Is Known and Needed

The tremendous emotional demands associated with the experience of caring for a loved one approaching the end of life are not easily understood by those who have not experienced them. Bearing witness to the illness, dying, and death of a loved one is a profoundly painful experience. Horowitz and Lanes (1992) have noted:

> Being witness has a peculiar property of being separate from the action, yet at the same time fully engaged. There is sympathy and empathy, resentment and compassion.... Often the patient's pain or distress is indirectly felt, transformed, vividly imagined, or distorted by thinking it is much worse than it really is. Witnesses are afraid for the patient and themselves as they, too, face change, while wishing for a return to normalcy. (pp. 13–14)

Furthermore, family members and caregivers can have their own unique ethical dilemmas and decisions, especially when providing home care. For example, family caregivers report dilemmas related to their involvement when assessing patients' pain and participating in their loved ones' pain management (Ferrell 2001; Johnston-Taylor et al. 1993). They face difficult decisions on a daily basis regarding which medicine to give, how much, and when to give analgesics. Family members struggle with titration: when to increase the dose, how to balance relief with side effects, fear of overdosing, and fear of addiction. Family caregivers feel responsible for unrelieved pain and often have difficulty weighing possible benefits of procedures against the anticipated pain. They feel responsible for communicating with healthcare providers, with balancing goals of comfort versus care, and with causing pain while providing care. They feel responsible for pain relief at home and often report spiritual and existential conflicts and a fear of the future.

Among the needs of family members of dying ICU patients, several directly pertain to the ethical decision-making process (Truog et al. 2001). These include the need to be assured of the patient's comfort, to be made fully aware of the patient's condition, to be informed of impending death, to ventilate emotions, to be accepted, and to be supported and comforted by health professionals. Family members may neglect their own physical and emotional needs to the detriment of their ability to participate in decision-making and care.

Simple actions can begin to address many caregiver needs. Professional caregivers can validate how difficult the situation is for the caregiver; express understanding and sympathy; maintain open and ongoing communication; explain the physiologic process of dying in concrete terms, while avoiding medical jargon; provide reassurance that the healthcare team is focused on the patient's comfort; routinely assess the patient's signs and symptoms of discomfort; and assure patients and caregivers that pain-relieving medications and interventions are continually available. It may also help to anticipate, ask, and answer questions that the family appears to be afraid or unable to verbalize, reassuring caregivers about the decisions already reached, and emphasizing that the responsibility for these decisions is shared between the family and the healthcare team. Relatedly, professional caregivers can provide additional support by making referrals to other members of the healthcare team, such as chaplains, psychologists, and social workers who can also be of great practical and emotional help to the caregivers.

Conclusion

The goal of this chapter has been to create an ethical framework that supports quality care of cancer patients and addresses issues faced by their caregivers. Major elements of this framework include guiding ethical principles, standards for decision-making, advance care planning, decisions at the end of life, and conflict-resolution strategies. Healthcare professionals working with and supporting caregivers—and caregivers themselves—should find within this framework parameters and guidance for identifying, analyzing, addressing, and resolving the many and varied ethical issues that arise in cancer care.

References

Abbott, K. H., Sago, J. G., Breen, C. M., Abernethy, A. P., & Tulsky, J. A. (2001). Families looking back: One year after discussion of withdrawal or withholding of life-sustaining support. *Critical Care Medicine, 29,* 197–201.

Aulisio, M. P., Arnold, R. M., & Youngner, S. J. (Eds.). (2003). *Ethics consultation: From theory to practice.* Baltimore: The Johns Hopkins University Press.

Back, A. L., Anold, R. M., & Quill, T. E. (2003). Hope for the best, and prepare for the worst. *Annals of Internal Medicine, 138,* 439–442.

Beauchamp, T. L., & Childress, J. F. (2001). *Principles of biomedical ethics* (5th ed.). New York: Oxford University Press.

Callahan, D. (2004). Bioetics. In S. G. Post (Ed.), *Encyclopedia of bioethics* (3rd ed.). New York: Macmillan.

Crawley, L. M., Marshall, P. A., & Koenig, B. A. (2001). Respecting cultural differences at the end of life. In L. Snyder & T. E. Quill (Eds.), *Physician's guide to end-of-life care* (pp. 35–95). Philadelphia: American College of Physicians.

Dunkell-Schetter, C., Feinstein, L. G., Taylor, S. E., & Folks, R. L. (1992). Patterns of coping with cancer. *Health Psychology, 11,* 79–87.

Emanuel, L., Danis, M., Pearlman, R., & Singer, P. (1995). Advance care planning as a process. *Journal of American Geriatric Society, 43,* 440–446.

The EPEC project: Education in palliative and end-of-life care. (1999). Chicago: Northwestern University. www.epec.net

Ewer, M. S., Kish, S. K., Martin, C. G., Prince, K. J., & Feeley, T. W. (2001). Characteristics of cardiac arrest in cancer patients as a predictor of survival after cardiopulmonary resuscitation. *Cancer, 92,* 1905–1912.

Faber-Langendoen, K., & Lanken, P. N. (2001). Dying patients in the ICU: Forgoing treatment and maintaining care. In L. Snyder & T. E. Quill (Eds.), *Physician's guide to end-of-life care* (pp. 139–158). Philadelphia: American College of Physicians.

Fagerlin, A., & Schneider, C. E. (2004). Enough, the failure of the living will. *The Hastings Center Report, 34*(2), 30–42.

Ferrell, B. (2001). Pain observed: The experience of pain from the family caregiver's perspective. *Clinical Geriatric Medicine, 17*(3), 595–609.

Fohr, S. A. (1998). The double effect of pain medication: Separating myth from reality. *Journal of Palliative Medicine, 1,* 315–328.

Foley, K., & Hendin, H. (Eds.). (2002). *The case against assisted suicide: For the right to end-of-life care.* Baltimore: The Johns Hopkins Press.

Freedman, B. (1993). Offering truth, one ethical approach to the uninformed cancer patient. *Archives of Internal Medicine, 153,* 572–576.

Grisso, T., & Appelbaum, P. S. (1998). *Assessing competence to consent to treatment, a guide for physicians and other health professionals.* New York: Oxford University Press.

Groenewoud, J. H., van der Heide, A., Onwuteaka-Philipsen, B. D., Willems, D. L., van der Maas, P., & van der Wal, G. (2000). Clinical problems with the performance of euthanasia and physician-assisted suicide in the Netherlands. *New England Journal of Medicine, 342,* 551–556.

Hagerty, R. G., Butow, P. N., & Ellis, P. M. (2005). Communicating with realism and hope: Incurable cancer patients' views on the disclosure of prognosis. *Journal of Clinical Oncology, 23,* 1278–1288.

Hendin, H. (2002). The Dutch experience. In K. Foley & H. Hendin (Eds.), *The case against assisted suicide: For the right to end-of-life care* (pp. 97–121). Baltimore: The Johns Hopkins Press.

Horowitz, K. E., & Lanes, D. M. (1992). *Witness to illness: Strategies for caregiving and coping.* Reading: Addison-Wesley.

Johnston-Taylor, E., Ferrell, B. R., Grant, M., & Cheyney, L. (1993). Managing cancer pain at home: The decisions and ethical conflicts of patients, family caregivers, and homecare nurses. *Oncology Nursing Forum, 20*(6), 919–927.

Karlawish, J. H. T., Quill, T., & Meier, D. E. (1999). A consensus-based approach to providing palliative care to patients who lack decision-making capacity. *Annals of Internal Medicine, 130,* 835–840.

Kissane, D. W. (2002). Deadly days in Darwin. In K. Foley & H. Hendin (Eds.), *The case against assisted suicide: For the right to end-of-life care.* Baltimore: The Johns Hopkins Press.

Kristajanson, L. J. (1989). Quality of terminal care. Salient indicators identified by families. *Journal of Palliative Care, 5,* 21–30.

Kuczewski, M. G. (1996). Reconceiving the family: The process of consent in medical decision-making. *The Hastings Center Report, 26*(2), 30–37.

La Puma, J., Orentlicher, D., & Moss, R. J. (1991). Advance directives on admission, clinical implications and analysis of the patient self-determination act of 1990. *Journal of the American Medical Association, 266,* 402–405.

Leikin, S. L. (1983). Minors' assent or dissent to medical treatment. *Journal of Pediatrics, 102,* 169–176.

Leland, J. (2001). Advance directives and establishing the goals of care. *Primary Care, 28,* 349–363.

Levinsky, N. G. (1996). The purpose of advance medical planning—autonomy for patients or limitation of care? *New England Journal of Medicine, 335,* 741–743.

Loscalzo, M. J., & Zabora, J. R. (1995). Care of the cancer patient: Response of family and staff. In E. Bruera & R. K. Portenoy (Eds.), *Topics in palliative care* (Vol. 2, pp. 209–245). New York: Oxford University Press.

Marquis, D. K. (2001). *Advance care planning: A practical guide for physicians.* Chicago: American Medical Association.

Meisel, A., Snyder, L., & Quill, T. (2000). Seven legal barriers to end-of-life care, myths, realities, and grains of truth. *Journal of the American Medical Association, 284,* 2495–2501.

Miles, S. H., Koepp, R., & Weber, E. P. (1996). Advance end-of-life treatment planning, a research review. *Archives of Internal Medicine, 156,* 1062–1068.

Molley, D. W., Clarnette, R. M., Braun, E. A., Eisemann, M. R., & Sneiderman, B. (1991). Decision-making in the incompetent elderly: The daughter from California syndrome. *Journal of the American Geriatrics Society, 39,* 396–399.

Morrison, R. S., Morrison, E. W., & Glickman, D. F. (1994). Physician reluctance to discuss advance directives, an empiric investigation of potential barriers. *Archives of Internal Medicine, 154,* 2311–2318.

Oregon Department of Human Services. (2005). Seventh annual report on Oregon's Death with Dignity Act. http://egov.oregon.gov/DHS/ph/pas/docs/year7.pdf.

Patient Self-Determination Act of 1990, Omnibus Budget Reconciliation Act of 1990 (OBRA). (1990). PL 101–508, Section 4206 and 4751. http://thomas.loc.gov/cgi-bin/query/D?c101:29:./temp/~mdbshAVp2O.

Pentz, R. D., Lenzi, R., Holmes, F., & Verschraegen, C. (2002). Discussion of the do-not-resuscitate order: A pilot study of perceptions of patients with refractory cancer. *Supportive Care in Cancer, 10,* 573–578.

Puchalski, C. M., Zhong, Z., Jacobs, M. M., Fox, E., Lynn, J., Harrold, J., et al. (2000). Patients who want their family and physician to make resuscitation decisions for them: Observations from SUPPORT and HELP. Study to understand prognoses and preferences for outcomes and risks of treatment. Hospitalized elderly longitudinal project. *Journal of American Geriatrics Society, 48,* S84–S90.

Quill, T. E. (2000). Initiating end-of-life discussions with seriously ill patients: Addressing the "elephant in the room." *Journal of the American Medical Association, 284,* 2502–2507.

Quill, T. E., & Battin, M. (Eds.). (2004). *Physician-assisted dying: The case for palliative care and patient choice.* Baltimore: The Johns Hopkins Press.

Quill, T. E., & Dresser, R., & Brock, D. W. (1997). The rule of double effect: A critique of its role in end-of-life decision-making. *New England Journal of Medicine, 337,* 1768–1771.

Quill, T. E., Lee, B. C., & Nunn, S. (2000). Palliative treatments of last resort: Choosing the least harmful alternative. *Annals of Internal Medicine, 132,* 488–493.

Reid, C., & Jeffrey, D. (2002). Do not attempt resuscitation decisions in a cancer centre: Addressing difficult ethical and communication issues. *British Journal of Cancer, 86,* 1057–1060.

Rousseau, P. (2004). Palliative sedation in the management of refractory symptoms. *Journal of Supportive Oncology, 2,* 181–186.

Sulmasy, D. P., & Pellegrino, E. D. (1999). The rule of double effect, clearing up the double talk. *Archives of Internal Medicine, 159,* 545–550.

Sulmasy, D. P., Terry, P. B., Weisman, C. S., Miller, D. J., Stallings, R. Y., Vettese, M. A., et al. (1998). The accuracy of substituted judgments in patients with terminal diagnoses. *Annals of Internal Medicine, 128,* 621–629.

Truog, R. D., Cist, A. F., Brackett, S. E., Burns, J. P., Curley, M. A., Danis, M., et al. (2001). Recommendations for end-of-life care in the intensive care unit: The ethics committee of the society of critical care medicine. *Critical Care Medicine, 29,* 2332–2348.

Weir, R. F., & Peters, C. (1997). Affirming the decisions adolescents make about life and death. *The Hastings Center Report, 27*(6), 29–40.

Weithorn, L.A., & Campbell, S. B. (1982). The competency of children and adolescents to make informed treatment decisions. *Child Development, 53,* 1589–1598.

Part IV
Conclusions

Chapter 16
Cancer and Caregiving: Changed Lives and the Future of Cancer Care

Ronda C. Talley, Ruth McCorkle and Walter F. Baile

Cancer is the plague of our generation. The leading cause of death worldwide, cancer accounted for 7.6 million deaths or 13% of all deaths in 2008 (World Health Organization (WHO) 2011). Cancer is a leading cause of death worldwide and accounted for 7.6 million deaths (around 13% of all deaths). In 2012, 577,190 U.S. citizens or 23.3% of all deaths in the United States were attributed to this deadly, invasive disease (American Cancer Society (ACS) 2012; National Center on Health Statistics 2010). In their 2010 (ACS 2012) report, ACS projected that 1,529,560 new cancer cases would be diagnosed that year. For each of those numbers, a team of professional caregivers (physicians, nurses, hospice workers, aides, technicians, etc.) and from one to dozens of family caregivers provide life-sustaining support to the individual with cancer (Nijboer et al. 1998, 1999). With this domino effect, the numbers of patients and family caregivers, plus the numbers of impacted professional caregivers could be added to determine the pervasive impact of cancer on the states and the world.

Federal Support in the War Against Cancer

While progress has been made in the fight against cancer, advancements have been painfully slow. In 1971, President Richard Nixon launched a "war against cancer" in his State of the Union address:

R. C. Talley (✉)
Western Kentucky University, 1906 College Heights Boulevard, GRH 3023, Bowling Green, KY 42101-3576, USA
e-mail: Ronda.Talley@wku.edu

R. McCorkle
Yale University School of Nursing, 100 Church Street South, New Haven, CT 06536-0740, USA
e-mail: Ruth.McCorkle@yale.edu

W. F. Baile
University of Texas M.D. Anderson Cancer Center, Houston, TX 77230-1402, USA
e-mail: wbaile@mdanderson.org

R. C. Talley et al. (eds.), *Cancer Caregiving in the United States,*
Caregiving: Research, Practice, Policy,
DOI 10.1007/978-1-4614-3154-1_16, © Springer Science+Business Media, LLC 2012

I will also ask for an appropriation of an extra $ 100 million to launch an intensive campaign to find a cure for cancer, and I will ask later for whatever additional funds can effectively be used. The time has come in America when the same kind of concentrated effort that split the atom and took man to the moon should be turned toward conquering this dread disease. Let us make a total national commitment to achieve this goal.

Despite the President's proclamation, funding for cancer research has remained a challenge. As recently as 2005, Andrew C. von Eschenbach, NCI director, pronounced "Our challenge goal to the nation... Eliminate the suffering and death due to cancer by 2015" (NCI 2005). However, federal funding for cancer research has remained level at approximately $ 4.9 billion from 2005 to 2010 (NCI 2011b) and while cancer research has yielded remarkable advancements, these accomplishments have been made against a backdrop of less than adequate funding to accomplish Director von Eschenback's laudable goal. More recently, NCI reports: "Cancer research today, especially on the frontiers America's cancer researchers are renowned for spearheading, requires investment at a scale unimaginable 40 years ago" (NCI 2011a, p. 4). Yet, again, at a time of economic uncertainty caused by the national deficit and debt, it appears doubtful that the full gains possible in cancer research will be made over the immediate years to come.

Cancer is Personal

However, to the patients and those who care for them, a single incident of cancer is one too many. One incident of cancer can destroy lives and families. If you are the one diagnosed with cancer, your world view changes forever. If you are the person who loves them, your life will never be the same. Unfortunately, cancer is deadly in too many cases and for each death, we know the life lost is irreplaceable and the love lost is devastating. And, for the physicians, the life lost is considered a failure.

While prevention and early intervention are helping to reduce the numbers of individuals who die from cancer, there are still far too many fatalities from this horrific disease. The following scenarios depict cancer's far-reaching effect:

When Dad told Mom that he had cancer, her world crumbled. He tried to be strong for her, but it was not enough. Why, she thought, hadn't his doctor done more? For years, he had been told by the physician that he just had stomach problems and to take over-the-counter medicine. When he finally talked the physician into giving him a test, the test was read as "inconclusive," but Dad was told it had shown nothing wrong. I told him it didn't matter what the test said, he was still sick and needed help. I tried to get him to go to my doctor for a second opinion. His loyalty to his long-time physician kept him from asking another physician for help. Finally, after the physician had a colonoscopy for himself, he ordered one for Dad. Cancer was found.

At the time of surgery, the colon cancer has metastasized to one lymph node. He had every treatment available to him, radiation and chemotherapy, so many kinds that we lost count. He lost weight, lost his hair, had cracks on his feet, was nauseated and tired, and couldn't eat. We counted calories of all he ate each day to try to get him to eat more. We bought nuts and set them by his chair so he could get calories and protein at the same time. We did, my mother did, everything one human being could do for another.

Finally, the treatments stopped working. Dad lived another year, and after Christmas, one year after Mom had lost her own father, he died. There was no bottom to the pain. Mom had almost killed herself taking care of Dad, and she was sick. For me, there was no way I could work now.

When I look back on this five years later, I am acutely aware of the pain that endures. While the passage of time does help, the loss of my father's living presence is a forever thing. I do believe in God and the hereafter, and that gives me hope that I will be with him again in the future. Yet, how much I would give to have him here, now, in the flesh, to share the grand events and small, daily routines of our family?

This is just one story of many that could be told about the toll cancer takes on families. Of particular concern is the caregiver, the loved one who is left behind to grieve, get financial and personal affairs in order, refocus on their own health, and begin to live a new life without the person they love. Completing tasks that are basically logistical ones, such as finances and housekeeping, can give the caregiver a sense of immediate purpose and some closure as they move through the mourning process. However, when it comes to living life anew without your life partner or loved one, no milestones or guidance fit all individuals left behind to cope with the incredible loss. We all, in our own way, must struggle with a new reality of life that is forever changed.

The previous account chronicles a family's multiple year struggle with a father's cancer. The next story tells the story of a hidden cancer that reoccurs in a man 56 years of age, then produces immediate, devastating results:

I loved him. He was the love of my life.

It looked like a mole under his chin. I told him I didn't like the way it looked. When he went to see the doctor, he was told it was melanoma. Surgery followed and the doctors said, "All clear." It had been dealt with quickly. We celebrated and went on with our lives.

Thirteen years later, I received a call. "Honey, I have cancer," he said. "What!?!," I exclaimed, "NO! We took care of that years ago." He went on to tell me that the cancer had returned even though we couldn't see anything on the surface of his skin. It turned out that the weight loss and night sweats were our clues. "Oh, no, oh, no, the cancer is back," I wailed.

What followed broke my heart. My loved one started on a series on tests and doctors' visits that lasted for months, and then, finally, he had a 16 hour surgery to remove the lymph nodes in his neck. A few weeks later, radiation was begun and took its awful toll. He couldn't eat and couldn't sleep; he was in increasing pain. The radiation was too much. He told the radiologist that he wanted to stop treatment, but the doctor talked to him and he continued. He was 98 pounds when he finished radiation, with radiation burns on the inside and outside of his throat. He was almost too weak to hug me.

Two weeks later, I convinced him to make the doctor check him into the hospital for nutrition. I was scared; he couldn't eat and threw up when he tried. I remember it was right before Christmas. In the hospital, he had every test you can imagine, but no treatment. The tests made him weaker, draining what was left of his energy. Nine days after admission, he died.

Despite the deadly outcome recalled in the previous two cases, people do survive cancer and thrive. The next first-person account tells this story:

It's Thanksgiving, my favorite holiday of the year. It's a day of reflection and a time to enjoy family and friends without all the hustle and bustle associated with the end of the year holidays. Even the weather cooperated today: in shirtsleeves, under sunny, warm, clear blue skies, we were able to rake the last of the leaves off the grass and plant tulip bulbs in the front garden. Two years ago at Thanksgiving we already had a blanket of snow! Last year, well, that is altogether a different story. By Thanksgiving last year, I had completed 12 of 35 radiation treatments for cancer and I was feeling awful.

The cancer saga started seven months earlier in April. While riding my bicycle home from work one day I discovered a tiny hard spot deep in my left thigh muscle. There was no discoloration, swelling, or pain, just a little hard spot that would occasionally rub against my bicycle seat. In fact, it was so small and seemingly innocuous, that I ignored it for almost three weeks. Then within a period of a few days, it grew from the size of a pencil eraser to almost half the size of my hand. That was the end of my doctor avoidance! Four days after first showing this "hard spot" to my primary care physician, I met with my cancer team, which still tracks me today, nineteen months later: an oncologist, a radiologist, a surgeon and support nurses. An MRI and biopsy confirmed that I had a high-grade malignant fibrous histiocytoma sarcoma subtype myxoid. This is a fairly rare cancer compared with breast, lung, colon, or prostate cancers. However, it is very fast growing and deadly if not treated quickly. Within days, I had a dual access port surgically installed in my chest for chemotherapy and several days later, started the first of four three-week rounds of chemo. These were followed by surgery in August to remove the tumor, which had now grown to be larger than my hand, two more rounds of chemo for good luck, and 35 sessions of radiation. Eight months of being poked, cut, poisoned, and radiated. Not fun.

The good news is I returned to teaching (at the university) full-time in January, two weeks after finishing radiation. I resumed bicycling in early February, got my swimming back up to a mile a day by April, and am cancer free almost a year after finishing treatments. Aside from a lingering fatigue, I feel fine. I'm glad to be above ground and actively engaged in life.

There are a number of ironies about this whole affair. One is that the cancer never caused any pain. (I wish I could say the same of the treatments.) Another is that two suspected causes of this cancer are exposures to toxic chemicals (e.g., dioxin) or to high doses of radiation. Well, I was exposed to more lethal chemicals during one session of chemo and more rads (grays) in one radiation treatment than I received during the entire prior 60 years of my life! Fighting fire with fire seems primitive, but it is the state-of-the-art today. A third is that the emotional toll on my family was greater than on me. (Perhaps I wasn't the perfect patient I thought I was.) The fourth irony is that I have always taken care of myself. I never smoked or used drugs, I exercise regularly (bicycle year-round, swim 5–7 miles a week, use stairs instead of elevators, etc.), and I was raised by a health-conscious mother who focused on organic foods. The only risk factor I am aware of is I grew up in a city well-known for its air and ground pollution from chemical manufacturing plants.

Lucky? You bet I am. Thankful? You bet I am. Firstly, I live within ten minutes of a world-class university hospital, one of the few in the country that has a sarcoma center. My medical care has been first-rate, delivered by professionals who really care about the individual. Secondly, I have excellent health insurance. Bankrupting my family or worrying about paying for my expensive treatment was not a concern for me, unlike for many of the people I met last year. Thirdly, I didn't lose my job. My colleagues and administrators were incredibly accommodating to give me time to heal and adjust. Fourthly, for my entire life, I have been blessed with a supportive, loving family and wonderful friends. The awareness of this gift has never been far from my daily consciousness, but it became front and central last year. Technically, what I received is called Care Giving, but I call it Love Giving. Family members, neighbors, colleagues, past students, current friends, and even high school friends I don't normally communicate with between five-year reunions lent their support through prayers, e-mails, letters, visits, prepared meals, freshly cut flowers, chauffeuring to the hospital, jokes, and just plain vanilla good vibrations. One of my sisters and a dear friend of mine each gave up a week of their lives to live with us when I was particularly sick to lend a hand to my wife who was supporting me 24/7. All of this is incredible!! I'm the luckiest guy in the world!

Thanksgiving Day is over. It's time to wrap up this epistle. But, it certainly isn't time to stop giving thanks. John Donne's quote sums this experience for me: No man is an island, entire of itself; every man is a piece of the continent, a part of the main; if a clod be washed away by the sea, Europe is the less. . . any man's death diminishes me, because I am involved in mankind. Brian (personal communication, January 17, 2007)

These three accounts tell different stories of the way cancer manifests and impacts the diagnosed individual and their families. While the pathways to and through the disease are different, there is no question that cancer takes an enormous physical, emotional, financial, and spiritual toll on both care recipients and caregivers.

Authors' Reflections

In this book, McCorkle and Given (Chap. 3) offer a number of suggestions for the future. Since we know that factors such as disease stage, patient's age, gender and emotional adjustment, coping and social support and other factors can affect distress levels in caregivers, clinical interventions can be targeted to cancer caregivers who are at high risk for physical and emotional distress. They note that primary care providers and other health care professionals need training and education in the assessment of patients' caregiving needs as well as caregivers' capacity to provide care. Policy recommendations include: (a) establishing advocacy groups to champion the needs of family caregivers; (b) developing policy initiatives that address financial support and legislative action at the state and federal level; and (c) establishing community initiatives, including establishment of local support groups, respite programs, and mental health services for caregivers.

Wilkie (Chap. 2) contributes to the dialogue by stating that an important goal for cancer care is eradication of disparities, both for patients and caregivers. This has implications for future research, practice, education, and policy. Research must be specifically targeted to investigate cancer family caregivers. Family support services must be tailored to specific needs of ethnic minority groups and accommodate their various language and cultural needs. Policy initiatives should explore creative initiatives to address disparities in cancer care. There is also a great need for multicultural education training among health care professionals.

Baile et al. (Chap. 6) introduced a strategy for establishing an alliance, which they call PERKS: determining patient Preferences for caregiver involvement; Engaging the caregiver; establishing caregiver Role and Readiness; providing Knowledge and information; and providing Support and Strategies. In each of these areas, emphasis is placed on providing ongoing, dynamic assessment of caregiver and patient needs and considering the individual needs and quality of life of the caregiver. Health care team members can take an active role in identifying patients' needs and instructing family members in implementation of patient care activities.

Bergamini and Hendrickson (Chap. 7) noted that the number of youth caring for older family members with cancer is growing, and although the tasks assigned to these youth may not involve direct patient care, there can still be a significant burden placed on these children and youth, which can impact their emotional status, education, and social interactions. Schools are typically supportive of these students; however, there are no formal protections in place for youth caregivers through methods such as Individualized Education Plans or Section 504 health plans, which are needed. (For more information on children and caregiving, see forthcoming book in this series on *Intergenerational Caregiving* 2012).

Puchalski (Chap. 11) suggested that extensive educational program development and research are needed in the area of providing spiritual support to caregivers while Smith and Paulk (Chap. 15) discussed the difficult issues of withholding and withdrawing life-sustaining treatment, comfort care that could hasten death, palliative sedation, physician-assisted suicide, and euthanasia.

Baldwin (Chap. 12) defined the various areas of cost associated with cancer as direct and indirect costs. These factors contribute to the difficulty in obtaining comprehensive care for cancer patients and their families. Kaufman et al. (Chap. 14) noted that federal policy initiatives such as the Family Medical Leave Act allow 12 weeks of unpaid leave Stromborg (Chap. 13); however, many caregivers are excluded and other initiatives focus on caregivers of specific populations that do not include cancer. National health care accreditation organizations also do not specifically address caregiver needs and this has forced states to take a larger proportion of responsibility for addressing family caregiving needs.

Reasons for Hope

Despite the staggering statistics regarding cancer morbidity and mortality, there are new reasons for hope. Prevention efforts are increasing. Early-detection campaigns are increasing public awareness of the importance of identifying affected cells at the start of their mutations from normal to cancerous. More people are emphasizing prevention behaviors, while early diagnostics and treatment are helping others who have existing disease. Therefore, individuals with cancer are generally surviving longer. The American Cancer Society (2011) reports that the 5-year relative survival rate for all cancers is increasing, up from 50% in 1975–1977 to 68% between 1999 and 2005.

Despite all the challenges faced by caregivers of individuals with cancer (Gilbar and Ben-Zur 2002; Given et al. 2001), there are few who would say that the battle is not worth the most ferocious fight possible. Despite all odds, the nation is advancing in its efforts to fight this disease, even if the pace of advancement is not all that we would wish. Public awareness is increasing and individuals appear to be taking more personal responsibility for behaviors that are protective in avoiding cancer and life-affirming when they are diagnosed. More attention is being given to the needs and health of family and friend caregivers who stay by the sides of their loved ones for days, months, and years as they fight to survive and thrive (Goodheart (Chap. 4); Jacobs (Chap. 8); Raveis (Chap. 10)). Professional caregivers, such as doctors, nurses, psychologists, and clergy, are increasingly recognizing that they need the support of other care team members as they plan the best course of treatment possible for their patients; they are also offering more thoughtful support for the family members who are often responsible for implementing the care plan once the family leaves the doctor's office. And, very importantly, more cancer victims are becoming cancer survivors and enjoying that precious extra time that early treatment and loving care makes possible (Balducci and LaCoursiere (Chap. 9); Glajchen (Chap. 5); Laubmeier et al. 2004).

Family caregivers make a difference in the quality of life of their loved ones with cancer. Their thoughts, feelings, and preferences are important variables in the care equation. For the best possible outcomes in cancer prevention, research, and treatment, families must be considered deserving the attention of cancer researchers who are working hard to find ways to help families survive and beat this disease. One day, hopefully soon, scientists will find the elusive "cure" for cancer. That will be a time when we can rejoice together that the pain of losing a loved one to this dreaded disease will never touch another caregiver's heart.

References

American Cancer Society. (2011). *Cancer facts and figures*. Atlanta: Author.

American Cancer Society. (2012). *Cancer fact and figures*. Atlanta: Author.

Gilbar, O., & Ben-Zur, H. (2002). Cancer and the family caregiver: Distress and coping. Springfield: Charles C. Thomas, Ltd.

Given, B. A., Given, C. W., & Kozachik, S. (2001). Family support in advanced cancer. *CA: A Cancer Journal for Clinicians, 51*(4), 213–231.

Laubmeier, K. K., Zakowski, S. G., & Bair, J. P. (2004). The role of spirituality in the psychological adjustment to cancer: A test of the transactional model of stress and coping. *International Journal of Behavioral Medicine, 11*(1), 48–55.

National Cancer Institute. (2005). The Nation's investment in cancer research: A plan and budget proposal for fiscal year 2007. Washington, DC: U.S. Department of Health and Human Services. http://www.cancer.gov/PublishedContent/Files/aboutnci/budget_planning_leg/plan-archives/nci_2007_plan.pdf.

National Cancer Institute. (2011a). Cancer: Changing the conversation: The nation's investment in cancer research, an annual plan and budget proposal for fiscal year 2012. Washington, DC: U.S. Department of Health and Human Services. http://www.cancer.gov/PublishedContent/Files/aboutnci/budget_planning_leg/plan-archives/nci_plan.pdf.

National Cancer Institute. (2011b). Fact sheet: Cancer research funding. http://www.cancer.gov/cancertopics/factsheet/NCI/research-funding.

National Center on Health Statistics. (2012). *Deaths: Preliminary data for 2010*. Atlanta: Centers for Disease Control and Prevention.

Nijboer, C., Tempelaar, R., Sanderman, R., Triemstra, M., Spruijt, R. J., & Van Den Bos, G. A. M. (1998). Cancer and caregiving: The impact on the caregiver's health. *Psycho-Oncology, 7*(1), 3–13.

Nijboer, C., Triemstra, M., Tempelaar, R., Sanderman, R., & Van Den Bos, G. A. M. (1999). Determinants of caregiving experiences and mental health of partners of cancer patients. *Cancer, 86*(4), 577–588.

Nixon, R. (1971). Annual message to the congress on the state of the union. http://www.c-span.org/executive/stateofunion/nixon1971.pdf. Accessed 2011.

World Health Organization (WHO). (2011). *Cancer* (fact sheet #297). Geneva: Author.

Index

R. C. Talley et al. (eds.), *Cancer Caregiving in the United States,*
Caregiving: Research, Practice, Policy
DOI 10.1007/978-1-4614-3154-1, © Springer Science+Business Media, LLC 2012

Printed by Publishers' Graphics LLC